THE JOURNEY

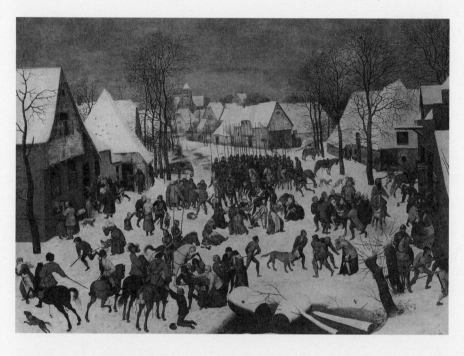

The Massacre of the Innocents *by Pieter Brueghel the Younger, from the Kunsthistorisches Museum in Vienna. King Herod had learned that somewhere had been born the King of the Jews. These Spanish soldiers and Flemish mothers and children are the universals of History: Germans in Poland, Americans in Vietnam.*

CHARLES MERRILL

THE

JOURNEY

Massacre of the Innocents

Kenet Media
Cambridge
1996

Kenet Media, Inc., 380 Harvard Street, Cambridge, MA   02138
© 1996 by Charles Merrill

Printed in the United States of America

ISBN 0-9644798-4-2

Cover lithograph *ARKA*, by Krysztof Skórczewski
Photograph of author by Frank Cordelle.

This copyright page continues on page 344

Our war booty is the knowledge of the world
   Wisława Szymborska

While the innocents were being massacred who says
   that flowers didn't bloom
      Julia Hartwig *Who Says*

Preface

"American authors have perfected one hundred sixty-five ways of describing the act of making love, but show less skill in examining the way an individual exists within the changing framework of history" was a statement by Czesław Miłosz I remember from sometime in the early '60s.

Well, I had my first exposure to life within that framework as a boy of 18 walking across Berlin, Warsaw, Vienna, and Prague in the summer of 1939. It was an adventure: disobeying my father who had other plans for my summer, exploring a part of Europe as far away as Romania and Bulgaria, seeing with my own eyes what I had read about in college on Hitler's National Socialism. And all of this lay under the threat of war due to break as soon as the harvests were in. For a disobedient adolescent, there was the side issue of the relation between attitudes towards Jews within my family's world and what I saw in Vienna of Jews wearing a yellow armband with a six-pointed star or seated on a yellow bench, and then the relation between that yellow bench and the special benches for Negroes that I had seen in Mississippi where my father owned a 3000-acre cotton plantation. A historian's fascination with unwanted comparisons began on that journey.

Later on the journey involved two years as a soldier in Italy and a dozen visits to postwar Prague and Warsaw to ask what *was* a Communist police state. How did individuals survive History and retain some sense of identity and integrity? I kept returning to what became "my" Europe, gradually making a few close friends through whose eyes I acquired a sense of this world from the inside. Out of the untidy suitcase of observations and conclusions from a lifelong career as history teacher came souvenirs like the similarities between Franz Josef and Ronald Reagan, the different ways of looking at abstractions like Staatsmacht, which needs no translation, the self-righteousness and self-delusions of nationalism. The heroic Pole stands up to the brutal German and then humiliates the Jew who does the same to the Palestinian who blows up a busload of housewives and schoolchildren. The Germans cheer their victories over Poland, Norway and France, the Americans theirs over Grenada, Panama and Iraq. There is no escape.

On a night of late November 1989, I was part of a crowd in the streets of Prague cheering the end of Communism and the coming of freedom with Vaclav Havel, one of the great joyous moments of my life. Then over the next half-dozen years I saw what came of those hopes in one post-Communist country after another, which included tangible tokens of freedom of speech and travel, of becoming one's own boss instead of a lifelong state employee. And also wildly widening the gap between rich and poor, unemployment and corruption, and a society run by and for go-getters, computer experts, journalists, Mercedes salesmen, sex queens and gangsters.

What is happening in the new democracies sadly parallels what one sees at home: the same gap between rich and poor—which alarmed American reformers a hundred years ago, the shrugging off of concerns about public education and health and the long-range future of the natural environment. How can a book like this, reflections coming out of long walks through the streets of Kraków, Olomouc, Vienna, Boston, stimulate or irritate useful thought about the way we measure our past and our future and what we mean by a decent society.

The Journey also allows me a dedication to my brother James, who died a year ago, and to my friend of almost 40 years, Jacek Woźniakowski, through whom more than anyone else I came to know and care about his country. The poet and the cavalry lieutenant, journalist, professor and mayor of Kraków led quite different lives but shared the same aristocratic concern for tradition, culture and language as independent of conformist self-indulgent mass culture as of police censorship.

Acknowledgments

My first acknowledgement for material on wartime and post-war Poland that led to these journeys and therefore to this book is to Czesław Miłosz, the stories I listened to at his home in Brie Comte Robert outside Paris. Then to Jiři Kořinek, to members of the Woźniakowski and Grocholski families in Olomouc, Warsaw and Kraków, who helped me gradually to feel that I was seeing their world from the inside. There are the people I've talked with over the past 40 years or so on matters large and small: Ralph Freedman, Josef Jařab, Richard and Irene Pipes, Edward Keenan, Krzysztof Kowalski, Krzysztof Skórczewski, Anna Kulczycka, Candida Mannozzi, Romana Vysatova, Nell Znamierowska. Much of the pre-1918 material on Moravia and Olomouc came from Dr. Jaroslav Pepernik of the Palacky University faculty.

The friends who have enjoyed hunting through the old man's chapters for errors of judgment, fact, grammar, style and spelling. The most rigorous, most helpful editor was, as always, my wife Mary, who disciplined and sharpened the language, pointed out the redundant and pretentious. Former students such as Lynn Nyhart, Müge Galin, Jacqueline Veal, Amy Ansara. My brother James. As editor, translator and poet himself, Stanisław Barańczak was my guide to Polish poetry, the richest, most tangible I have explored in its portrayal of the relations between human beings and war, police, politics, fear, hope. Frank Cordelle helped me in preparation of the illustrations. Lubos Cech was the map draughtsman. Judith Lessard was a resourceful, precise typist who made the endless process of rewriting bearable.

For the book's actual production, I had at the *Znak* office in Kraków a helpful, tolerant publisher in Henryk Woźniakowski, a sensitive translator and responsible, energetic author's representative in Andrzej Pawelec. For the American version I enjoyed collaborating with Alwynne Wilbur as editor and felt particularly fortunate in Brian Kenet as publisher. His specialty is dermatologic textbooks, but in some lonely impulse of delight gambled on my manuscript. It has been a joy to work with a professional as knowledgeable, practical and courteous as he.

To the many, many editors who turned down this manuscript, it is too late for you to say you're sorry. Have a nice day.

Charles Merrill

Pronunciation

Polish and Czech are difficult. Grammar, vocabulary, and pronunciation combine to make a foreigner quit after Lesson 3. The heavy bramble patches of consonantalized syllables scare off the American who loves Italian, and there is a disheartening subtlety of accent marks on both vowels and consonants. Nevertheless, a certain number of basic rules allow a grade B pronunciation that shows Pan Szczepanski in Warsaw and Pani Sevčiková in Prague that you're trying.

Basic rule: in both languages, c, whether hard or soft in English, is always pronouced ts.

Basic difference: Polish is always pronounced with the stress on the next to last syllable. In Czech, stress is always on the first syllable, but often with an accented elongated vowel that can be confusing.

Szczepanski: sh–cheh–*pan*–ski

Sevčiková: *sev*–chi–ko–*vá*. If you stress ko, the name becomes Polish. The vá, elongated rather than stressed is reasonable in that word, but with Janáček, the composer, stressed and elongated vowels next to each other become so subtle that you simply hit the accented syllable.

Remember that the rolled Czech r, as in Serbo-Croat, is a legitimate vowel: čtvrty means fourth.

Polish cz and Czech č become ch

Polish sz and Czech š become sh

Polish rz and Czech ř become rzh, as in Dvořak

Polish ż or ź and Czech ž become soft j, as in azure

Polish nasals are softer than in French: Lech Wałęsa (ch, as in German ach or ich). Soft ł is w, thus Lekh Va-wen-sa. Dokąd (where to?), is pronounced dokant.

Łódż = woodj, Lwów = L-vuf, Olomouc = O-lo-mouts.

J = y in both languages. German Schweik becomes Czech Švejk.

Maps

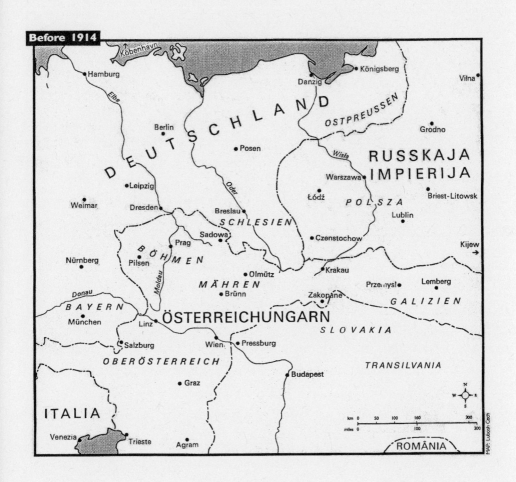

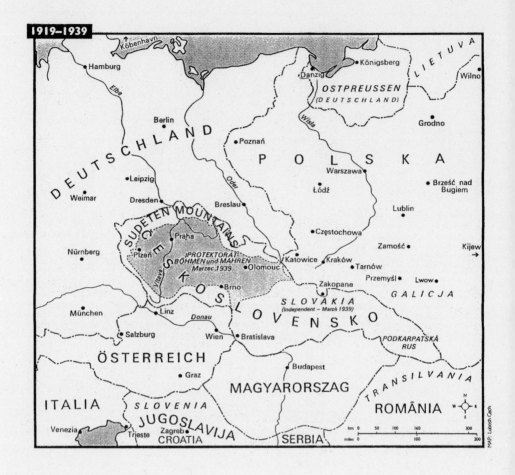

XIV

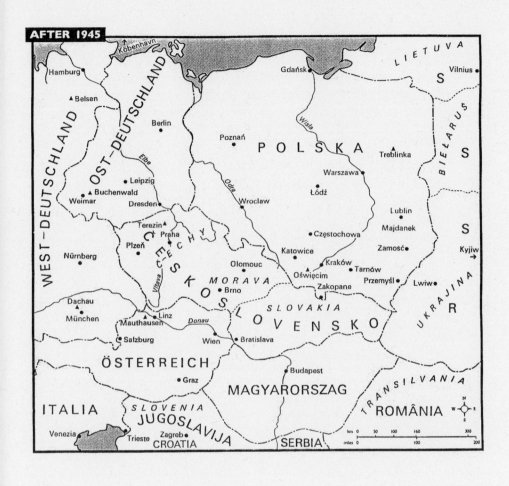

Contents

THE JOURNEY

PART I

~

THE GERMAN APPROACHES

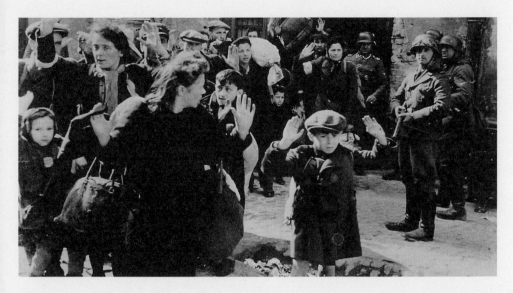

Massacre of the Innocents—German Warsaw, 1943. Cleaning out the ghetto, probably to Auschwitz. Those unimpressive Germans are not the handsome, young, supremely confident soldiers who entered Warsaw in September 1939. By then most of them had been killed in Russia. Courtesy of Yivo Institute for Jewish Research, New York City.

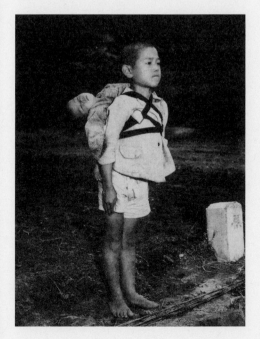

Massacre of the Innocents—Japan, 1945. "I had never before witnessed the obvious military influence on the young until I watched this boy bring his dead brother to a cremation site at Nagasaki. Every kid I knew in America would not have been able to cope like this boy did. He stood rigid, no emotion seen except for the terrible unshed tears." Picture and words by Joe O'Donnell, a young Marine Corps photographer who landed in Japan on September 2, 1945. From his book Japan 1945, Images from the Trunk, *published in Japan 1995 by Shogakukan, Inc.*

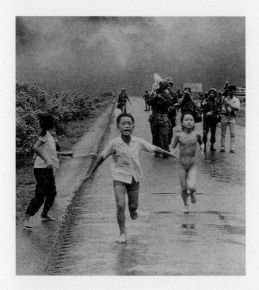

*Massacre of the Innocents—
Vietnam, 1972. Children fleeing
burning village near Saigon
accidentally bombed by South
Vietnamese plane. The
photographers in the background
find this an interesting picture.
Courtesy Bettmann Archive, New
York City UPI/Bettmann.*

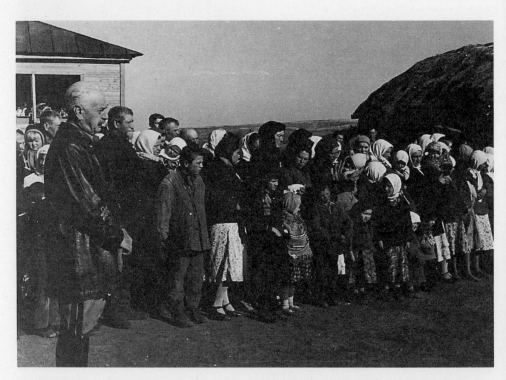

*Ukrainian peasants who have walked all night to attend an Italian army
mass, 1942. This action will not be forgotten when the Red Army returns. A
poor picture but historically valuable, taken by Lt. Chersi.*

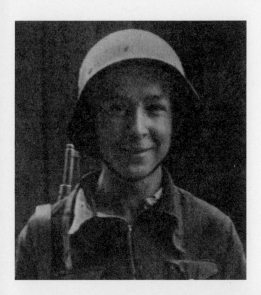

Polish soldier, Warsaw, August 1944. From Dni Powstania (Days of the Uprising), *Instytut Wydawniezy Pax, Warsaw 1984, Copyright by Stanislaw Kopf.*

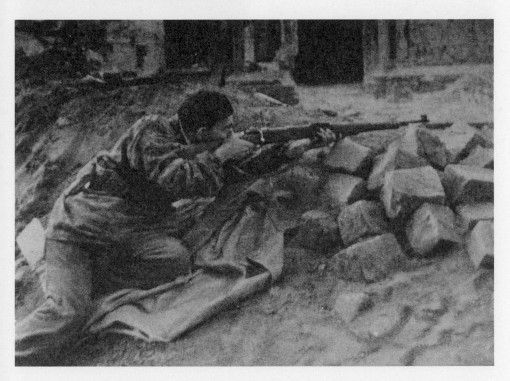

Home Army rifleman against tanks and dive bombers, Warsaw, August 1944.

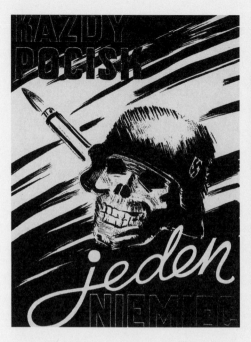

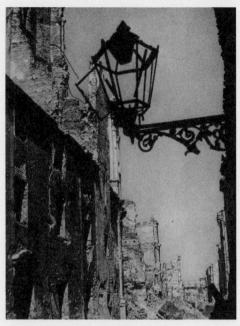

A poster from the Warsaw uprising of summer 1944. "Each bullet—one German": ammunition is running low.

Warsaw street, October 1944.

Berlin 1939, 1960

Truly, the world I live in is bleak.
The guileless word is foolish. A smooth brow
Denotes insensitiveness. The laughing man
Has only not yet received
the dreadful news.

And yet we know well:
Even hatred of vileness
Distorts a man's features.
Even anger at injustice
Makes hoarse his voice. Ah, we
Who desired to prepare the soil for kindness
Could not ourselves be kind.
        Bertolt Brecht *Three Elegies*

"Die Amerikaner lieben die Deutschen aber nicht die Nazis."

HOW MANY TIMES, in how many variants was that simple sentence worked over in those years? A boy at a gas station somewhere beyond the border of Luxembourg where we had spent the night had asked the standard question. I gave him the standard reply, my first step in international communication.

Now we were at a pension in Berlin. The landlady, pleased to have gentlemanly young guests like my friend Bruce and myself, had beamingly showed us a newspaper photo of Hermann Goering with his handsome family.

"How nice."

We were at the heart of the land of Oz, in a residential quarter, looking for a cheap restaurant, waiting impatiently for the first way in which the Evil Empire would reveal itself. Yes, a dentist's yellow sign on the gate to a front yard: "Dr. Oskar Nehemiah Weintraub, Zahnartz" beside a black Star of David. Yes, it was true. Even the middle name from the Bible.

And, of course, every encounter was framed by the obligatory Heil Hitler. To Bruce and myself, eighteen-year-old Americans, that was ridiculous, from the "Eilitler" of the out-shopping housewife to the full formal, heel-clicking explosion of the true believer. Did you repeat it when you kissed

Mom good morning? A hundred times a day it reminded you where and who you were. If you loathed the gesture, your impotence was rubbed in your face each time. It was also a source of mischievous merriment to the young alien who, armed with his passport's magic shield, could stroll into a shop, hands bravely in pockets, say "Guten Tag" and defy the whole system.

The uniforms in every mix of brown, black, gray, and summer white; the swastikas on flags and armbands; the strut that a pair of black boots gave to any man in uniform—their Germany was all around us. At a little ceremony—they were easy to come upon—we stopped to watch a trio of soldiers goose-stepping to lay their wreaths upon a shrine. It was exciting, a visit to a movie set. No expense spared for verisimilitude.

Arguments both complicated and simple had brought Bruce and myself to Berlin. As liberal, if adolescent, intellectuals we felt personally threatened by the Nazis. They wanted to eliminate people like us. The unprotesting conformity of our lives at Deerfield Academy, the rule of its kindly despot, Frank Boyden, and the storm-trooper spirit of schoolboy athletics were not totally unlike certain aspects of Germany. The parents of our friend Fritz were Jewish musicians from the world of Munich, Vienna, Prague, Zurich; when we were invited to Sunday dinner at their house in Northampton we listened to the stories they told. Their world, except in Zurich, had been destroyed, and we were conscious of that loss in every city we visited.

Berlin was also tied up, more obliquely, with my father's home on Long Island. *The Orchard* was the most beautiful house I have ever known. Damask curtains, polished antiques, silver and china with Sauternes and Rhine wine, Emma the maid arranging tomato-colored gladioli in the great Chinese vase, the vast lawns, the apple trees, the fragrance of boxwood—that supreme elegance was far above the rather ordinary people who moved around it.

> *Tel and Tel executives,*
> *Heads of cellophane or tin,*
> *With their animated wives*
> *Are due on the 6:10.*
> James Merrill *Days of 1935*

To leave that stage-set for Berlin on my way to Warsaw was, like having Jewish friends at Harvard and calling myself an atheist socialist, an expression of Oedipal defiance harmless to myself, exasperating to my father.

Charles E. Merrill was the ruling prince. When he had arrived at Amherst College from small-town Florida—5'5", with little money, a Southern accent, accompanied by his mother—he had been a totally marginal youth who supported himself by selling second-hand clothes and serving as business manager of a boarding house; after two years, unable to accept the humiliation of being poor at such a self-respecting institution, he had dropped out. That was long past. Wall Street encouraged an aggressive, hardworking young man who could be very charming, make a clear, rapid analysis of any complicated financial problem, and make firm decisions without fretting over his errors. He was a millionaire before he was 30.

His wife Hellen, my stepmother, had polished *The Orchard* into a smooth-running mechanism which presented him with no problems, and he was free to enjoy well-dressed guests who played bridge and golf and laughed at his stories. Back in West Palm Beach Dad had been a semi-pro baseball player; neither my brother nor I could catch, throw or bat a ball. That failure helped turn James into a poet and me into a Democrat. Sometimes during an empty afternoon I was drawn into his bedroom by two taboo icons that represented his authority: a fist-sized wad of $20 bills on his dresser and in the drawer of his bedside table a monstrous Colt automatic 45. My pre-occupation with Power in all the ways it showed itself and tried to disguise and fool itself (and its limits: I was there while he was dying) was connected with that beautiful house and its master.

President Roosevelt was the supreme foe of *The Orchard's* guests, threatening their fortunes and their status, but inescapably part of their hatred of him was the contempt they felt for Jews. They all had Jewish 'friends,' of course—and they liked to tell stories about how these friends had been humiliated when they had pushed too hard at the wrong doors. Now New York was full of Jews who had been driven out of Europe by Hitler, working in Macy's basement or occupying the biggest suites at the *Carlyle*.

Our family doctor's definition of psychiatrists: "Kikes with dirty minds."

After the unquestioning homogeneity of Deerfield, Harvard had made a traumatic impact upon me. There were so many classmates smarter, more radical than me, with a harshness of criticism that made me feel cautious and timid. And as a student's first exposure to Freud opens a door to the magic realism of sex, so my freshman course on Fascism and Communism had opened the door to political analysis of *The Orchard*.

I would not call *The Orchard's* dinner guests pro-Nazi, as people like them were in London and Paris. My father was instinctively anti-German, a holdover from 1918, when he had trained in Texas to be a combat fighter pilot, and he had a sincere respect for the English and French. Hitler was a vulgarian, a bit like Roosevelt perhaps, and my father's crowd, despite its whining, had not been pushed hard enough to follow such a radical path. Nevertheless, I felt obliged to see with my own eyes what was the end station of the prejudice taken so much for granted.

∾

Now in July 1939 we were in Berlin, on the first leg of our two-month trip. Bruce's involvement in the adventure was rather different from mine. His father had been a pioneer of the new Madison Avenue as mine was of the new Wall Street, rebuilding post-crash Merrill Lynch and Co. upon largeness of scale, open records, and democratic mass marketing. Mr. Barton had revolutionized advertising into the creation and marketing of desire—in fact had written a book on Jesus as God's salesman—until he had made a sufficient fortune and status to go into politics, becoming the Republican Congressman for Upper East Side Manhattan. His economic beliefs were as sternly conservative as my father's, but because his district included a large Jewish population, Mr. Barton found himself, to his surprise, an outspoken defender of the needs of refugees from Hitler's Europe. For Bruce to go with his friend to Berlin and Warsaw was proof of the whole family's concern for this terrible tragedy.

For me, the formal reason was to obtain a Gestapo permit to visit Prague. Prague had become a tragic city for me, betrayed by its allies so that the West, including myself, could enjoy a few more months of peace. I had heard President Beneš speak in Boston. I had pored over pictures of its towers and spires, its castle high above the Moldau. So, once in Berlin we must go first to the American Embassy for an introduction to the Gestapo. The officer we met was not sympathetic: "You're just going to get yourself into a lot of unnecessary trouble, and then you're going to expect us to get you out of it."

Outside the Embassy stretched an endless, motionless line of Jews waiting to apply for immigration visas, due perhaps in 1984. Across the avenue, on a large wooden box, stood a rigid, brown-shirted guard of the Arbeitsfront, holding a spade, watching that line of Jews. Every so often he turned his head from side to side like a wind-up machine. He was watching them. They would never escape.

In London, somehow, Bruce had been given the name of a Jewish tailor. We should call upon him; perhaps we could be of help. We tracked down the address, Teich, Schneider, (tailor) on the list of names outside the front door. Herr Teich, his wife, and a boy our age lived in an absolutely bare apartment. They had sold all their furniture to raise money for a Cuban visa, only to learn it was false, a scam, a joke. Now they had nothing. We spoke, with what German I knew and a smidgen of English from the son, in whispers.

The room might be bugged. (Did the Nazis—as later on the Communists—have the compulsion and resources to place tiny microphones, and listen to them, in every single room in Berlin and Warsaw and Prague?)

"I will get to England and join the English army."

Did Frau Teich offer us coffee? I forget. Should we have offered them money? That was not a gesture I was yet accustomed to. Bruce and I were already counting our bills and checks every day to see if we'd have enough cash to take us to Bucharest and Prague and back to Paris.

They were doomed. They didn't have a chance. The boy would never get to England. Even we could see that.

As I came to know a half-dozen cities that I trudged through later in Communist Poland and Czechoslovakia, I never saw a spectacle like that line of Jews, also doomed, stretched around the American embassy, and I never witnessed a personal agony (although they existed, I knew) as hopeless as that of the Teich family.

> *Say this city has ten million souls,*
> *Some are living in mansions, some are living in holes:*
> . . . .
>
> *Yet there's no place for us, my dear, yet there's no place for us.*
> *Went to a committee; they offered me a chair;*
> *Asked me politely to return next year:*
> *But where shall we go today, my dear, but where shall we go today?*
> . . . .
>
> *Saw a poodle in a jacket fastened with a pin,*
> *Saw a door opened and a cat let in:*
> *But they weren't German Jews, my dear, but they weren't*
>   *German Jews.*
>   W. H. Auden *Refugee Blues*

How would you compare the Nazis with the Communists? Jacek Woźniakowski, a friend I would make later in Kraków, saw it as duplicity: "The Nazis said they would destroy us and they did their best to. The Communists said they came as our friends and they acted just about as badly."

Beyond symbols and rhetoric, the Nazis sought primarily to destroy the outsider, whereas the worst brutality of the Communists was directed towards groups and individuals within the body politic. If you were not a Jew, a Gypsy, a homosexual, a Communist, an abstract artist, a Pole, a compulsive Christian, a senile or insane marginal (who were quietly put to sleep that fall as an economy measure), a flat-chested bluestocking with horn-rimmed glasses, and showed some sense in what you said and did, the very anti-intellectualism of the Nazis might have left you alone. Karl Marx, unlike the myth-rapt progenitors of Fascism, was an intellectual. His endless hours of study in the library of the British Museum meant a legacy which his heirs endlessly kept recycling. It was not so much the member of an evil category that the Communists sought to extirpate as the heretic. That statement, of course, is false: the five million uncooperative peasants, called kulaks, who died in Stalin's collectivization of the Ukraine formed a category. If your parents were bourgeois. If, as usual, you were a Jew, though it was anti-Semitic, fascist, to attack Jews as such; they must be punished as Zionists. Nevertheless, as the party line swung back and forth, searching out revisionists today or dogmatists tomorrow, those who made jokes about moustaches and did not praise poems about the Eagle of the Caucasus, who did not understand that yesterday's truth had to be quietly changed to conform to today's reality, the heretic became the traitor and had to be treated as such. The further up the ladder one climbed, the more dangerous any possible deviance appeared.

The German customs officials on the Luxembourg border dismissed Bruce's copy of Freud's *Moses and Monotheism* with good-natured contempt. A Communist with the slightest sense of duty would have confiscated it.

To die of cold and exhaustion at Vorkuta or Karaganda was better or worse than to die in a gas chamber at Auschwitz or Majdanek? Was a Harvard-Oxford-Sorbonne intellectual who ignored the one more or less guilty than a Southampton houseguest who ignored the other?

Bruce and I did reach the correct office at Gestapo headquarters and received a letter for the Gestapo in Vienna requesting them to issue us a three-day permit to visit Prague. I remember a poster of a kindly policeman helping an old lady and a couple of blond children cross the street while in the background a colleague blew a whistle to halt a mean thin dark young man running away with a bundle under his arm.

Then we got in our Renault and set out for Danzig.

2

Danzig/Gdańsk, 1939, 1968; Poznań 1960, 1964, 1968

Die Fahne hoch! Die Reihen dicht geschlossen.
SA marschiert in ruhig festem Schritt.
Kameraden, die Rotfront und Reaktionen erschossen
Marschieren im Geist in unseren Reihen mit.

The banners high! The ranks fast closed,
SA marches in calm firm pace.
Comrades shot by Red Front and Reaction
March in spirit in our ranks
    Horst Wessel Lied

BRUCE AND I had misjudged our supply of marks. There weren't enough for even the cheapest hotel. From Berlin we had driven through the pine forests and sandy potato fields of northeastern Prussia, through the uninteresting towns of whitewashed brick, but, as dusk slowly turned into night, we became too tired to travel further and shortly before the Polish border parked the car off the road.

A Renault makes an inadequate bedroom—Bruce folded into the back seat, I curled around the steering wheel—but we fell into enough sleep to be awakened at dawn by the tramp of boots and the marching song of a column of soldiers. Our stopping place turned out to be at the edge of a motor park, and we were given the privilege of observing a Wehrmacht unit begin its morning duties. The soldiers knew what to do: checking the gear, starting the engines, moving off without the slightest confusion to a sergeant's barks, and the column roared off correctly for some excursion along the Polish border. If French and British staff officers had been watching in that Renault instead of a couple of cold, cramped, hungry, unwashed New York teenagers, they might have learned something useful.

Eventually, the red-white-black swastika flag appeared in front of the guard post, and the black-clad, moustached official inspected the car—"French. Not very good, is it?"—and stamped our papers. (How much easier it was to get in and out of Nazi Germany than in and out of the Deutsche

Demokratische Republik.) He pointed proudly to the patch of medicated sawdust for Polish cattle to shuffle their feet through against the spread of hoof and mouth disease.

"Why do you want to visit a country like that?"

Fifty, a hundred yards ahead flew the white and red flag. A soldier in a khaki uniform, with a diamond-shaped cap and a rifle slung across his back, guarded the white-red striped Schlagbaum across the road. Both of us were too choked to speak. We had come for this: The white eagle on the red shield, the portraits of the aristocratic president and the iron field marshal on the wall, the signs and sounds of Polish, even the Gothic typewriters. Poland was the nation that would stand and fight. No compromise. No retreat. It was an honor for us two pilgrims to drive along this road, past men in their shabby suits, potato-shaped women, flaxen-haired children, heroic soldiers.

In London a couple of weeks earlier I had run across a long article in the *Times* on the Polish army that tried to be both analytical and optimistic. True, they were under-equipped, with not even enough rifles for their infantry, but they made up for it with their toughness, able to march 35 miles a day, farther even than Stonewall Jackson's men. Perhaps the Poles did rely on doubtful assumptions: German tanks were built out of plywood and lacked reserves of gasoline, the rains of September would wrap their treads in mud and free the cavalry for flexible counter-attacks. Perhaps it was not true that Polish lancers would trot through the suburbs of Berlin within six weeks, but.... That cavalry had defeated the Russians in 1920, a war forgotten by everyone else, and of course the forceful but rational French offensive—it wouldn't be like 1916—on the Western front would tie down the bulk of the Wehrmacht.

Back in Paris Bruce and I had watched and cheered the last sunset march-past of 14 juillet: Chasseurs Alpins with skis, Algerian Spahis in flowing white robes, a company of the Foreign Legion with their heavy tread, Senegalese ("bravo les noirs!"), Grenadier Guards, Royal Navy sailors, RAF fighters overhead, heavy tanks ungainly as, little faster than, beach cottages, simple infantrymen as had fought at Verdun.

> ... the plumed troop and the big wars
> that make ambition virtue ...
> ... the neighing steed and the shrill trump,
> the spirit-stirring drum, the ear-piercing fife,
> the royal banner, and all quality,
> Pride, pomp, and circumstance of glorious war!
> Othello (act III, scene III)

In Gdynia, in the bright new Poland that had come to life in 1919, we had breakfast. The very butter and jam we smeared on our rolls were signs of the country's peasant wealth. Toilet doors were marked panie and panowie. I chose the wrong one. No matter; one pays the price for adventure.

By noon we reached Danzig. The city had a confusing legal status. In a way, with its own postage stamps, it was a 'free city' accepting some paper supervision by the League of Nations and under the suzerainty (whatever that meant) of the Polish republic. The authority of the streets, however, was National Socialist. Berlin might be the official center of German power, but the front line was here, Danzig. Here the war would begin and crush that inferior enemy: "Suppose the Mexicans tried to seize Texas!" Voices were louder in Danzig. Every pair of boots made a proud German noise. The Hitler salutes were even more phallic than in Berlin, the women's eyes more flashing, their bosoms richer.

That winter I had read *Buddenbrooks*. Danzig was the same sort of Hanseatic trading city as Thomas Mann's Lübeck. Its buildings had the same sharp-edged brick sobriety, the same stepped gables, and stood for the same German Fleiss. Fleiss, translated in the dictionary as diligence, industry, application, assiduity goes beyond that and encompasses promptness, cleanliness, the respectful (but not servile) bow to your superiors followed by the reprimand to your inferiors, neatness, order, serious attention to food, self-respect, accurate filing systems, well-oiled tools. Anxiety? The personage at the top of one's ladder is suddenly replaced. The bank one deals with in Rio fails. One's daughter falls in love with a musician.

Danzig lived off its Polish hinterland, exporting the grain that had been rafted down the Vistula, reshipped at Lublin from as far as the Ukraine, timber from the Carpathians, amber and garnets. Its labor base, lovingly portrayed in Günter Grass' *Tin Drum*, was the Kashubian under-class, half-Polish, half-German, which supplied the vegetable women, carters, servants, prostitutes, dock workers.

All these details were hidden from Bruce's and my perception by the flagged and swastikaed excitement of the coming war.

September 1. It came. A gang of amateur soldiers made a suicidal defense of the Polish post office. In the film version of *The Tin Drum*, while the building is under a hail of machine-gun fire moments before the Germans wheel up a fat little cannon to blow in the entrance, a postal clerk runs across the office, rifle in hand, and stoops to pick up a sheet of stamps. When the building surrenders, its defenders are hustled out against a wall and shot. Perhaps they were the fortunate.

No rain. The tanks were made of steel, not plywood. They had fuel enough. The beautiful horses were machine-gunned. Any defense was smashed by dive bombers. Danzig's surviving resistance, which lasted almost as long as the Polish army's ten or twelve days, was the Westerplatte fort on the curving strip of sand outside the harbor. Every so often one of its guns fired back at the aged heavy cruiser, *Schleswig Holstein*, which leisurely shelled it day after day. Warsaw itself held out until September 28, broadcasting Chopin's *Polonaise* over and over.

What joy the war must have brought to the burghers of Danzig. A shame that they could not enjoy it on television, but there were newsreels of marching infantry, broken bridges and burning towns, Stukas gracefully peeling off towards their targets, endless lines of shuffling prisoners. The Poles would be placed forever in the helot roles fitting for them: cabbage growers and coal miners. A Pole with a little education might become a primary school teacher or a postal clerk, but it would be dangerous—as it was for Negroes I met in 1941 Mississippi—to aim higher. A priest was tolerated if he taught submission, to be rewarded later on, of course, in Heaven.

In the Hohenzollern provinces of Pomerania and Posen west of Danzig, the Nazis intensified Bismarck's old policy of pushing the Polish peasants off their lands so they could be given to Germans. (History forces ugly comparisons: thirty, forty years later Israeli police and settlers were pushing Arabs off the lands that the God of Abraham had reserved for Jews. Arab workers I saw in Jerusalem were there to repair streets and clean toilets.)

Danzigers were proud, I am sure, to join the Wehrmacht and share its quick victories after Poland: Denmark and Norway, Holland and Belgium, France, above all, and the defeat of the British army (as Americans enjoyed the defeat of the Marxist regime on Grenada—celebrated by postage stamps of Mickey Mouse and Donald Duck, the overthrow of the corrupt dictator of Panama, and the destruction of Iraq's army with lines of shuffling prisoners as long as Poland's).

The first weeks of Hitler's invasion of Russia, which had begun June 22, 1941, must have seemed glorification of the German historic right to total victory. There was no more beautiful beginning of a military campaign in all history. The maps trembled as the armored phalli thrust ever deeper into Russia and the Ukraine.

At what moment did each individual German come to the private conclusion, staring at the ceiling at three o'clock in the morning, that his side, no matter how often victorious, was going to lose? When Wehrmacht troops in summer uniforms (winter uniforms implied a longer war) were caught by the first Russian snows? When America entered? When the 6th Army surrendered at Stalingrad? When Hamburg was obliterated?

The bill for those good times was presented to Danzig in January 1945. The Red Army was moving almost as fast now as the Wehrmacht had in 1941. Rokossovsky's army reached the suburbs, and the glorious war turned into house-to-house fighting for each street while its citizens huddled in the cellars and argued about how to burn their swastikas, how to store their excrement, how to chop off the girls' hair and smear their faces with ashes to discourage rape.*

In February of 1968 I came a second time to Gdańsk, its postwar name, by train from Poznań. I am fascinated by Polish architecture, so little known by parochial art historians of the West. Where does it reflect German and Russian influences, even French and Italian, where, in qualities even of fantasy—the prickly spires of its church-tower, the adventurous towers of each ratusz (Rathaus), the colors of its gentry town-houses—is it absolutely itself? How does Poznań, like Breslau/Wrocław, reveal itself as a Hohenzollern city? Passing those humorless buildings of heavy brown stone one can smell the beer and cigars, hear the distant thump and blare of a regimental march, the rustle of its hospital nurses' starched uniforms, and the whistle of the express from Berlin arriving, as it should, at exactly 1:13. If they could be disciplined anywhere and learn Prussian promptness, thrift, cleanliness, up to whatever limits their flawed genetics permitted, the Poles in Hohenzollern Posen were.

---

* An odd detail was the Russian soldier's delight in throwing a piano out of a window. In the last months of World War II when a city like Danzig, Poznań, or Breslau had been liberated, the Red Army commander granted his men two days to drink, rape, and destroy. Their ultimate joy was to locate a piano in some looted building and then tug, push, grunt, sweat it up the stairs, crash it into the apartment at the top landing, and then, after smashing the window frames with gun butts, to shove it out the window and let it drop to the sidewalk below.

Imagine if you can the fall of a piano from a four-story building, the explosion when it hit, the unbelievable sound of shattering wood and torn wires in a hundred different tones. If you met someone whose soul had been ravished by the same experience, you would know that he knew, and together you might set out to recapture the moment, like the perfect high, the perfect orgasm, the perfect rock concert, that those who had not shared could never grasp in a thousand years. One absolute moment of creation and destruction, both as one, that the Eastern mind could comprehend and the Western, fettered to sterile rationalism until the student uprising of the 1960s, could not.

Posen was the fortress city built to defend the Eastern approaches to Imperial Germany against a Tsarist invasion, and indeed did hold off the Red Army until February of 1945. There is a story that the secret details of that fortress were completed by French war prisoners in 1871, rewarded by a lavish banquet of all good things to eat and drink, then quietly executed.

Poznań became a leading industrial center for post-1945 Poland, its ruins rebuilt, especially its glorious ratusz, and its annual trade fair a way to show Western buyers what Polish industry could produce. It was also the first city where, in June of 1956, savage rioting (as in East Berlin in 1953) revealed the proletariat's rejection of Communism. Because the riots occurred at the time of the fair, they could not be hidden, and the new Gomułka government took the risk of open trials with Western journalists admitted. In a Communist state the first priority has to be education so that young people grow up to be disciplined workers and loyal citizens. The sullen hoodlums in the dock told of an entirely different upbringing. Father was dead or so exhausted by work and brutalized by vodka that he held no place in the family. Mother was away ten, twelve hours a day, at her job and standing in line for soap and sausage. If any supervision came it was from babcia—grandmother. No one bothered about these kids.

The riots at Poznań forced whatever liberalism Gomułka was willing to risk, which might have amounted to something structural if the revolution in Hungary had not frightened every apparatchik, and if the Anglo-French-Israeli attack on Suez had not distracted world attention.

My train reached a rainy, shabby Gdańsk early Sunday, 1968. One should travel in Poland during February or November when the awful weather matches reality.

The excited German crowds with their boots and Heil Hitlers were gone. The city had been pretty well rebuilt since 1945, when it had been fought over and then burnt out by either the Wehrmacht or the Red Army, take your pick. The original dignity and richness of the old city now restored did not have to be attained for the new city, but I found a bare, clean hotel and a large tourist restaurant with the regulation pork chop. Although it was to no one's interest to serve any customer with courtesy or diligence, sometimes my Polish would elicit a smile.

In the afternoon I happened upon a small historical museum that presented an elegant, three-dimensional floor display of the Vistula system running from the Baltic to the Carpathians. At the border of the Soviet Union, a few miles to the north of Gdańsk and then Lithuania, everything became blank, taboo, as if it were on the far side of the moon. Under Stalinism all the barriers between the socialist lands became impermeable. It was easier to travel from Warsaw to Paris than to Prague or Vilnius. Travelers should not be encouraged to make contacts or compare notes.

The argument of the museum was that Danzig had originally been founded by Poles and then brutally Germanized. The German argument is that Poles were people of the fields and that only Germans possessed the social structure, construction skills, and discipline with which to build the cities of Eastern Europe. A month later I would be motoring down the Dalmatian coast with my wife and two sons, and in the beautiful white cities of Zara/Zadar, Spalato/Split, Ragusa/Dubrovnik, there was presented the similar question of whether they were originally Venetian or Croat. One remembers Plato in the *Crito*: I choose the theory that makes the most sense to me and then employ the facts that conform to it.

That February morning, still groggy from the Poznań train, I had attended mass at the great cathedral, St. Mary's, built with a noble brick Prussian austerity that gives it a dignity unlike any other Gothic church I know. I seldom go to church at home. Perhaps it is easier abroad, isolated by language, undisturbed, left to make one's own reflections on society or one's own moral reality. The power of the building's architecture together with the choreography of the service at the distant altar, the unanimity of this crowded congregation, with whom I obediently rose and sat, protected us from the muddy streets outside and the mechanics of the Communist state.

Gdańsk would become famous twelve years later as the center of Solidarność, the united force of workers at the Lenin shipyards led by a young electrician named Lech Wałęsa, who insisted that a labor union should speak for the workers and not for the state. It was a simple message that rapidly included other arguments and led to the seizure of power by General Jaruzelski and eventually to the presidency of Poland for the former electrician, who had become a rather different man by then.

My own contact with that Baltic city last came in 1980 at an exhibit of the treasures of Danzig at the Jewish Museum in New York. The congregation knew they were doomed, so in early 1939 they sold the land of their synagogue and graveyard for whatever it would bring, and, packing up all their ceremonial objects (including a memorial to the loyal soldiers who had given their lives in 1914–1918 for the Fatherland), shipped them to the Jewish Theological Seminary for safekeeping. Along with the Torahs and prayer shawls were picture books of shtetl life, the annual forest picnic of the Sons of Zion, and Rabbi Myersohn's new academy in Bialystok whose thirteen-year-olds had the faces of boys and girls I taught.

3

Nuremberg 1939, 1945

Und so werden wir marschieren,
Wenn alles in Scherben fällt,
Denn heute gehört uns Deutschland
und Morgen die ganze welt!

And so we shall march,
Though everything falls in pieces,
For today Germany belongs to you
and tomorrow the whole world.
    Adolf Hitler

IN ITS WAY, Nuremberg was also on the approach to Warsaw, even if Bruce and I reached it at the end of our trip, after Prague. We had lunch in Dresden, at a pretty restaurant looking across the Elbe to the Zwinger Palace. We kept checking our watches, waiting for the war to arrive, and could not spend time there, a pity. Later on the Dresdners would fool themselves that there was a sort of tacit agreement: We won't bomb Oxford, They won't bomb us. It was a charming city, of no military importance, and by February of 1945 crowded with refugees from the fighting in front of Breslau. General Harris, head of the RAF Bomber Command, saw no reason, however, not to kill Germans, anywhere, and in 24 hours wave after wave of British and American planes wiped out the city.

My second visit to Dresden came in late November 1989, when I stayed at the *Neva*, a standardized Russian-style hotel, with a Leningrad Restaurant and a Pushkin breakfast room, and in the morning a view from my bedroom down the Pragerstrasse, a formless avenue that posed the question not simply of what century was I in, but what continent: Pittsburgh? São Paulo? Singapore?

In 1939 Bruce and I spent the night in Leipzig, an unmemorable city where we heard Verdi's *Masked Ball*, and then took the autobahn southwest to Nuremberg. With war so close, the Parteitag with all its hundreds of thousands of boots and salutes had been canceled, but just the same the city was jammed with excited visitors. I remember the brown-stone gabled houses

with their green and white shutters, restaurants with red and white checked
tablecloths and folksy beer mugs. Shops for toys and clocks, swans swimming in the moat before the castle walls. Every window box was bursting
with pink and white petunias. There were no soldiers, no SS, they were away
on the borders, but their beefy fathers wore party uniforms or lederhosen,
their younger brothers wore Hitlerjugend* brown, their sisters and mothers
gay dirndls. Everyone was clean, wholesome, sparkling with health and
energy—no wonder many French and English envied the German spirit that
their own citizens lacked.

The spiritual mentor of Nuremberg was Hans Sachs. That bluff, forthright,
16th-century shoemaker of the medieval guilds, hero of *Die Meistersinger*,
which Hitler saw again and again, was eternal Germany, now at last reborn.
All doubts and smudges had been cast aside. Every boy in Hitlerjugend shirt
and boots could now grow up to become, as best he could, Hans Sachs. Every
one of these well-formed, laughing girls in their dirndls would eagerly be his.

Nuremberg's other mentor was the Iron Maiden, star of the torture chamber in the Schloss. She was an ingenious machine designed to excite the males
and frighten the females. The client was fastened inside, the works wound
up, and tock tock tock, three pairs of spikes would gradually pierce his eyes,
chest and groin. Germans were good-natured, generous people, but don't try
to put anything over on them.

Bruce wanted to buy a mother's medal for his mother, so we went into a
shop that displayed patriotic souvenirs. Mrs. Barton had only three children,
and thus fit into the lowest category of medal wearers, but all her son's
friends were very fond of her and she clearly deserved the honor. The shop-
keeper, not liking our American accents or untrustworthy faces, refused to
sell us one. A Hitler picture instead? There was every sort: in shining armor
on horseback holding the Banner, staring straight ahead like one of Schiller's
heroes to the Ideal, to Truth, to Death. With a loyal dog. Graciously accepting a bouquet from two little girls. Saluting, staring straight at you so you
would not dare even think an ambiguous thought. I bought a bayonet.

Danzig had been exciting, like walking along the streets of Madison just
before the Michigan game, but Nuremberg was sexy. Tonight would be a
date not with that blonde from Sigma Chi but with War, when the Wehrmacht in self-defense invaded Poland. You didn't have to be a Freudian to
know what those salutes and tanks and bombers stood for. Boy oh boy!

---

* Years later I met a Pole who knew a former Hitlerjugend from Silesia, who described the
initiation ceremony of being handed a rabbit or kitten, and told to kill it with one's hands in
order to learn the discipline of cruelty.

I returned to Nuremberg six years later, part of a guard detail escorting Obergruppenfuhrer Wolff, formerly supreme SS commander in Italy, to the site of the War Crimes tribunal. The 88th Infantry Division, headquartered at Lake Garda, was responsible for the control and repatriation of all German PWs, and this jaunt was a pay-off for twenty or so long service GIs.

At the airfield we stood around to stare at our prisoner: tall, hard, more arrogantly military than our own generals, unapologetic in his immaculate uniform though its jacket was pocked with little holes where his medals and badges had been removed. Next to him stood a Jewish infantryman from the 10th Mountain Division, originally, he told us, from a village in southwestern Germany where his family, the only Jews, lived surrounded by silence. On Saturdays he used to bicycle to a town nearby with a few more Jews where he played table tennis. Now he was General Wolff's interpreter and guard.

Our plane flew over the Alps, through passes where our wingtips almost brushed the pines; over Munich, whose houses seemed untouched until one noticed that none of them had any roofs; and landed outside of Nuremberg. The general was taken away. We 'Italians' were billeted with a headquarters unit at a Siemens' electrical appliance plant. After supper I set out alone to explore the city center. Because the city stood on a hill in the middle of the great Bavarian plain, any Allied raid that could not reach its primary target dropped its bombs on Nuremberg on the flight home. There was a full moon, and the piles of rubble that used to be houses and the Schloss might just as well have been the mountains of the moon. Because this was Germany the stones bordering the streets were arranged neatly. In Naples and Milan, later in London, I had walked across cities where every block held a bombed-out building. Here, though one might see distant lights where someone had constructed a shelter under a piece of corrugated iron, entire blocks lacked a single building upright.

At a crossroads separating those hills of moonlit rubble, two housewives were bidding each other goodnight with the same little German formulas of sociability as if they had spent an evening of coffee, cakes, and radio at a home of a mutual friend, decorated with lace curtains and rubber plants. Ridiculous wind-up toys or tragic heroines of civilization? As I grew older I became more sorry for those two women and what they had lost.

Many years later I understood the metaphor for Nuremberg: Disneyland. More than any other city, Nuremberg, for Hitler, was Germany. Berlin had perverts. Hamburg had reds. Munich had artists. Frankfurt had Jews. Nuremberg, by God, had Germans! Hans Sachs and the master singers were both reality and myth. The symbol of re-awakened Germany, the Third

Reich that would last a thousand years, without any marginal people or ideas to confuse matters. The strength of our soldiers and their weapons, the purity of our girls and those pink and white petunias. Unless Nazis are dressed up as sadistic and stupid prison guards or as cold-blooded officers harassing beautiful, half-Jewish girls named Anna, it was hard at that time for Americans to grasp why the system was so bad. The mountains, the village churches, the symphony orchestras, the efficient policemen, the clean, courteous children, those petunias—what was so wrong with all that?

Another charismatic mythmaker, Ronald Reagan, sold Disneyland as America. While he did not go back to the Middle Ages, his comprehension of history was not all that different: a band parading down Main Street, a boy and a girl, hand in hand, coming out of a soda fountain, Dad in shirtsleeves, Mom with her shopping basket, the kindly cop, no Jews, a couple of cheerful darkies playing their banjos on the river boat, petunias in the front yards.

To be sure, Mickey Mouse lacked Hans Sachs' moral vigor. Minnie Mouse had a personality unlike the Iron Maiden's. Nevertheless, each pair expressed in the deepest possible way the true spirit of their race, untouched by today's headlines or the criticism of rootless intellectuals. The German boys beat those slovenly Poles in a couple of weeks as the American boys beat those Iraqis. No one saw the faces of the men they killed.

This section on Germany, however, should not end here.

When Bruce and I reached Munich the evening after we left Nuremberg, I was a foolish enough 19-year-old to think it might be fun to witness the coming of war from inside Germany—which would also postpone a meeting with my father I wasn't looking forward to. We were driving a Renault with a French license, however, and I did not want to show up at the car rental office in Paris and whine that the Germans had confiscated it. Because rumor said that the French border was already closed, Bruce and I, with a couple of American students we'd run into, headed towards Zurich. "Stay off the Autobahn—it'll be crowded with convoys," someone warned.

As we drove along the side roads, we passed columns of sad, heavy farm horses being led to their mobilization posts. (One forgets how much military transportation was horse drawn in that war—the first Russian soldier to enter Graz, where I later taught in southeastern Austria, was on horseback.) Just before the Swiss border we stopped for supper. Might as well use up our last marks.

At the table next to ours sat a thin young man, a reservist from the suitcase by his chair, silently eating. Opposite him, unable to touch her food, sat his wife, weeping into her handkerchief. The war had come.

Waves of anger and fear
Circulate over the bright
And darkened lands of the earth,
Obsessing our private lives;
The unmentionable odour of death
Offends the September night.
W. H. Auden *September 1, 1939*

4

War 1941–1943

What passing-bells for these who die as cattle?
Only the monstrous anger of the guns.
      Wilfred Owen *Anthem for Doomed Youth*

Wish me luck as you kiss me goodbye,
Cheerio, here I go, on my way.
Give me a smile I can keep all the while
In the years I'm far from you.
Wish me luck as you kiss me goodbye,
Cheerio, here I go, on my way.
      Song 1939

Mississippi 1941

BEING A SOLDIER in wartime is a bit like being a visitor to some strange city with its own architecture and language.

It is hard for my children and students to understand how firmly I was directed all during my boyhood towards becoming a soldier. My earliest grown-up novel was Remarque's *All Quiet on the Western Front*, a story of the life and death of a German infantryman. For years afterwards when my pals and I played war games in Central Park, I was the Germans. When I was ten, my father took me to a shattering performance of Sherriff's *Journey's End*, set in a dugout where some English officers were awaiting the last German offensive of 1918. Years later I met a young man who had served in the Abraham Lincoln Brigade.* Why hadn't I been old enough to fight for Spanish democracy, as Dad had wept that he hadn't been old enough to fight in Cuba?

When Bruce and I returned to Paris in the last days of August, was it my duty (and the way to avoid my father, angry at this unauthorized adventure) to join the French army? The friend of his whom I asked for advice knew the correct reply: there would probably be little real fighting soon and nothing

---

* 3000 men of whom 500 were black, the first racially mixed American combat regiment.

in the world could be more boring than life in a French barracks. How hungry young men are to look for opportunities by which they can throw away their lives. Less so now.

With the war devastating Europe, I was serving no useful purpose at Harvard, I thought after a while, so in the early summer of 1941 I went down to the Marines' recruiting station in New York. The nineteen-year-olds waiting around were such a scruffy lot, not my social class, that I left. Probably 80% of them were dead by the end of 1942. I even wrote to headquarters of the Polish army in Canada for enlistment papers.

Instead I might fight fascist aggression by working for a Christian Socialist cooperative farm — Kolkhoz — in Mississippi. There I kept books for the creamery and the credit co-op, and at ten cents an hour sold corn meal, snuff, rifle cartridges, pickled pigs' feet, and women's underwear in the general store.

"They sure looks large, cap'n."

"They'll shrink, ma'am."

"They pretty small, cap'n."

"They'll stretch, ma'am."

Sam Franklin, my boss — the only man of our community with a library, a piano, a flush toilet, and no gun — had been a Presbyterian missionary in Japan until he was expelled for combining discussion sessions for university students with a settlement house for Korean and Formosan slum children. Tragedy in Mississippi, he said, was cold, slow and ungrammatical. Even worse than the poverty was the sense of repressed violence ready to explode if any white man lost his temper.

The Japanese attack on Pearl Harbor came over the radio the Sunday afternoon that my fiancée traveled from Chicago to see Providence Farm where she was to live. She arrived just before we had our weekly service in the little frame building that the stricter white families boycotted because dances (clutch-and-hug dances) were held there on Saturdays. Sam spoke about the Christians he had worked beside during his years in Japan and closed the service with a prayer for the Americans and the Japanese, who were to suffer so sadly before they could be reconciled.

Canada 1942

Mary and I were married in her parents' living room, we took a week's honeymoon in Cuba, and then I left for Toronto. To serve in the Canadian army would preserve the international quality of fighting the Nazis that I considered important. They had a smarter uniform. At basic training outside

Chatham, Ontario, a town about 70 miles east of Detroit, we were issued rifles stamped 1902, surplus from the Boer War, and at night we removed their bolts, a British custom, so that barefoot Afghans would not creep into the barracks to steal them. Our bayonet instructor, an English corporal who had served at the Somme, told us that the early morning sun glistening off our steel blades terrified the Germans, who would throw down their machine guns and run away. We took long route marches made bearable by old-fashioned songs (American soldiers rarely sang), the favorite being cheerfully unprintable, from a harmless Scottish tune: "Nelly put your belly up to mine."

After a couple of months at Chatham I was sent to the artillery camp of Petawawa, a tarpaper waste among sand and pine trees up the Ottawa River. F battery was anti-tank, but because Canada had been too poor, too complacent to buy arms in peacetime, we drilled on wooden guns. When the gunner pulled the imaginary lanyard we shouted "bang!"

Canadian troops had reached Britain too late to involve themselves in the debacle at Dunkirk. The big event of 1942 was the massive raid on Dieppe, a test of German defenses and of Allied assault techniques, and a massacre of the Canadians, though it had some long-range value in persuading the Germans that the ultimate invasion would come on the Channel coast around Calais and not, as it did, in Normandy. The men I served with probably fought and died along the endless Adriatic coast as part of the 8th Army, and later in the liberation of Holland.

Having applied for officers' training, I was kept on at Petawawa as a bombardier (two stripes) in the instructional cadre and after a few months began referring to Americans as "them." On a bunk near mine lived a withdrawn, older lance bombardier who while cleaning his gear used to drone away:

> *There'll always be a Ningland*
> *And Ningland shall be free,*
> *If Ningland means as much to you*
> *As Ningland means to me.*

In words and melody it was the world's most banal piece of 'music,' but for some soldiers there still remained the conviction from that terrible summer after Dunkirk that Britain, plus some Canadian and Australian units, scatterings of French and Poles, could rely only on herself. Russia and America were seated on the sidelines. Whatever the world became rested, for a while, upon British shoulders alone, and that tedious little song brought one close to tears.

Nothing remains unchanged. After the war, that memory of lonely courage, when everyone else had surrendered, kept Britain from playing any leadership role in the efforts to unify Europe. "There'll always be—" became the hymn of beery hooligans at Brussels and Amsterdam soccer stadiums to work up fighting spirit before they staggered forth to brawl with the natives.

As a training battery, gradually with guns made out of steel and with enough ammunition so that we could fire them once or twice a month, we handled a new draft of recruits every ten weeks. Sometimes it didn't seem proper to observe someone else's country so intimately: the desperately poor villages in Nova Scotia and mining towns of northern Ontario, the wretched schooling.

> *When this bloody war is over,*
> *Oh how happy I will be.*
> *When I get my civvy clothes on,*
> *No more soldiering for me.*
>
> *No more rising at reveille,*
> *No more asking for a pass.*
> *We will tell the sergeant major*
> *to shove his passes up his ass.*
>   Melody *What a Friend We Have in Jesus*

Every so often we received a draft of French-speaking soldiers from Quebec. Conscription was universal, but the French deputies in Parliament had insisted that no one be sent overseas except voluntarily. Then he had the right to wear a Canada badge on his shoulder. The soldiers who did not were called 'zombies.' There was no effort made to explain these two groups of resentful, ignorant men to each other. The fellow who took the upper bunk next to mine ate sardines in bed and spat on the floor.

"Eh, vous, ne crachez pas sur le plancher!"

"Va te faire foutre!"

How wide should the windows be opened? Every Frenchman knows that night air is deadly. We English-speaking soldiers might win the Ukrainians from Manitoba or Saskatchewan over to our side window-wise, but the permanent barracks staff of latrine-cleaners and stove-feeders were French, and after everyone was asleep they would shut all the windows so that we gasped awake each morning in a mustard-colored fog.

My wife was renting a room in Petawawa with a French family whose man worked as carpenter in the camp. If the war lasted long enough, Madame explained, they'd be able to pay off the mortgage. Mary made friends with an officer's wife next door. We would call upon them on Sundays, he and I taking off our jackets so that the difference in rank wouldn't be too evident. As a Harvard man, with my father owning that great house in Southampton, you might think that I would believe myself the equal of those callow lieutenants from the University of Toronto, but I didn't.

She's got hair between her knees
Like the branches of the trees,
Nelly put your belly up to mine

USA 1943

My hopes of becoming a Canadian officer, wearing a moustache and carrying a swagger stick, were going no place, so when a last notice came that any Americans still in the Canadian army could apply for transfer, I put in my name and by January found myself in Fort Knox, Kentucky, preparing to be a tank driver. To go through a second basic training was like seeing a bad movie twice.

The ethnic mix was different—Italian, Irish, Jewish soldiers from the cities, hot-tempered country boys from Southern towns. Juke box songs were filled with self-pity:

Low and lonely, sad and blue,
Always thinking of little you.
Always trying
To keep from crying . . .

You swore to be true till the end of the world

Seven beers with the wrong woman

I had first heard that on the jukebox of the *Blue Moon Café* in Webbers Falls, Arkansas, while hitchhiking across the country in the summer of 1940.

Our equipment and expenditure of ammunition were lavish by Canadian standards, our training much more professional: "With your left hand turn the cotter pin 45 degrees counterclockwise while with your right withdraw the alignment flange one half inch." Everyone else in the world was our inferior, not a Canadian concept. It was fun to ride in a tank with the hatches open, like the Germans rolling across Russia, but I suffered a terrifying claustrophobia when we had to close them: flames, fumes, exploding ammunition, and then the gas tank would catch and the whole machine blow up in a fire storm.

I was given a pass to Chicago to see our daughter Catherine, and Mary had me change her diapers so that I knew she existed. Then by train to our staging area, Camp Campbell on the Tennessee border, with an action-filled day of combat training: crawling through barbed wire under machine-gun fire, learning how to bury excrement, and sticking a hypodermic needle in an orange so we would know how to administer morphine to a wounded buddy. The day ended with a lecture that we shouldn't be afraid of combat because statistics proved that a surprisingly small percentage of soldiers were actually killed.

Algeria 1943

There's a star-spangled banner waving someplace
In a distant land that's many miles away.
   Song 1942

Our troop ship zigzagged from Newport News to Casablanca, and after a week or so we were stacked in a museum-grade freight train—8 chevaux, 40 hommes—for a slow trip across Morocco to Oran. Senegalese soldiers guarded the railway bridges with antique Hotchkiss machine guns, an Arab sheik wearing a scarlet cape galloped up to watch us roll past his black tents, from the other direction rolled trainloads of light-hearted Italian prisoners from Tunisia. "Hey, Joe, gimme the address of your girlfriend!"

The 36th Division had gone into a staging area at Arzew, an Algerian town about thirty kilometers east of Oran, before embarking for the invasion of southern Italy. The heavy equipment—tanks, guns, trucks—was parked wheel to wheel beside the road as far as the eye could see, and in the stubblefields framed by the long green bars of vineyards, the infantry regiments were bivouacked. It was twilight. The hill slopes were dotted with little campfires, and one could hear music from the guitars and harmonicas. The 141st had originally come from San Antonio, and one of its rifle companies was entirely Mexican, with all commands given in Spanish, and as I walked past the lines of tanks I could hear someone singing in Spanish. Beyond the mountain rose a scarlet curve of tracer bullets where the anti-aircraft guns were shooting at a German reconnaissance plane over the harbor of Arzew, but the puptents, the campfires, the sound of guitars seemed to be from some American past only slightly in touch with this particular war. The men and much of the way they spoke weren't much different, despite all the tanks and artillery, from what one would have found with Pershing or with Lee and Sherman.

I turned off the road until a rise of ground cut off the military paraphernalia and I was back in North Africa. I wasn't alone, however, for in a hollow there stood an Arab boy with a couple of dozen grazing sheep and a restless dog. He was clad in a cotton shift, bare-legged, and playing a flute. He could have been King David.

Salerno 1943

Our line of landing boats had begun to attract shellfire, and the excited sailors yelled back and forth to each other that we'd better pull off to the left. That was their business. We were passengers and enjoyed the bright Italian colors—the mountains still purple with the sun rising over their tops, the pink and yellow houses and dark green umbrella pines beyond the beach, bordering the sparkling blue of the water, the action of our boats, the bustle on the beach where the first barrage balloons were being put up, a truck in flames, and the incoming German shells. They whined and burst and indignant soldiers yelled, "Hey, we're being shot at!" just as they did in the movies. As our truck rolled off the ramp and through the surf, grinding across the beach, we passed a group of advancing infantrymen holding out their rifles and bayonets with self-conscious aggressiveness, glancing at each other sideways, bit players in this extravaganza not yet sure if they were playing their parts right.

Away from the beach, our truck full of gasoline cans and ammunition was a fat target. I dropped off the back. A shell burst so close I could see its orange center. Something cut the top of my shoulder and I fell to the ground. The wide-screen Hollywood epic narrowed. What I saw now were blades of grass, a couple of ants walking past my face. What I heard were the shells coming one after another and exploding a few yards away. There was nothing to be done. No magic wall protected me, only the inch-high defenses of the track I lay in. I remember a sad process of trying to bargain with God. If He kept me from getting killed, I would never again ask anything more of life. I would become a postal clerk and be grateful for each day. The Germans stopped firing. I, however, went back on my end of the agreement.

My cut was bandaged, my truck had vanished, I was a tourist, costumed with helmet and rifle like all the other extras. German prisoners passed me, some of them wounded and helped along by their comrades, thinner than we were, with sharp, tanned faces and long hair. To my left appeared a Doric temple (the temple of Nettuno at Paestum), but right in front of me was a smashed German tank and a few feet away from it a soldier, face down in his own blood, one leg moving slowly back and forth. In a half circle nearby stood a dozen American soldiers watching him, neither callous nor compassionate. They were in combat for the first time and they had never seen a man die.

The 36th was being hit by desperate German tank attacks from a Panzer division that had just moved in from the Russian front. Their infantry had lain in the dunes, letting our own soldiers walk past them in the darkness, and then had opened fire in both directions. There is quite a difference between what one does in training and what one does under fire. Many American soldiers and their officers became very private people, concerned only to dig holes and wait quietly in them until the war went elsewhere. It was out of this background that the most important story—at least for me— came of the landing at Salerno.

A badly wounded American was being bandaged by a medic in the middle of an open field when a German tank, siren at full blast, emerged over the stone wall. There was nowhere the medic could hide or run and he had his duty, so he stood up beside his soldier, pointed to his Red Cross armband, and thumbed the tank out of the way. At the last minute the German tank driver swerved to one side, passed the two Americans, and continued down the field. Here were two soldiers who shared the same respect for duty and courage, who, in all the murderous polytheism of war, obeyed the same god. Years later as a teacher I came across these verses, rarely quoted, from Chapter 19 of *Isaiah*:

> *The Lord shall smite Egypt, He shall smite and heal it; and they shall return even to the Lord . . .*
> *In that day shall Israel be the third with Egypt and with Assyria, whom the Lord of Hosts shall bless, saying, Blessed be Egypt my people, and Assyria the work of my hands, and Israel mine inheritance.*

Whether they liked it or not, the three peoples were brothers.

San Pietro 1943

By November the 36th Division was locked into the valleys and hills in front of San Pietro, a town between Naples and Rome, on the other side of Venafro and Mignano, before one reached San Vittore and Cassino. The 141st Infantry Regiment made up part of all this and set up an observation post on Monte Rotondo in order to comment on the gradual destruction of San Pietro, which crumbled under our artillery like Miss Havisham's wedding cake. Our hilltop world was a prairie-dog village where we sat on the edge of our burrows, cautiously socializing, until the first German mortar shells fell across our ears again and we dove underground. It was a dangerous post. When we reached the base of the hill to start our climb, there were always two or three blanket-covered bodies lying next to each other, one I remember with an arm in the air, frozen in some last agony, a glove clasped in its fist. We manned our post in twenty-four hour shifts, two men on duty, two sleeping under a tent dug into a second slit trench. My partner was a taciturn soldier from Dallas named Karpan, and we stood silently, and as I reflect now, uselessly, beside our telephone to regimental headquarters, in the rain of every day where it seemed important to be sure that something was kept dry, even if just a pocket handkerchief, and at night, a part of the dark without thought or a sense of time, shifting a little from foot to foot, every so often hearing a truck motor, a burst of machine-gun fire, three or four shells, ours or theirs, landing in the valley. We enjoyed the beauty of dawn, the line of brown and then yellow over the hills, the mist silver in the valley. After that, though, it was just another gray dangerous day.

On one day's shelling we heard again the whine and crash of mortars working their way up the slope, and then as they got closer, with Karpan and me lying back to back in our trench, the size of a grave, his boots against my neck, the screams of the shells became more insistent until just on top of us they turned into a sort of flutter, as if someone was drawing in his breath, and one felt the ground shake and smelt the powder and I could feel Karpan's body tremble. I wasn't afraid of being killed, I repeated, I just didn't want one of those shells to strike against a tree branch and burst down and tear me up. It was like being in a dentist's chair with the drill going deeper and deeper, this rehearsal for death. I remember a feeling of intense resentment. I was twenty-three. I had a wife, a distant sort of fact, named Mary. I had a daughter, whom I had seen once, named Catherine. It didn't seem as if I had done much with my life. I heard a man cry out in pain, but I was too close myself to being hurt and I felt only anger. Then we saw him stumbling down the hill, his hands against his face, blood running through his fingers. We found out later that he had been hit because he was standing up in his trench. He was an artillery observer and had seen the muzzle blasts of these German mortars, phoned back their grid points on his map, and was registering in our counterfire when a shell splinter splashed everything with blood.

Another day, while we were again targets, I heard outside our trench a different sort of noise. It was a soldier repairing a telephone wire. The whole purpose of this hill was to relay messages back to whatever switchboards we were attached to. The mortars tore up the lines and this man's job was to move up and down and find the breaks and repair them. When a shell fell nearby he just squatted closer to the ground, scraping the insulation away from the ends of the broken wires, twisting the copper filaments together, covering them over with rubberized tape.

"You've got some job," I remarked from our fortress of infinite safety.

"Soldier, ring up your switchboard and see if the phone works."

I turned the crank. It worked. He moved off till he came to another wire and followed it, hunched over, ducking whenever a shell came near.

᳹

That was life on Monte Rotondo. After a while the Germans abandoned the wreckage of San Pietro and both of us dug in around another town. I was transferred to army headquarters, and had no further contact with the 141st Infantry. I suppose that most of the soldiers I knew there were killed or wounded in the crossing of the Rapido, the fighting around Velletre, in Southern France, in Alsace, or wherever the slow-moving regiment was employed again and again. The director who made the epic film about Salerno wouldn't have bothered with Monte Rotondo. It was just one of 5th Army's hills and I just happened to be on it for a while. How do I know? Is that hill any more real than the field of Cold Harbor I read about, where Grant's soldiers were so demoralized that they pinned their names to the backs of their greatcoats so that their bodies could be easily identified, and an hour after the Northern attack had begun, you could walk across the field stepping from body to body and never set foot on the ground? I talk about Monte Rotondo and the words make the reality. I have some snapshots in my mind: the man stumbling down hill with blood running through his fingers, the side of the slit trench Karpan and I shared, the blurred stones three inches from my eyes, the curve of my helmet rim. It would be a waste of time to invent details like that. Does it add up to anything? For what it is worth I shared something that other men also shared. When radical students vilified American soldiers for the way they acted in Vietnam, I could believe it because I had seen the way Americans had acted in the far more civilized environment of Italy. But I thought of the linesman on that hillside. He had been the Good Soldier and looked after his telephone lines under fire. If other men misused his sense of duty he could not be blamed. I had gone through a rehearsal for my own death and, when I have to, I will be able to face that. I learned some appreciation for being alive. Some things can be managed—not always well. Some things simply have to be endured.

Say that they mattered, alive and after;
That they gave us time to become what we could.
    Richard Wilbur

5

War 1944–1945

JUST BEFORE CHRISTMAS I was transferred to 5th Army Headquarters, mercifully without warning, so that my acceptance of daily life was not poisoned by hope. Perhaps, someone hinted, through contacts of my father's. . . . The system looks after its own. I never asked.

In the rapid stages back from the frontier, civilization was marked by changes in caliber: from mortars to 155 mm. howitzers, from dressing stations to hospitals, from division and corps headquarters to army until I was dropped at the Bourbon palace of Caserta in time for Christmas dinner. I remember a middle-aged French soldier (General Juin's French Corps was beginning to arrive from Algeria and Morocco) wishing me 'bon appétit' as we sat down and a Wac silently weeping.

My first job was translating Italian and French police documents, mainly about the savagery of those Arab soldiers towards Italian civilians. Then, a week or so later, I was installed in the tents compound of the G-2 section, set among the firs and palm trees of the palace gardens. It was a large office with many scary personalities, headed by fat frantic Colonel Howard, chief of 5th Army intelligence, always on the verge of hysteria for fear that someone would make a mistake he would be blamed for—and who once pointed at Yugoslavia on a map of Europe and said, "That's Finland, isn't it?" I was assigned as assistant to the two draftsmen in charge of the giant situation map of every German unit up and down the entire front. From prisoner interrogations, documents on corpses, occasional civilian reports and—top secret—British radio intercepts, we could place just about every division, regiment, and battalion, and have a reasonable picture of their strengths and capabilities. A second-rate mountain division implied a holding pattern, an armored or SS division moving down a highway, its convoys picked up by our reconnaissance planes, meant trouble. The map revealed all of that.

Next door was the G-3 section, which set the operations plans for allied units, the corps and division generals being its agents, fruit of the meticulous staff organization of Field Marshal Helmuth von Moltke directing his beautifully rationalized Prussians against the Austrians and the French.

Many of my new colleagues were Jews originally from Hamburg, Berlin, Leipzig, and Vienna, involved with documents and PW reports. Other sub-sections, connected with decoding or photo interpretation, were British, and there were British officers (a New Zealand lieutenant for months) in and out of our tent. General Eisenhower had insisted on American-British command integration, followed still by General Clark, 5th Army's head, even by distraught Colonel Howard, who insisted that any enlisted men's party should always include our allies.

As the front line moved, at high cost, northwest of the towns around San Pietro, headquarters left the gardens of Caserta for the olive groves before a hill town named Presenzano. Every so often I felt ashamed of being safe. Shouldn't I ask to transfer back to my regiment? In January, however, the 36th was committed to a disastrous effort to cross the Rapido River flowing south from Cassino. The rifle companies of the 141st were slaughtered—one started the crossing with one hundred twenty soldiers and came back at the end of the day with three men and one officer—and I was afraid.

My best friend was a sergeant from Hamburg. Not until he was thirteen, when Hitler assumed power and his father, a banker like my own, was briefly imprisoned, did he realize that he was not a fully accepted German, free to enjoy Christmas trees and Easter eggs like everyone else. His father became a clerk, his mother started a dry-cleaning establishment. Ralph continued for a while at his Gymnasium, and though he was subjected to often intolerable hazing by his classmates in their Hitlerjugend costumes, he took all the tests, and most of the time his teachers gave him As when he deserved them. (It was possible to find teachers, loyal Nazis, who, still, as veterans of 1914–1918 gave some protection to Jewish students whose fathers had also been soldiers then, as Ralph's was.) He joined a Zionist youth group that studied Hebrew (few Gestapo understood Hebrew) and farming in preparation for Palestine. At vacation they cycled as fast as possible from Hamburg to Denmark and freedom. Once a group of Danish Nazis cornered them and weren't prepared for how fiercely these Jews fought back.

In 1937 all Jews were expelled from German schools, and Ralph transferred to an old-fashioned orthodox school whose citizens believed that reform Jews were godless materialists who deserved what they got. On Kristallnacht in November 1938, when Nazi mobs sacked Jewish stores and broke their windows to avenge the murder of a German diplomat in Paris by a young Polish Jew, and teachers in his school were being arrested in front of their classes, Ralph was in charge of a classroom of terrified children, telling them stories, leading them in songs till it was safe to go home. Eventually he got to England as a farm laborer, then to New York, then to Tunisia as a combat interrogator with the 9th Division. When stubborn prisoners refused to answer his questions he would threaten to send them to a Polish camp always a few kilometers behind the line. Ralph and I shared the same puptent in the olive grove and at night used to talk about poetry and history.

We visited Presenzano once a week with our laundry, which we paid for with the lire that the army printed and with food, soap, cigarettes, and sometimes a piece of clothing. My laundress had spent eleven years in Boston; we used to repeat street names to each other. The signora owned a bathtub, though no water ran in it. Except for that tub, the town had been untouched for a hundred years. The animals had always lived in the houses (the street was everyone's toilet—in hot weather the smell must have been fantastic). There had always been too many babies, even if a lot died. There had never been enough rain (when it was needed), enough food, enough jobs. And during these years the war scraped over Italy like an iron rake. I was always glad to start off on the laundry trips, to leave the tents and see human life again: houses and animals, women and children, but I always came back heavy hearted.

At each mealtime twenty or thirty children appeared to collect our leftover food. They waited between the garbage pit and the washtubs with their empty cans and cracked china bowls for us to empty out the beans, bread and pancake scraps, soup, coffee, and fat. Mothers or grandmothers would reheat the slop back home and that would be the family's meal. "Hey Joe, please, hey, hey Joe?" called the boys with their wise, grown-up voices, elbowing, smiling, their sharp eyes calculating who had a good messtin, who looked generous—real little businessmen. The little ones, holding the cans over their heads, struggled to keep their footing in the tussle. The shy ones stood in the rear, and you had to push through the pack to make sure that they, too, had something to carry home. It was a nuisance, and some of the soldiers were irritated enough to throw their garbage into the big pit. Still, we were grown men in boots and a dozen different pieces of wool clothing, and many of the little girls were wearing only dresses and sandals without socks, while the boys stood before us in shorts and ragged sweaters with maybe an old army cap pulled down over their ears.

The hubbub offended the company's administrative officer, Captain Sutro, and one morning an order was posted on the bulletin board by the chow line saying that henceforth, in the interest of sanitation and discipline, leftover food was not to be given to unauthorized civilian personnel. I'm glad to say no one paid any attention. After breakfast we doled out the same cheap charity of oatmeal slops and half-eaten french toast. An MP stood guard by the washtubs at lunchtime, a stupid young man, but the children were agile, and if he attempted to enforce law and order at one spot, we would scatter a bit further, leaving him to complain, "Hey, fellas, don't do that," and be laughed at. Only the littlest children, whom even he could frighten, lost out.

By suppertime Captain Sutro had fixed up the system. Three strands of barbed wire, thirty yards long, had been strung behind the washtubs. Two MPs with Tommy guns had been set on guard. The boys and girls and one old woman stood on the other side of the wire with their empty tin cans and watched us throw our food into the pit. We were angry, we were ashamed before those silent children, and we grumbled about this swollen example of discipline. But that was all. No one spoke to Captain Sutro about it, no one complained to the other officers. A soldier is accustomed to injustice and each man occupies himself only with his own cares.

⚬

Fifth Army landed a corps of Americans and British at Anzio in order to outflank the Germans, but that surprise was so slowly exploited that nothing came of it. American, British, New Zealand, Indian, Algerian, and Moroccan divisions bloodied their heads trying to capture Cassino and the monastery behind it, to no avail, and when finally taken by the Poles, it no longer stood for much. When the big offensive came in June, General Clark might have gone straight north and cut off Field Marshal Kesselring's army on the Cassino front, but was led astray by his longing to be the liberator of Rome. There was his jeep, the distinguished American general in his simple uniform beside the driver, surrounded by deliriously happy Italians, cheering, reaching out to touch his arm. Mark Clark was handsome and knew it: tall, forceful, graceful, with a noble profile, and if fate had been kinder he might have made a career like Gary Cooper or John Wayne's. He showed diplomatic skill, however, in dealing with his multinational troops, skill that an impulsive general like George Patton lacked.

From Rome the battle front moved rapidly north. Perhaps the Germans would be unable to re-establish a firm line. Perhaps the July 20th assassination attempt on Hitler by anti-Nazi aristocrats might mean an end to the war. In the rumors that reached us below-stairs employees, this was not entirely good news for the high command. A lot of careful planning and career enhancement was involved in formal military victory. A comic touch appeared in a panicky cable from Washington that the newly arrived Brazilian division was to be immediately committed and 'bloodied.' This was a large, not particularly effective unit that suffered more casualties from jeep accidents than from German fire, and spent its time among quiet mountains.

Its presence in Italy was important more for diplomatic than for military reasons. If Brazilian soldiers fought (with tangible losses) in the great crusade against Germany, that would raise their prestige in South America and lowered that of Argentina, which was sympathetic to the Nazis, and the rival of Brazil (and the United States). That whole undertaking would be jeopardized if the war irresponsibly ended.

Our luck held.

Every so often the moving front brought partisans up to headquarters, wild rather than domesticated soldiers. A few were British, in civilian clothes, who had walked out of their prison camps when Italy left the war just before the Salerno landing back in September of '43, and who had lived and worked with peasant families until the resistance built up. The Italians called themselves Communists, the name that had the most prestige then, and were scornful of the royal troops like the regiment paired with the 141st at San Pietro. We envied their lack of rank and salutes, the old-fashioned bandit quality of their ambushes. They were not popular with other Italians, though, for the Germans were willing to arrest and shoot 50, even 100 local civilians for every soldier killed. Then there were Russian deserters from the Wehrmacht's Cossack division raised to fight partisans in Croatia and later in Italy. Whether they had been brave anti-Nazi guerrillas or not made no difference. When delivered back to Russian authorities they were ceremoniously welcomed so long as Allied officers stayed present. When those departed they were bundled together as traitors and sent to Siberia or shot.

In August, of course, came the invasion of southern France with soldiers of the American II Corps (including the 36th Division) and the French Corps, which ended Churchill's fantasy that 5th and 8th Army divisions would punch through northeastern Italy into Slovenia and invade Austria while establishing a barrier to prevent the Red Army from overrunning central Europe. The two divisions of the Canadian Corps were withdrawn as well in order to start the liberation of the Netherlands. The 5th Army sought some salvage out of this by making enough commotion with trucks and ships and rumors to con the Germans into fear of an end-run landing at Genoa (this had been done in Sicily and at Anzio), so they would pull some units off the front.

A weakened 5th Army and a stiffened resistance slowed our advance as we neared Florence. To protect the city the Germans destroyed all the bridges across the Arno except for the precious Ponte Vecchio, though they blew up the buildings at both ends to stop the Jew-manipulated Negroid Americans from exploiting this cultural sensitivity. Both sides pulled back from a Stalingrad house-to-house devastation, and the city was liberated by Communists fighting the Fascists with rifles and hand grenades. General Clark

wanted to formalize his victory by immediately putting in 5th Army Headquarters. His engineers warned him away from the obvious location in the
heavily mined park at the western edge, but he waved them off and his subordinates obediently set up their tents. Back from breakfast Ralph and I
watched in horror while a soldier stepped on a mine 30 feet from where we'd
slept. An explosion, a burst of smoke, and there he lay with a black stump
below his knee instead of a leg. A British soldier ran up to help him only to
step on a second mine. The bystanders froze. The two men were carried off,
I forget how, and then an Englishman (they had steadier nerves) showed up
on a tiny steamroller to chug back and forth across our turf hunting for further mines. For some days we walked in careful single file, setting foot
exactly where the man ahead had put his.

The soldiers who fought on Tarawa and Iwo Jima scorned the undeserving
tourists who relaxed in a city like Florence. The gently educated trotted off to
the Duomo, others made friends with undernourished young women. As a
privileged adolescent on the Grand Tour I had visited Florence in 1937,
strolled past the Palazzo Vecchio by moonlight, listened to a lecture on Dante
and Machiavelli at Santa Croce, stayed at the *Excelsior*, closed now to anyone
less than a major. My sister had spent a year at a finishing school in Fiesole.

Somebody must have stuck around to keep 5th Army functioning, for the
fighting still went on in the hills north of the Arno, guns were shot off, men
were killed, and the engineers were working very hard to put together steel
bridges across the river. Nevertheless, had the Germans possessed the
resources to launch a serious counterattack, no one at headquarters would
have paid much attention.

It was easy for an Allied officer to run across a friendly aristocrat in soft,
worn English tweeds whose earlier politics would be overlooked as he overlooked the major's friendship with the contessa. Ralph met a painter from
Hamburg who had been employed by the German Naval Art Protection
Abteilung. Bargheer was too cautious to be anti-Nazi, but 'working' for this
strangely titled group had allowed him more freedom as an artist, and he
now supported himself by selling watercolors of city monuments, in gradu-
ations from literal to impressionist according to the rank of his customer.

One of our Viennese colleagues discovered an overlooked Jewish children's home, and supporting it with all the toothpaste, food, toys, and
underwear he cadged from us (mailed from home) became the purpose of his
life. A twelve-year-old boy selling his father's English library, Aldous

Huxley and D. H. Lawrence, for cigarettes. A desperate woman introducing herself as a French teacher, 'no one wants to learn French' and she wouldn't feed herself *that* way.

Such a collage of wartime life, and here and there a trip up to the Boboli Gardens and a view over the city that was, if you focused your eyes exactly, still *Florence* was exciting, but exhausting—were you missing something?—and I for one was relieved when headquarters moved north to Futa Pass on the highway to Bologna.

The same hills, protected by the same mines, mortars, machine guns, barbed wire, were given the title of the Gustav Line, which the Germans had vowed never to give up. For map makers there was nothing of interest in this, the same Allied units grinding out frontal attacks against the same Germans. The regiments leached away while the priorities for more men, more guns and ammunition were Patton's, Bradley's, Montgomery's armies on the borders of France. Nothing was arriving for the British divisions. When a man fell, the space remained empty. That led to extreme caution which led, of course, to angry remarks by the Americans. Their vehicles were so cumbersome and slow, and of course at four o'clock their drivers liked to stop by the side of the road, fill up a can with gravel and gasoline and make tea, that a number of highways had signs saying, "Off limits to non-American vehicles." 'White niggers' was the comment of a trashy dame in one of our sections. Casualties mounted so high that an urgent appeal went out for blood donors, promised $10 and a shot of Four Roses.

Mary and I wrote each other just about every other day, the minutiae of existence, a slice of gossip, a book read, dumb remarks of comfortable friends—"Charlie is so close to Venice maybe he'll be able to get there—I'd give him the address of a really wonderful shop for embroidered linen." What filled our letters and filled our lives was the daily activities of our daughter Catherine. She was one and a half, and each day she had some new response, a new word, adventure, friend. For Mary, to see a safe acquaintance stepping out with her husband was always painful, but we had Catherine. We knew how lucky we were. Still it was November, which meant a second winter of separation. Sometimes we just felt dried out. Almost everything had been used up.

Truscott, our new general (Clark had moved up to Army Group, 5th and 8th, back at Caserta), had abandoned the make-believe of an offensive. Office life was regular enough so that I had a weekly day off. Often I didn't bother about Florence, but just slept late and then went for an afternoon's walk along the cart tracks through the woods of oak and firs (telling myself I wouldn't worry about mines), over the hills, and past the stone farm houses, exchanging greetings with the peasants, enjoying the silence and the wind and the harmony between the landscape and the people who lived in it with a dignity that ignored the war.

Once a month or so I felt obliged to take a truck down to the city. I should know what was going on, visit the Duomo which in its vast stone winter darkness became a place of renewal or protection for me as St. Stephen's would be in Vienna or the tall black Mariacki church in Kraków. A couple of times I called on Ralph's friend, Bargheer, the painter from Hamburg. He offered me tea and I looked at his art books. I used the Catholic Center, the sole facility where British and American soldiers were equally welcome, as headquarters; it had books to read and sometimes showed films like Lawrence Olivier's *Henry V*. A lightweight Viennese clerk at headquarters had worked his way into the affections of a beautiful woman of distant Rothschild and musical background, and once she invited me to tea at her apartment. She called herself Communist and Catholic and as her war service had negotiated a job as secretary to a major in German intelligence (she spoke perfect German, little English). He was working up a list of agents that would be left behind for espionage and sabotage when the Wehrmacht withdrew. Leli stole the list, crossed the lines, and handed it over to British counter intelligence. The Fascists were vulgarians; she despised them for that. The Americans had very limited ideas as to what a decent society was supposed to be.

I sought to hold on to that afternoon's conversation and all its wrestling with language as long as I could and even put it into a novel I tried to write. Leli and her room, my silent walks around the cathedral, the watercolors that Bargheer kept on painting—one of a flowered hillside at the Boboli gardens poignantly beautiful, though he was not a man I esteemed much personally—the frightened woman who taught French, made up some level of culture that seemed ever more precious and vulnerable. The streets in wintertime held none of the life they had appeared to enjoy when we first arrived. Florence was closer to Naples by now—soldiers and their women, sellers of bootleg liquor (drugs hadn't appeared yet) and stolen army gear, kids begging and pimping. An hour's truck ride would take you within artillery range of the front where Americans and Germans kept hacking pointlessly at each other. We came to hate Florence as we hated every other town we came upon—the stone buildings we hadn't chosen, we couldn't leave, were just a variant of the tar-papered barracks.

On the last hilltop I shared with my partner Karpan before my transfer, we could see through our glasses the walls of the Benedictine abbey of Monte Cassino. The issue of what overriding value did such a monument possess in wartime had been raised in the *Stars and Stripes*. The discussion angered Karpan. No pile of stones, he said, historical, religious, whatever, had more value than the lives of American soldiers trying to liberate this Godforsaken country. His life wasn't worth much but it was all he had. A few weeks later the abbey was destroyed by American bombers after reports (false) that it was being used by the Germans as an observation post.

Vienna and Kraków, two cities that came to mean much to me for their beauty and for the mixture in their streets of culture and misery, often seemed quite close to that winter's Florence. As a teacher all my life I worked with students richly endowed with awareness and tradition like Leli, or like Karpan angry and resentful at everything that touched them.

The day's pass ended at the large modern railway station on the north side of town where soldiers could pick up vehicles back to their units. Many men never left the station, hanging out with beer and snacks and loudspeaker music, unwilling to venture out on those foreign streets.

The first detail that would strike a visitor from today is that all the soldiers there were white. The one black division in Italy was the 92nd, located on the coastal flank above Pisa, a quiet stretch of front the other side of the Brazilians. The army command did not respect their segregated troops, in fact had cannibalized a previous division in the Mediterranean theatre from infantry (so badly needed) into quartermaster personnel—dock and road workers, truck drivers, prisoner guards, hospital orderlies. Port cities like Naples and Livorno held large numbers of semipermanent black soldiers who often, replacing the husband/father dead or a PW far away, became head of the Italian families they moved in with. They were less imprisoned by the white compulsion to despise civilians, and came to speak urban dialect fluently. I used to wonder how those black men would return from their wartime status as equals, superiors, back to their inferior caste. At least a lot of novels and Ph.D. theses would emerge from the experience. Not a trace. A black soldier would not have been welcome at the railway station in Florence.

The combat infantry were quite a different race from us semicivilians. Sometimes they showed up weaving drunk, mouthing about the whores they had bedded, but I remember their silence, the distant way they seemed to be locked within themselves, how young so many of them were, seventeen and eighteen, just out of high school and basic training. An interesting set of figures is that the average age of soldiers in this war was twenty-six; in Vietnam it was nineteen. Half the 58,000 names on the memorial in Washington are of boys killed at seventeen and eighteen. The soldiers in the railway station, like infantry back in 1916 and 1918 and like their sons in Vietnam, were marked for death.

One afternoon waiting for my truck back to Futa Pass, I remember watching two of these men dancing the Lindy Hop surrounded by a silent, unsmiling circle of soldiers, mainly privates. Maybe the music came from a radio, maybe there was no music at all, just the slap of their feet and gasps for breath, I forget. No one was beating time. The Lindy Hop or any other jitterbug variant makes you think of some carefree performance by high school seniors. But this dance and those two dark thin short dancers—Italians from Brooklyn?—spinning the other out, ducking, twisting, shimmying, no girls, and the totally silent circle of onlookers made the blood run cold. I thought of the 141st's rifle companies trying to cross the Rapido, one hundred twenty men in the morning, three men and an officer in the evening. Someone should have offered an apology.

> *Here dead we lie because we did not choose*
> *To live and shame the land from which we sprung.*
> *Life, to be sure, is nothing much to lose;*
> *But young men think it is, and we were young.*
> A. E. Housman

When Easter came (with ribbons and flowers we made fancy bonnets out of the wicker bottoms of Chianti bottles as gifts for our Wacs) there was to be a sunrise service above the mists—looking like a Japanese woodblock print—of our valley. The last Easter of wartime was worth an early rising, and I joined quite a number of other GIs on the hillside. Cameramen had got there first, however, and after some recognition of the simple religious values of American soldiers—"There are no atheists in foxholes"—they turned their machines on an olive grove out of which came an elderly peasant leading a donkey on which sat a young mother with her baby: Holy Family courtesy of the 5th Army.

Springtime brought the last great offensive. A beautiful new division, the 10th Mountain, had arrived from the ski slopes of Colorado and Alaska, ready to show our worn-down, introspective battalions just what fighting meant. 'Our' Italian government was making an intense effort to stimulate anti-German resistance in the Po Valley, their radio playing again and again *la Canzone del Piave*, the song that inspired the Italians to start fighting again after the disaster of Caporetto in 1917. Once we broke out of the mountains you'd see what our tanks could do. The Americans, spearheaded by the 10th Mountain, which took heavy losses, did break out of the mountains, but someone had neglected to read a large-scale map carefully enough to notice all the canals that cut through the plain, each one of which had to be crossed against German machine-gun and mortar fire.

The 5th Army moved headquarters to an apple orchard south of Bologna. We passed truckloads of British ex-PWs moving south, and young men with red armbands giving the Communist salute—they had already liberated their country, thank you. A lot of fascists were lynched on the spot—Mussolini and his mistress shot and properly enough hung upside down from a gas station outside Milan.

Vaclav Havel and his peers in Poland and Hungary were too legalistic in deposing the Communists gently at the end of 1989. It was too easy for the losers simply to change their clothes—as did ex-Fascists and Nazis in 1945. People who have been despised and humiliated need to believe that justice still exists. Forget about lawyers and judges, give the job to angry young men who will shove these soiled individuals against a wall and shoot them.

The war was racing to an end, in Italy, in western Germany, around Berlin. How unfair to step on a mine now. The exhiliration of victory got paid for, however, in an unexpected way. For 20 years the returning GIs kept telling and retelling the stories of 1945 to their sons and nephews. When war came again in Vietnam, and the army went out of its way to enlist these poor dumb kids too young to know anything, the boys shipped off to Saigon expecting to find the same flags and cheers and girls jumping up and down.

Another move, to the suburbs of Verona, and the German armed forces in Italy surrendered. The regiments and divisions which give a soldier his identity, were rapidly dissolved—what the Germans had done with every army they defeated—and warehoused together into prison camps. But if there was no more Wehrmacht, there was no more need for draughtsmen to mark down unit locations on their maps. I was unemployed. Panicked, I went to a friendly major to ask what chance was there in counter-intelligence. I was given a number of interesting, mildly useful jobs, mainly with prisoners, before flying home in September, but for years I remembered that when the war was done with and the guns were finally silent, all I could think of was that I had lost my job.

> And send, O God, the English peace—
>   Some sense, some decency, perhaps
> Some justice, too, if we are able,
>   With no sly jackals around our table,
>   Cringing for blood-stained scraps.
> Dorothy Sayers *The English War, 1940*

Well, what did I learn?

1. A deep respect for the Italian people, whose humanity shone in contrast to what the Americans, Germans, British were apt to practice: their courtesy, concern for children and old people, their valuation of people for what they were, not for their station, values that survived Mussolini's Fascism, now being eroded by American ones. A love for the Italian countryside, a partnership between humans, nature and time, eroded now by get-rich-quick concrete.

2. An acceptance of my weaknesses and strengths. It was just as well that I didn't become an officer, Canadian or American, lacking a 'follow me, men!' spirit and a readiness to justify the military ethic. "Live and let live" is not the motto for a combat officer.

3. In a small way I had shared the great crusade against the Nazis' domination of the world. The scar on my shoulder was my union card. To what extent were the Communists, with their own death camps, any better? The victory by the Western nations didn't work out altogether as we'd hoped. The slaughter and tyranny in Korea and Vietnam, in Algeria, Uganda, South Africa and Zaire, El Salvador and Afghanistan, Somalia and Bosnia make the victory retroactively less worthwhile. But I had taken part as a soldier, Mary as a soldier's wife.

PART II

~

POLAND

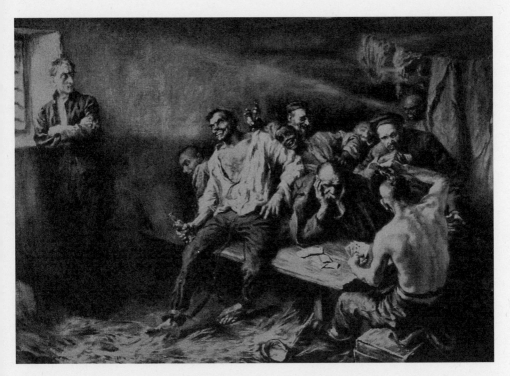

Aristocratic Pole and bestial Russians sharing Siberian prison cell, by Gorski. From Russia, Poland and the West, *Waclaw Lednicki, Roy Publishers, New York.*

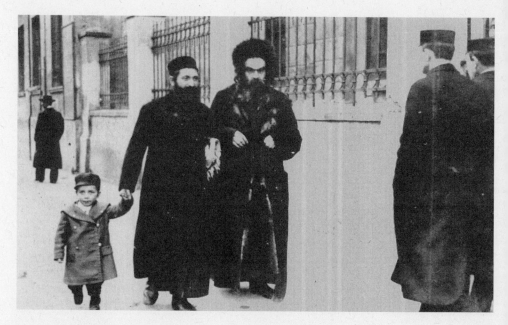

Jews of pre-1914 Kraków.

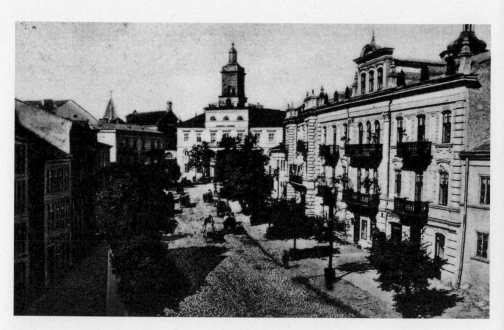

Lublin, Krolewska Ulica, 1907; a provincial city of Russian Poland.

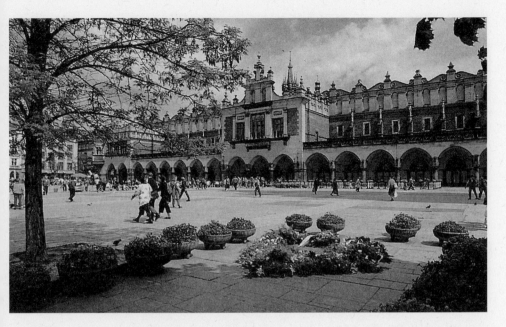

Kraków rynek in springtime, the Sukiennice or cloth merchants hall in background.

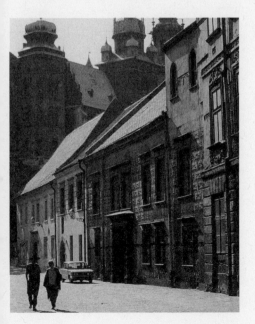

Kanonicza Ulica in Kraków with towers of Mariacki church.

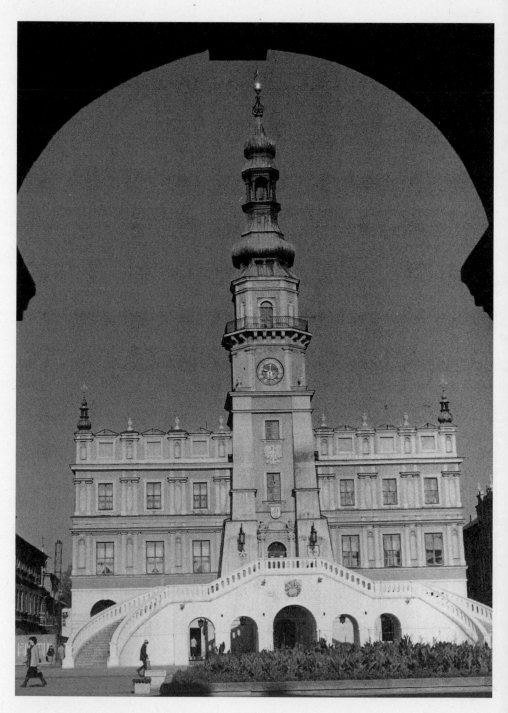

Zamość town hall (ratusz).

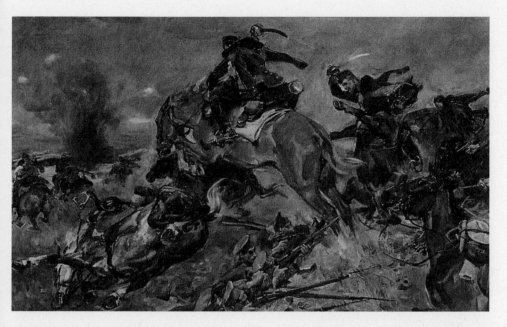

Polish cavalry attacking Russian trenches, a mythic picture of the totally forgotten war of 1919–1920.

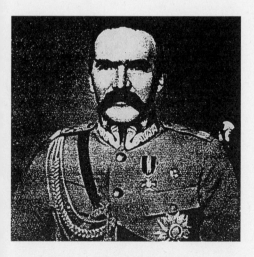

Marshall Joseph Piłsudski, 1867–1935, the elemental force that with sabre, horse, and mustache dominated Poland for almost 30 years.

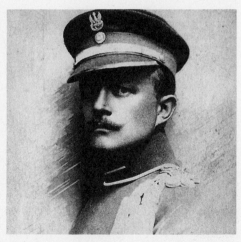

Remigiusz Grocholski as young cavalry officer.

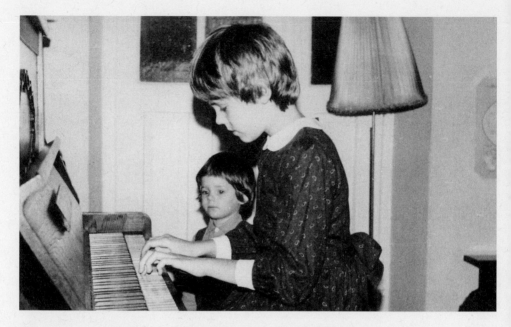

Eleven-year-old Justyna Woźniakowska watched by two-year-old Urszulka, Kraków.

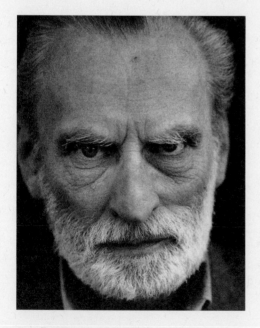

Jacek Woźniakowski.

6

Warsaw 1939 War

Riders gallop black horses, a tyrant composes
a sentence of death with grammatical errors.
Youth dissolves
in a day; girls' faces freeze
into medallions.
    Adam Zagajewski *Lava*

THERE ARE FEW cities that offer a more disappointing first impression than Warsaw. It is not simply that, with certain exceptions like the main square of the old city painted with such care by Bernardo Bellotto, the city's sprawl along the west bank of the Vistula is composed of buildings unimaginatively designed, poorly built, and sloppily maintained. The traveler himself carries such heavy emotional baggage arriving at this Paris of the East set at the edge of the Russian plain: a bulwark of patriotism, intellectual independence, and spirituality against heavy-footed brutality; the city that, along with Leningrad, suffered the most and fought back the most bravely in wartime, with its subtle but courageous independence against Communist oppression, that when he sees the charmless avenues, the presence of so few details to please the eye in this city he has been so eager to reach, when to reach Warsaw has become a sign of his own independence and judgment, of his insistence upon being quite different from the mediocrities satisfied with shopping at Harrod's—he might as well admit his mistake and go back to Zurich.

Buses are crammed, taxis are rare, and, in fact, if he found one where would he go? So, he sets out walking, without limits, like Hitler's tanks crossing the Russian frontier, measures the city with his feet, and when feet, legs, knees ache beyond measure, he knows where he is. Yes, as Warsaw's eastern borders have historically stretched to Siberia and its western to Chicago, the wasteland reminds one of the western moraine of Chicago. A city, for both Poles and Jews, to have come *from*.

For Bruce and me each swastika and Heil Hitler, each tomorrow-the-world German we had faced in Berlin and Danzig, made Warsaw our city of pilgrimage. In a steady rain we drove south from Danzig through the brick towns of what had been Prussia and then past the whitewashed houses that had been Russia. It was a shabby country, whether measured by the aged cars and trucks, the horse-drawn wagons with a peasant wearing a cap and a jacket soaked by the rain, or lunch at a hotel in Bydgoszcz of kotlet and kompot. By afternoon's end we drove through the nineteenth century fortifications—this would stop the Germans?—and then, as the buildings became higher and denser, we were in the middle of the city in front of a *Hotel Europejski* where we might as well stop.

What could we learn? How could we be more than tourists? The officers' diamond-shaped caps and olive green capes that fell from their necks to their black-booted feet transformed them into human bomb shelters. Small clots of cavalrymen on beautiful horses, some even carrying lances with little white and red pennons, trotted through traffic. In one church a man lay face down before the altar motionless—was he dead?—in the form of a cross. The two men at dinner next to us finished off a whole bottle of vodka between them. We drove down to the southern rim of the city to visit the rococo elegance of the Lazienki Palace with its busts of Voltaire and Franklin. Part of my preparation for Poland had been the great amount of reading I had done that first year at Harvard, each book from Widener Library leading to the next, particularly in the Yiddish writers Israel Singer and Sholem Asch. If we had seen the Nazi world, then we must see the world they had sworn to destroy. Accordingly, Bruce and I spent the better part of one day walking through the ghetto.

The streets, a frantic antheap of poverty, were frightening. "Come in," the store keepers begged, grabbing a sleeve. "Please, young gentlemen, come in and buy. You must buy!"—a shirt, pants, shoes. Down a step were the pushcart peddlers selling cheap candy, bagels, socks, celluloid combs, and mirrors; down another step were those who sold the same goods from a basket or a suitcase. The poorest were the porters, dragging carts, pushing wheelbarrows over the cobblestones. These were horses' jobs, but a horse needs more to eat than a Jew.

In the strangeness of these desperate streets, filled with the faces of 'anguished intelligence,' a phrase that came to my wife when we were trying to move along similar streets in Benares and Delhi years later, as well as the faces stunned by the fight for survival, to us the most alien were not the bearded men in kaftans with wide fur-bordered hats nor the middle-aged women in red wigs with wisps of gray hair escaping beneath, but the Yeshiva students our age with curled ear locks. Later on we learned the anthropologists' explanation of protection against exogamy, to frighten off gentile girls.

Nothing is so bad it can't get worse. In October of 1938 the Nazis expelled most Polish Jews from Germany. No one wanted them. They just sprawled in the no-man's land between the two borders—like the Arabs expelled from Israel in December 1992, memory insists, not allowed to enter Lebanon or return. After a while Polish soldiers shoved them into army barracks, but many of the fugitives slipped away to Warsaw, where they still had a measure of security. Since 1936 there had been a strictly organized boycott by the National Democratic Party to stop gentiles from patronizing Jewish stores, to convince store owners to dismiss Jewish employees, to encourage police and tax collectors to use harsher measures of harassment.

Traditional Polish society had been divided between peasants and landowners. Those who performed almost any trade in between were Jews. Roman Dmowski's National Democrats saw as their historic purpose the building up of a Polish middle class, or simply the insurance of its survival during the terrible years of the '30s. The Jews would be ground up and done with: "They can always go to Madagascar."

In their anti-Semitic policies the National Democrats had come close to the National Socialists, and with the ever-nearing threat of war some of them looked for a silver lining whereby Polish fascists might be tolerated by their German colleagues. Hitler had not the slightest interest in Polish anti-Semites. They were hardly better than Jews. As many Jews were eager to state after the war, the Germans simply finished off what the Poles had begun. The grandmother of one of my students had actually survived the war years in Warsaw. "What did she tell you?" I asked the girl. "Never trust a gentile."

In a middle-class section of the antheap we came upon a small park, and Bruce and I sat on a bench near some young women to watch their children play. A red-headed boy and three girls of five or so were racing about with a great deal of noise and laughter. Everyone was having lots of fun, and the two chatting, smiling mothers were obviously very pleased with their offspring.

I was not yet nineteen years old, Bruce a year and a half younger. Gradually, this little group of children was leaving us sadder than the terrible streets we had passed. Fifty years later I see us two as pretty naive kids, but even we knew how close war was. And we knew that these laughing children and their mothers would be the first targets.

Exhausted and troubled we found our way back to the *Europejski*. The friendly desk clerk asked us where we had been. When we told him, he replied, "Alors, mes jeunes messieurs, vous étiez parmi les animaux."

Among the animals, indeed.

The four little children playing in the park and their mothers were waiting for the Germans.

The BBC sells television dramas to the Public Broadcasting System for Sunday nights at nine, often with silly young men out of Edwardian times — striped blazers, ice cream trousers, straw hats, tennis rackets or cricket bats. After a while I found these programs unbearable. My first trip to England came in July 1936. It was the twentieth anniversary of the Battle of the Somme, and each morning in the front page 'agony columns' on the front page of the *Times* were little notices: "Dearest Bunny, forever young, forever loved, 2nd Lieut. Gloucestershire Somethings, killed July 12." This was Lord Kitchener's New Army employed by General Haig, who stressed the importance of perfect alignment of these lines of infantry. The officers of the first wave threw out soccer balls for their men to kick forward.

Mary and I go to the funeral of an old friend, an obstetrician who represented a Jewish ideal of skill, scholarship and service at its highest, who had had a mercifully rapid end to a long life that included delivering more than 6000 babies. He was an opinionated man with whom I shared anti-Republican jokes, and who when he meets the Lord of the Universe (blessed be His name) will probably remind the Boss of any number of occasions when He could have done a better job. All the people at the service, where Dr. Kasdon's nephew is the rabbi, accept Death's proper arrival. Two little girls are in tears, however, because they have lost their beloved grandfather. They are beautiful, their hair very dark — the dumbest German soldier would know they were Jews. "Because I was blond the Sisters took the risk (to shelter a Jew was punished by death) of sheltering me, and changed my name to Olga." I have read the almost identical sentence over and over. No one would have taken that risk with these two girls.

Almost the entire Polish air force was destroyed, mainly on the ground, within the first few hours. The French army, which Poles have always overvalued, risked a few cautious patrols on the Western Front. Within two weeks, the Polish army had been smashed. A few days more and what Churchill called 'the magnificent and forlorn defense of Warsaw' ended too. The Russians suddenly invaded and scooped up all Polish soldiers whom they found. Some of them eventually became Allied soldiers again, in Russia and by way of Iran and Palestine, in Italy, save for the tens of thousands who died of hunger, disease, and cold, and the 4000 or more officers murdered by

Stalin's security police, 1940, in the forest camp of Katyn.* By moving fast the top officials and rich people were able to scurry through Lwów across the Romanian border.

Then what? A ribbon perhaps 200 miles wide on the Eastern border becomes part of the Soviet Union. The area in all directions from Poznań becomes part of Germany as it had been in Hohenzollern times. Central Poland becomes the Gouvernement General under Wehrmacht-SS adminis-tration from Warsaw.

Again, then what?

In the spring of 1956 I met Czesław Miłosz, winner of the Nobel Prize for literature in 1980, at a lecture for Smith College students in Paris. He had been trying to explain the differences between wartime and the Communist era in Poland from what was true in Russia or any other Eastern European country, which I found so fascinating that I talked my way into an invitation. I made a series of pilgrimages to his home in Brie Comte Robert, a small town east of the city, asking so many questions about wartime and postwar life that at first he thought I belonged to the CIA.

Warsaw was the capital of a very centralized nation. When the Polish state ceased to exist, unlike what occurred in every other conquered country except Greece, no collaborationist government was either offered or permit-ted, and a large slice of the population suddenly found itself unemployed. They read Proust, Miłosz stated. That seemed furthest from the rainy days of October and November 1939. They made excursions by train to country villages in order to barter linen, glass, china, silverware for cabbages, pota-toes, onions, sausage. Sometimes, as in a children's board game, a German police control confiscated the suitcases of both those going and those return-ing, and the players had to go back to the starting line.

Cafés selling both vodka and real coffee to newly rich black marketers and older rich who still had things to trade became very popular. In the ghetto, even luxury was still available for a few, with restaurants, cafes, nightclubs and brothels. In the evening the atmosphere was glutinous with honey and soot, perfume and ashes, as beautiful, shameless Jewish girls sat eating rich food with their temporary German lovers, while corpses were thrown naked out into the streets so that their roommates could keep their rags.†

For the Poles the second blow came when that French army they had always counted on surrendered, after little hard fighting, in May of 1940.

---

* This death toll had been recalculated at more than 20,000 by the mid 1990s.

† John Lukacs *The Last European War — Sept. 1939–Dec. 1941*, Anchor Press-Doubleday, Garden City, N.Y., 1976, pp. 199–207. Here he is quoting G. Reittlinger, *The Final Solution*, N.Y., 1953. Lukacs' book is the best I have read for its picture of wartime life across Europe.

Back to Miłosz: the major resistance force, perhaps 80% of all combatants, was the Home Army, which received its orders from the London government-in-exile under General Sikorski. About 10% belonged to the hard-right National Army, mainly composed of ex-officers, with the reputation of being willing to finger Communists and Jews to the Germans.* Another 10% belonged to the Communist People's Army, which did not amount to much till the end of the war. After the great victories in the West, German divisions were increasingly being transferred to Poland in preparation for the attack on Russia. Many of their soldiers had picked up Allied side-arms as souvenirs, and were willing to sell these French and Belgian-Dutch pistols to Home Army fighters in civilian clothes for $5 bills dropped in packets at special points by Polish pilots of the RAF—a neat business deal. A secret hoard of American bills was considered good insurance by many Germans.

After the invasion of Russia began on June 22, 1941, Warsaw became a major rail center. The Home Army maintained a racket with the German crews of purchasing the last car of every train that passed through: sometimes with bad luck—a carload of pickled turtles from Greece bound for headquarters' mess tables, sometimes with good—a load of louse-proofed winter underwear. A German ate better in Poland than in other lands of occupied Europe, but life in 'Gangstergau' was more dangerous.

Jews might take Hitler at his word and know that this was Apocalypse. Or they might reason that any Jew living in Warsaw had experienced and survived generations of Polish anti-Semitism. In Kasrilevke one faced a drunken Easter mob yelling 'Christ killers!' who burned down the synagogue, sacked the stores, and killed any man who got in its way. So one left for New York. Or stayed and picked up the pieces and hoped for better luck next year. Or moved to the greater safety of Warsaw. One gained a sense, like Negroes of old-time Mississippi, of what were the rules, who were the officials to bribe, how to teach your children to behave. That very success at surviving traditional anti-Semitism allowed the Jews of 1941 to fool themselves that they could survive this new model; or they were simply human and believed that when the sun went down in the evening it would rise again next morning.

After the German armies were stopped in late November almost within sight of Moscow, Germans and non-Germans were visited by a whisper of thought, dreaded or longed-for, that Hitler might not win. One war he

---

* A Jewish writer like Lucy Davidowicz (*The Holocaust and the Historians*, Harvard University Press, Cambridge, MA, 1981, p. 94) does not confine guilt to these fascists, but accuses peasants of turning in Jews in order to collect German bounties and the Home Army partisans who murdered fugitives in the forests and marshes.

swore to win, however, was the annihilation of Europe's Jewry. The ghettoes of Warsaw, Łódź,* Lublin were simply a staging area for the death camps of Auschwitz, Majdanek, Belsen, Sobibor, Treblinka, Belzec, and on and on. An old-fashioned bribe might deflect the first blow, but not the second or third. In every social class some Poles were glad to observe and even help along the process. Others risked the threat of that automatic sentence of death.

A story I heard in 1957 was of a group of women who ran a home for little children whose parents were dead or imprisoned, in the underground, in hiding. The women were willing to take risks on the children's parentage. One day the knock came at the door, an officer and his sergeant. "Are any of these children Jewish?" The women were too frozen to reply. The two Germans entered the main playroom, which held a busy little crowd unaware of the new grown-ups. You could tell apart the two groups pretty accurately by hair color: Polish children have hair the color of straw, Jewish have brown or perhaps red. (Dr. Kasdon's black-haired granddaughters would not have been invited.) The Germans watched motionlessly. The Polish women hardly breathed. Then the officer turned without a word and, followed by his sergeant, left the building.

When I repeated this story to a Jewish parent of one of Commonwealth School's first students, her response was "I don't care for stories like that." She did not elaborate, but I suppose she felt that to talk about one decent German obscured the point that there weren't any.

By 1943 the pressure upon the Warsaw ghetto was becoming unbearable. It was as if the Germans were curiously testing how much humans could endure—like one of the scientific experiments at, I think, Belsen where prisoners were submerged for gradually lengthening periods in icy water, then put in bed with a naked gypsy to see if she could bring them back. Still, however, the lower-level administration was kept in Jewish hands, the police who kept the starving inhabitants from causing disorder, the officials given even the task of selecting who would be on the next list for Auschwitz. Finally, at Passover, whatever spark still remained burst into flame. Enough weapons had been stock-piled or smuggled in at great risk by Home Army soldiers for the Germans to need dive bombers in order to break the uprising.

(Arabs have compared the hopeless odds with the Intifada's fight against the Israeli army. "No!" There is, nevertheless, a whisper of truth to this.)

* Pronouced Woodj

Miłosz describes a group of Poles on the roof of their apartment house watching the German planes swoop down over the burning buildings: "You've got to hand it to Hitler, he's sure cleaning up Poland."

When, by early summer of 1944, the Russian army under General Rokossowski, made into a honorary Pole by Stalin for the occasion, crossed the 1939 border, there began an intense radio propaganda that Poles and Russians should forget past differences and fight shoulder to shoulder against the Hitlerite invaders. The Polish government in London was beginning to worry about the eventual Eastern border with the Soviet Union, in fact the eventual independence of Poland or, to be blunt, to the extent Churchill and Roosevelt would sell out the Poles in order to keep on good terms with Stalin. If, by a supreme effort, the Home Army itself could liberate Warsaw and then welcome the Red Army as its guests, that might alter the nation's future. As the Red Army came nearer and set up a pro-Communist 'government' in Lublin, it became clear how theoretical the concept of shoulder-to-shoulder comrades-in-arms and how real the probability of Poland's being turned into a docile client state.

On August 1 the uprising—the Powstanie—broke out, to last 63 days, at the cost of a quarter of a million lives. Small arms fire caught the Germans in the open, the first strong points were readily captured, and the Poles grabbed guns and ammunition. Russian soldiers reached the east bank of the Vistula, and there they stopped. It was possible for the Russians to state, as they did at the Slovak uprising that same month, that Rokossowski had run out of supplies and that his men were badly worn. True enough, but they gave no artillery support, ferried no supplies by night across the river. Russian officers clearly enjoyed seeing the non-Communist resistance liquidated.

For a moment the city had almost been theirs. Warsaw, despite the bombing and shelling of the first month of the war, the annihilation of the ghetto, and the bone-deep atmosphere of fear, hunger, and humiliation, despite the barricades across its streets, was still, in a way, a normal city. The picture books show Home Army fighters, often teenagers, with German helmets, carrying captured German rifles and machine guns, sometimes wearing the riding boots beloved of Poles, a civilian jacket, even glasses. Women were nurses, messengers, sometimes soldiers, in dresses as well as trousers, and with incongruously elegant hair stylings. It mattered how you looked. There were even weddings, with the bride carrying a tiny bouquet. As long as possible the dead were given formal burial, in a coffin, by a priest. There were children and grandmothers. When the gunfire fell silent for a moment, you could hear, I suppose, as in Sarajevo today, children crying.

Nevertheless, week by week Warsaw was turned into a rubble heap, a step-by-step descent into hell. Tank and artillery fire, rockets, air bombardment, an interesting little tank called a Goliath that could be directed by an electric cable up to a barricade and then exploded, were ending the city's life.

The defenders were running out of ammunition, the Germans were bringing in reinforcements: the Hermann Goering SS Division from Italy, sadistic anti-partisan units recruited out of prisons. The Germans gathered groups of civilians and made them walk in front of their tanks as protective devices. When they came upon wounded Poles, they doused them with gasoline and set them on fire. Captured doctors and nurses were shot. As their control of the city became more fragmented, resistance fighters could move about only by way of the sewers. The Russian propaganda changed: now the Home Army fighters, dupes of the reactionary opportunism of the London government in exile, were reckless, proto-fascist adventurers.*

At 5th Army Headquarters, late August 1944, some distance south of Florence, I met two RAF pilots, one English, one South African, who had paid a visit to look at our great situation map of German units. Their job was to fly supplies—machine guns, ammunition, medical gear, radio batteries—across Europe to Warsaw, then as low, as slow as they dared, fly above Nowy Świąt (the main pre-war shopping street), turn right at the corner of Jerozelimskie and parachute a parcel at number 127. Because the Russians would not allow them to refuel at their fields a few miles the other side of the Vistula, the planes were burdened by so much gasoline that the supplies, carried at great danger, were too limited to have much more than psychological value.

The desperate, largely useless courage of these pilots was a symbol of the Powstanie, which in its way was a symbol of too much of Polish history. The uprising formally ended in October. The Germans shot many of the surrendered fighters, but accepted some as prisoners of war or sent them to the camp at Treblinka. By then the Polish government-in-exile in London, desperate at reports of the massacre at Katyn, were making themselves an unbearable nuisance, in Churchill's eyes expendable. The Germans evacuated Warsaw at year's end, blowing up the city block by block to leave only, as Hitler proclaimed, a wasteland. Then the Russian army crossed the Vistula.

* John Erickson, *The Road to Berlin*, Vol. II, Weidenfeld-Nicholson, London 1983, pp. 247–290.

Too old to carry arms and fight like the others—

they graciously gave me the inferior role of chronicler
I record—I don't know for whom—the history of the siege
. . . .

I write as I can in the rhythm of interminable weeks
monday: empty storehouses a rat became the unit of currency
tuesday: the mayor murdered by unknown assailants
wednesday: negotiations for a cease-fire the enemy has imprisoned our
    messengers
we don't know where they are held that is the place of torture
thursday: after a stormy meeting a majority of voices rejected
the motion of the spice merchants for unconditional surrender
friday: the beginning of the plague
saturday: our invincible defender
N.N.* committed suicide sunday: no more water we drove back
an attack at the eastern gate called the Gate of the Alliance

all of this is monotonous I know it can't move anyone.
. . . .
Zbigniew Herbert *Report from the Besieged City*

---

* Abbreviation of the Polish equivalent of John Doe

7

Warsaw 1957

AMERICAN VETERANS and their wives who bought houses in the suburbs where they raised large families have received a glut of sociological condescension. Yes, we were quiet and conformist, mowed our lawns and feared radical ideas. Waiting ahead of us was History—Elvis, youth culture, drugs, black militancy, Vietnam; at the moment there was only the ceaseless movement of station wagons taking the kids to the swimming pool and their parents to PTA meetings. Of course. On the other hand, to build a marriage and a home on something more than letters and weekend passes, to build a family, a job; for me to learn responsibility for the boys I taught and the school I was helping to put together, to join a community in the outer suburbs of St. Louis, Missouri, was to learn how to act like an adult.

Raising small children can be limitlessly exhausting, adults confined under house arrest by the noisy little prison guards, and yet there are memories of these sweet smelling, hair-brushed creatures in their pajamas and nightgowns, climbing over a parent for their bedtime story—that became one of my links to history, to the children somewhere else who had never known, who had lost forever any evening hour like this.

One began with getting through each day: feeding and dressing the children, teaching classes of American history, Spanish, Shakespeare to those likable boys from Ottumwa and Dallas who knew just about nothing. Read *Macbeth*, take a test to show you know the facts, memorize "Tomorrow and Tomorrow and Tomorrow." Then into the station wagon on Sunday afternoon to hear your first Beethoven from the St. Louis Symphony.

That routine was played out against the changes of post-war America under President Truman's leadership, which had its own amateurish qualities. To what extent could that leadership plan, and the American people accept, the reconstruction of an exhausted, devastated Europe? How far could Americans understand the threat of Communist aggression—intellectual, political and ultimately military—without losing themselves in hatred and fear whipped up by a thug like Joe McCarthy? What price were we willing to pay to accept black Americans as equals?

Democracy starts with the way you act in whatever community you are dropped into. True enough. For me that meant leading a painfully artificial discussion group on "World Federalism." Then I worked to encourage local fundraising and propaganda to support Adlai Stevenson's hopeless 1952 campaign against General Eisenhower, was rewarded two years later by my being offered the Democratic candidacy for St. Louis County Council. I rang 3500 doorbells and won the support of Jews and Negroes, homosexuals and intellectuals and people who left rusty lawn furniture in their driveways; but people who kept their grass neat and their houses nicely painted voted as God meant them to.

Nevertheless, was this suburban order what I wanted? My loyalty was to the survival of the world I had seen in wartime Italy, in winter's Florence. The search for a role to play had expressed itself in three novels I wrote on the dialogue between Americans and Europeans, in a foolish idea of teaching in Prague, in a practical idea of being a Fulbright teacher in Vienna. It might be time to leave my classroom above the garage, remove my family from the house on Lincoln Road, and at least accept the gamble of living for a couple of years in Paris to become a professional author. The Paris we encountered, however, was not a stimulating environment, and the publishing industry was not interested in my fiction. I did find the reward of a series of long conversations about Poland with Czesław Miłosz, and so, before our final departure July of 1957 for Boston where I would start a school of my own, I ran away for a week to Warsaw.

⚮

*Whoever desires to found a state and give it laws must start with
assuming that all men are bad and ever ready to display their
vicious nature. Men act right only by compulsion.*
Machiavelli *The Discourses*

*I am twenty-four
led to slaughter
I survived.
   The following are empty synonyms:
   man and beast
   love and hate
   friend and foe
   darkness and light.*
Tadeusz Różewicz *The Survivor*

> *To kill in the name of the universal beautiful ideas*
> Czesław Miłosz *Bypassing Rue Descartes*

> *But of course you too would make a good martyr*
> *with that poor health of yours with your shortness of breath*
> *with your fussy habits*
> *and your liking for a hot bath every day*
> *But of course No one said anywhere*
> *that you'll always keep on walking deep in thought*
> *with that gentle smile of yours*
> *that one day they won't throw your books about*
> *that blood won't trickle from your beaten face.*
> Julia Hartwig *But of Course*

With ideas similar to George Orwell's in *1984* but with fiercer passion, Alexander Wat, a once enthusiastic fellow-traveler who spent years in Russian prisons, describes one quality of Communist Poland: "The loss of freedom, tyranny, abuse, hunger would all have been easier to bear if not for the compulsion to call them freedom, justice, the good of the people. Mass exterminations are not an exception in history; cruelty is part of human nature, part of society. But a new, third, dimension had been added that was more deeply and subtly oppressive: a vast enterprise to deform language. Had it been only lies and hypocrisy—lying is part of human nature and all governments are hypocritical. . . . But here all the means of disclosure had been permanently confiscated by the police . . . the viler the deed, the more grandiloquent the name."*

The rubble heap and corpses left behind by the Germans, the arrests and deportations that followed them are easier to comprehend by Americans than the intellectual qualities of Communism. Our presidents tell lies and are afflicted by similar vindictiveness and paranoia, but not on the same imperial scale. American lack of respect for abstract thinking also limits a president's ability to build a logical system as subtle and as thorough.

Miłosz's *Captive Mind*, which came out in 1951, is still the most brilliant analysis of Communist thought. He was condescending towards Americans, whom he dismissed as good natured idiots, impatient in the face of complicated facts and uncomfortable in the face of tragedy, their ability to reason crippled by their ignorance of history, and their comprehension of the relations between language and understanding muddied by their slovenly speech habits.

---

* *My Century, The Odyssey of a Polish Intellectual*, W.W. Norton, N.Y.-London, 1988, pp. 173–174.

Miłosz had even greater scorn for western European intellectuals, who believed that their knowledge of "Marxism" allowed them to grasp the reality of what went on in the lands conquered by the Red Army. As good Platonists they had received an education of such philosophical acuity that they could ignore what their senses told them, and they were sufficiently demoralized by the defeat of the civilized West by the Nazi armies that they were ready to abandon the moral traditions that gave birth to their culture. They did not grasp the full meaning of the poor hero's final torture in *1984*: the torturer holds up four fingers in front of Winston Smith and sends the electrical shocks higher and higher until Smith finally gives the desired answer— five.

What happened politically in Warsaw was about the same as what happened in Prague, Budapest, Bucharest: the initial toleration of a fragile coalition government under a democratic figurehead, and then within two or three years the collapse of this theater and its replacement by an unhampered Communist boss: Bierut, Gottwald, Rákosi, Pauker. The physical destruction of Warsaw was worse, of course, than that of any city outside Germany, but in some ways that was not entirely bad. Every hand was needed to rebuild it, to turn that vast rubble heap back into some sort of city. No, the untouched, ugly textile city of Łódź, near enough, is not a fitting capital. The cosmopolitan artificialities of plans drawn up in London will be discarded, and Warsaw will be rebuilt in Moscow's proletarian classic. Certain precious areas like the Old City and the Royal Palace will be rebuilt from Bellotto's paintings at enormous expense. To live, to have babies again, to come to terms with the nation's dead, six million, one in every five, to put stone on stone and restore the sewer system can let both sides work together, in a way, for a while.

In certain almost paradoxical ways, the atmosphere in Poland was better than within its neighbors. There were no collaborators to root out. The German contempt for all Poles, of any persuasion, meant that no one had been invited to come aboard. The pre-war Catholic church had been intensely anti-Communist, anti-Semitic, but unlike the church in Slovakia, Hungary, Croatia, it had not sided with the Germans. The solidarity between Church and Nation in those terrible years, the deaths of thousands of priests, won it dignity and loyalty. The Home Army, fighters in the Powstanie, received the blanket sobriquet of fascists, but nobody believed that. An aristocratic family might be granted a small apartment within the building they once had owned. Their child might grow up to make a low-profile career as art historian.

The supreme metaphor of Communism, the heart-stopping knock on the door at 4 A.M., still existed, of course, and a small packed suitcase waited in every man's bedroom closet. In an image given me by Miłosz, if a man in some office was rumored to be suspected by the police, his colleagues' desks and chairs spontaneously distanced themselves a little bit further each day (as with an AIDS suspect 40 years later?) until one morning his desk stood all by itself in the middle of the room. The next day he was missing.

> *He that is ready to slip with his feet is as a lamp despised in the*
> *thought of him that is at ease.*
> Job 12/5

Wladysław Gomułka, first secretary of the Party when I visited in 1957, had been first secretary in 1943, then imprisoned for three years in 1951 for rightist deviations and Titoist nationalism. In any other 'people's republic' he would have been executed. Perhaps the massacres suffered under the Germans limited the Polish Communists' readiness to kill. The skeptical realism of the Polish mindset immunized them, to a fair extent, from the 'Sieg Heil!' unanimity of totalitarianism. And the hatred of intellectuals by the Polish working class immunized them against the Communist leadership, as well as the contempt of all Poles for Russians. In the conclusions, once more of Alexander Wat,* the cruelties and deformations of Nazism may not inevitably drive the onlooker to Communism. It may instead open his eyes to the similarities of the two and propel him in an entirely different third direction.

Jews. Probably 90 to 95% had perished during the war years, but the cruelty toward those who remained did not stop. Nearly fifty survivors were massacred by Poles, July 4, 1946, in the industrial town of Kielce (northeast of Kraków) on their return from concentration camps.† By the time the Communists took power, some Jews had been so alienated from anything to do with Poland that they willingly served as judges and prosecutors in the Communist courts, even as guards in the prisons for counter-revolutionaries.

1956 was a year of change in Poland. The whole Communist world had been shaken by Khrushchev's reading of the crimes of Stalin at the 1956 Party Congress. Boleslaw Bierut, the hard-line Stalinist, had been replaced by Wladysław Gomułka. The July riots in Poznań by workers and rootless 'hooligans' revealed a nihilistic underside of Polish society that the Communists had never suspected. The rapidly intensifying uprising in Budapest was

---

* Wat, *Op. cit.*, p. 83

† Dawidowicz, *Op. cit.*, p. 94, "After all, the experience of the German occupation had demonstrated to the Poles that Jews could be murdered with impunity." Arabs, sadly enough, might say the same of Israeli soldiers. And in the free-fire zones of Vietnam any American soldier, in the air, on foot, was legally free to kill any Vietnamese.

meanwhile pushing the party in opposite directions. For liberals this was the example of what Poles could also hope for in demanding freedom; for hardliners this would lead to the betrayal of every truth of Marxist Leninism, if any concessions at all were allowed. Nevertheless, when Khrushchev aimed Russian tank columns at Warsaw in October as the ultimate threat if the Poles continued to insist upon independence of action, Gomułka received unanimous support from the Party as well as the army and public opinion. Perhaps the old-timers remembered the way that Stalin had murdered the leaders of the Polish Communists, in Moscow exile, back in 1938, when, of course, neither Khrushchev nor any other apparatchik had uttered a word of protest.

> *What is poetry which does not save*
> *Nations or people?*
> *A connivance with official lies,*
> *A song of drunkards whose throats will be cut in a moment,*
> *Readings for sophomore girls.*
> Czesław Miłosz *Dedication*

There was also in 1956, as Miłosz explained, the particular Polish phenomenon of the impact of *A Poem for Adults* by Adam Ważyk, earlier a hard-line Communist, who could no longer tolerate the lies that he had been force fed and forced to write year after year. One still had to speak obliquely, but that, after all, is the function of poetry. In the over-charged atmosphere of a police state, to write 'I believe that a table has only four legs' challenges the reader to supply the words that are not said.

> *It was dawn, I heard the whistle of jet fighters*
> *Which cost us so much and yet we must have them —*
> *When we do not wish to speak of the earth with simplicity*
>   *with truth,*
>   *with loyalty.*
> *We say 'The sky is not empty!'**
>
> *Nourished in the desert of big words . . .*
> *When the vultures of abstraction eat our brains,*
> *When one shuts up students in books without windows,*

---

* A slogan for building ever larger the Polish air force

76

When one reduces language to thirty incantations,
When one extinguishes the lamp of imagination,
When the good gentlemen who've come from the moon (Russians)
Refuse us the right of taste
    Yes, that's the truth: the threat then is stupidity.

Years later, in the cheerful days of Ronald Reagan's "It's morning in America!" anyone who offered facts contradictory to his was stamped as a gloom-and-doom, tax-and-spend liberal. The Communists were even easier to offend. The poem continued:

The dreamer Fourier* exquisitely predicted
that (under socialism) the sea would run lemonade
Doesn't it?
They drink the sea water/and cry/"It's lemonade!"
They return home on tiptoes/to vomit,/to vomit.

Forbidden words about the women who become old so quickly, the fifteen-year-old prostitutes, the boredom and stupidity of these inhuman cities as common as the rubbish and dirt, the dead weight of clock watchers and slogan mongers and paper shufflers . . .

Take from me the rags of dogma
Clothe me in a simple cloak

We demand here, on earth
For harassed humanity,
Keys that fit the locks,
Lodgings, poor perhaps, but with windows . . .
The simple difference between what is said and what is done . . .
We demand the fires of truth, the wheat of liberty
The spirit in flames.
    Adam Ważyk *Poème pour Adultes*

Lines that were easy to remember, to write on a piece of paper and hand to a friend, that could be recalled a dozen times a day.

---

* Jean Baptiste Joseph Fourier (1768–1830), a French sociologist of the early nineteenth century.

We were permitted to shriek in the tongue of dwarfs and demons
But pure and generous words were forbidden
    Czesław Miłosz *A Task*

❧

"I am interested to know how the human spirit survives under totalitarianism."

"I am the richest man in Poland. I am the father of ten children, none of whom was killed in the war."

That pair of introductions, in French, must win some prize.

From Miłosz I had received a letter of introduction to an elderly priest whose commitment to social justice had won him distrust from both Party and Church and who should be a useful door opener. Father Zieja's rectory was only a couple of blocks from the *Hotel Bristol*, but he was ill and his housekeeper referred me to a Colonel Remigiusz Grocholski who lived nearby.

Colonel Grocholski invited me into his apartment, crowded with old furniture from a far larger home. He was an erect, aristocratic gentleman, close to 70, clearly used to receiving guests in gracious surroundings. Madame, more reserved, the worker who supported this claim to elegance, offered us tiny cups of coffee. Who was I?—a teacher, a writer, a visitor to Poland before the war, a soldier on the Italian front. The Colonel had some free time today. Perhaps he might show me around the city.

Proust, of bourgeois origin, was awed by meeting aristocrats whose names were the history of France. Colonel Grocholski's history was the history of Poland. From that balcony a great uncle had thrown a bomb at the Russian viceroy at the start of the 1863 insurrection. The little street shrine to Lieutenant Zbigniew Szczepanski—there seemed to be one every block: a pair of candles, a withering bouquet of red carnations, a photograph, a notice on cardboard with his name, 1944, age 23, and the words I caught of Hitlerite Fascists—was a man he knew. In that direction, beyond the broken teeth of ruined buildings, in a cellar of the Stare Miasto (the old city), Madame had run a dressing station, her assistant an Ethiopian who had found his way from Athens. A cousin had swum the Vistula at night with a map of German positions, easily within artillery range, but still the Russians did nothing, and no one heard again of the swimmer. Yes, he used to have an estate in Podolia, by the Eastern frontier, but when war came he had left to join his regiment. He had commanded a partisan battalion east of Lwów, in the Polish Ukraine, but was in Warsaw when the Powstanie broke out. His unit was the last to surrender.

Would I be interested to visit the next day an institute for the blind in the woods west of Warsaw? The Colonel presented me to the bus driver: although an American, I was intelligent and sympathetic and had been a soldier. He showed his card to a young man in the seat reserved for wounded veterans, who respectfully yielded it. As we walked through the forest of birch trees—laski—he quoted Adam Mickiewicz on Poland as the Christ of the nations, which as a boon for its sufferings could ask God for the redemption of the Russians. Home Army fighters outside Warsaw, Partisans, had held the woods during that terrible summer of '44, and he had sent off his daughter Anna—who would think an eleven-year-old girl to be carrying papers in her underwear?—as a messenger. She had been wounded but survived.

The institute for the blind was a collection of little wooden houses with blank-faced children walking uncertainly along its paths. Some had lost their sight from measles or meningitis, some from playing with the grenades that littered every field. Its plump, bald director, Anton Marylski, who, like the Colonel, had been an officer in the Tsar's army, when the sopranos at the Petrograd opera wore necklaces of real diamonds, ruled a little empire. Tiny, eager-to-please nuns brought us chłodnik—beet soup (barszcz) with sour cream and crayfish tails—and chocolate éclairs. The post-war needs were so great, the resources so few that the Communists allowed the church to operate these shelters for the blind and the insane, which, after all, were funded mostly from abroad.

A few days later I returned to Laski and spent the night in a tiny, scrubbed room, with straw mattress, wash stand, crucifix. The chapel bell, a few crows made the only sounds. A nun was pointed out as Jewish, a former Communist. I was introduced to a priest who had just returned from exile. In 1946 and 1947, when the Russians were grabbing just about any man they could find to labor in the factories of Siberia, he had taken off his robe and stood in the way of one of their press gangs, then was shut into a freight train that crept across the Urals. He was assigned to a factory of old, grinding, wasteful machinery, with the duty he set himself to prove that wherever His people were sent, Christ would be there too. With a tiny glass of homemade wine, a little bread saved from the mess hall, he said a secret Mass. Gradually other prisoners learned he was a priest, a fact the guards never discovered. He heard confession from the men working beside him, to forgive the sins of anger, hatred, and despair.

"Were you effective?" I asked, an American question I immediately became ashamed of.

"I don't know."

I was the outsider, the witness they had been waiting for, and I listened to more people that week than throughout two years in Paris.

"You know what I think of the Communists," said the lady who was Pan Marylski's assistant, "but in the old days before the war, the poorest peasant children could not go to school in the winter because they had no shoes. Now, no matter what else the Communists have done, every child in Poland has a pair of shoes."

(In the winter of 1991-1992 the new Republican governor of Massachusetts, William Weld, sought to balance the state's budget by ending the clothing allowance for welfare children. Among the many letters I received pleading for help were appeals for money to buy shoes so the children could go to school.)

Gomułka was still enjoying his reputation as a liberal. The theatrical performances that had been given, dangerously, in living rooms, were now, for a while, appearing openly. I formed one-sixth of the audience for one silly celebration of freedom that included a clown posturing in a boxing rink among dolls and potties. Sold out all spring, however, had been a production of Beckett's *Waiting for Godot*.* It is a play that never meant anything to me: pretentious, empty, boring, but for a Polish audience it was overwhelming. Beckett's picture of life, the two lost tramps on a barren stage waiting for someone who will never come, was a totally honest picture of the world they knew, and the audiences sat through the performances in tears.

As he once would have invited me to spend a week, a month on his estate in Podolia, Colonel Grocholski insisted that I must feel free to drop in at any time. In the crowded apartment, set within an intricate university compound on the great avenue of Krakowskie Przedmiescie there seemed always to be space for a mattress to be put down, for one of the ten children (I collected them: the Olympic ski champion, the one fatally attractive to women, the one who had served time for mistakes with currency regulations, the art historian, and on and on), a cousin, a friend's friend.

After my over-exposure in Paris to French self-protection, I was moved by the uncomplaining, unquestioning responses of Count Remi, the first nobleman I had ever met, unaffected by the principles of 1917, even those perhaps of 1789. He had been in more than one prison but was free. He had no money but something always turned up: his suit came from a cousin in Belgium. In Poland the rents were low. The Communists were corrupt vulgarians but not people he was afraid of. What he missed most were his horses. There were drawings (some by himself), photographs, paintings of horses in every room.

---

* Presented in 1993 also by Susan Sontag in beseiged Sarajevo, the stage props representing 'hope' were empty United Nations provisions boxes.

On a theater poster I had figured out that *Cyrulik Sewilski* was *Barber of Seville*, and I invited the Colonel and Madame and the ex-messenger Anna, a beautiful art student with whom I immediately fell in love, to accompany me. It was a sparkling performance in a single, two-story set that allowed easy switches of action, and the old gentleman was delighted that his head was filled with Rossini and not the garbage of propaganda.

Traveling alone one can move towards any object that the radar screen picks up. On a loudspeaker I heard the repetition of "Hemingway-Faulkner-Steinbeck" and tracked the words to a sound truck where a group of students were selling a magazine (*Wyspolczesnosc*) of American writing. Yes, the new Gomułka liberalism—a pity that Hungary had alarmed the conservatives. Nevertheless, one should be grateful. Whom would I consider the most significant new writers? After two years of scorn from any French intellectual for my reactionary, racist, semi-literate nation, what a treat!*

My radar led me to a sophisticated cocktail party (Hungarian vermouth), and afterwards to a café with the French cultural attaché and a journalist from Kraków. What made Poland so different from both France and America was the fact that nothing was taken for granted. The reality of the streets, the lines in front of any provisions store, what one knew of wartime statistics and the reality of Communist control (invisible, except for the border and customs police, to any foreigner who remembered Berlin, with its uniforms, swastikas, salutes) gave special value to the crackers and vermouth at the party and this conversation at the café.

The Pole, Jacek Woźniakowski, a slender, dignified gentleman with a scarred face, was to become one of my closest friends. His personal history, like the old Colonel's, was the history of Poland. His father had been a landowner; totally in love with horses, he had created a highly reputed breeding establishment that was destroyed within a couple of hours of the arrival of the Red Army, and had finished his days teaching art history to coal miners in Katowice. When war came, Jacek was a junior lieutenant in the 8th regiment of Uhlans, and a specialist in horse-mounted machine guns. Always retreating, he fought in one rear-guard action after another, then, after the surrender of all Polish armies, he joined a group of cavalrymen

---

* A proletarian French spectator sport at that time was roller skate racing and in some working class quarter of Paris was being held a match between a French and an American team. The Americans were a loathsome crew who maddened the audience with obscenities and foul gestures but at first were far ahead because they cheated so outrageously. Finally, however, speed, skill, and courage allowed the French to win, to thunderous applause. In fact, the 'Americans' were French, carefully coached in transatlantic vulgarity, and were raking in the francs as the barbarians who always almost won.

headed for Hungary (the Hungarian seizure of Czech Ruthenia east of Slovakia, in March 1939, had given the two countries a brief common border) in hope of continuing to fight from abroad. On the way his band ran into Ukrainians, heavily armed by the Germans but building triumphal arches for the Soviets—Hitler and Stalin would liberate them from Polish oppression—and in one violent combat he was badly wounded. Saved by loyal Polish peasants, proud to be the humble descendants of medieval knights, Jacek recovered and became an officer in the Home Army (jobs: sabotage of German rail facilities, distribution of arms and ammunition to partisans, aid to clandestine secondary schools, sheltering of Jews). When peace came, he studied at Jagellonian University in Kraków, and eventually worked as a writer and editor at *Tygodnik Powszechny (Universal Weekly)*, the mouthpiece of the liberal Catholic establishment. Like his father, he also taught art history—a man of his background would not be allowed to teach real history.

What Jacek remembered most intensely of those war years was *trust*. You could knock on any Polish door, regardless of class, and ask for help. People treated each other honestly. It was not like what came later, the rule of lies. They weren't necessarily believable. Perhaps the Communists were so cynical that they didn't care whether they were believed or not, but it seemed that no fact could be presented without a framework of deceit. One example was the press response to the uprising in Budapest, during which the crowds killed many of the hated security police who, as everyone knew, were recognizable by the white shoes they wore. Yes, the Polish papers printed a front-page photo of one of the hanged victims. But they all cropped it at the knees (Woźniakowski had seen the original in a French magazine—forbidden reading matter entered quite easily inside the diplomatic pouches of friendly embassies) so the caption could be of Hungarian workers lynched by fascists. Pasternak's *Dr. Zhivago* was a favorite piece of contraband. The Polish translation, printed in Paris, of *1984* had the cover title of *Fighters for Freedom* and showed a heroic soldier bayoneting a capitalist paw.

Woźniakowski also worried about the Asiatic ant heap (typically Polish, always threatened from the barbaric East, the mechanized West?) of Mao's China. The European Communists had to regard this mass democracy with favor, though ambiguity might be detected, but Poles were already asking silently what level of integrity could be retained under their own variety of Communism; how vulnerable were they to the faceless numbers of these blue-clad ants?

The dimensions of the difference between life in Warsaw and life in Paris took me a while to understand. The *Barber of Seville* was a bright, brainless opera whose sparkling performance that evening would have delighted any audience in either city. In Warsaw there was the extra, wordless appreciation that the costumes worn by Rosina and the Count, the sweetness of their songs existed at all. Paris had been worn down by the war, dirtied by collaboration—French policemen not unwillingly rounding up French (Jewish) children to be handed over to the Germans to be murdered, humiliated at being liberated by primitive American soldiers and rebuilt by rich American women buying fabrics. Nevertheless, there was a difference between being liberated by the Americans and by the Russians, which a twelve-year-old could see clearly but a Parisian intellectual would not.

Every nationality has its favorite image of naively arrogant American ignorance—that goes without saying—but for Poles, as for Miłosz, the most oppressive ignorance was that of Parisians: "Yes, we know the realities of European life." Of course, but for Western Europeans those realities were too often verbal, analyzing the precise slice of Marxist theory acceptable and ignoring what theory turned out to be in practice. Integrity was based less on intellect than upon character. Woźniakowski's *Tygodnik*, unlike other Polish magazines, refused to publish an idolatrous obituary of Joseph Stalin and for a while was simply shut down. In the face of this reality, that Parisian pretense of understanding was harder to bear than ordinary American vulgarity.

On my last day in Warsaw I happened upon the great granite monument to the *Heroes of the Ghetto*. It was set amidst a waste of rubble and had obviously cost a lot of money. The heroes were generic Stalinism: noble, muscular, full-bosomed, holding their weapons and obviously crying out that it was better to die on one's feet than to live on one's knees—the products of some Heroic Memorials factory. I am not trying to be obtrusively cynical, but the nobility of the actual Jewish warriors was exactly that they were not monumental. They were poor, malnourished, desperate amateurs armed with a few rifles and grenades they had scrounged here and there, or smuggled in by Home Army volunteers; and the miracle was that this riffraff had forced the Germans to employ tanks and dive-bombers to break them. Now the monument had been erected in a wasteland of the city—without a flower on it, in a city where the slightest memorial was always marked with flowers—and that was that.

(By the way, there was no monument anywhere to the dead of 1944. For Communists the Powstanie was an irresponsible episode of a criminal gang, however 'heroic' its fighters might have been.)

I flew back to Paris (planes flew lower then and I remember the giant cumulus castles we passed) with a turbulent wash of feelings inside me. On the flight out I had been reading Simone de Beauvoir's *The Long March* about Mao's struggle to build a new China through Communism. It was an interesting book, but this French intellectual's arguments now seemed both superficial and complacent. In Warsaw I had shared talk with strangers all day long about what was most important: war, freedom, religion, the meaning of art, until I went to bed in my tiny room at the *Bristol*, with the French and English phrases, the background sounds of Polish rolling through my head like freight trains, and above all I had been allowed to share this intense conviction of the value of the *Will*—of standing up to the Germans, who had wanted to wipe out the city, and to the Russians, who had seen it as a docile provincial capital within the Soviet Union. One held to a faith in human spirit when there was little else to hold.

By that time I had abandoned the fantasy of becoming an international intellectual, seated over my vermouth at *Les Deux Magots*, discussing last week's interview at Gallimard, the review in *Figaro*. Putting one more manuscript on a closet shelf, I would start a school, in Boston, where neither my wife nor I had a family member to eat Sunday dinner with, and would choose the Warsaw mermaid as its symbol. She used to sit on a rock in the middle of the Vistula, exchanging comments with the raftsmen sailing their cargoes of wheat, timber, and furs down to Gdańsk on the Baltic. People would ask me questions, and I would tell them about her and History.

> *It didn't require great character at all*
> *our refusal disagreement and resistance*
> *we had a shred of necessary courage*
> *but fundamentally it was a matter of taste*
> > *Yes taste*
> *in which there are fibers of soul the cartilage of conscience*
> . . . .
> Zbigniew Herbert *The Power of Taste*

> *I never really felt the cold, never*
> *was devoured by lice, never knew*
> *true hunger, humiliation, fear for my life*
> *at times I wonder whether I have any right to write.*
> Stanisław Barańczak *A Winter Diary*

8

Warsaw 1960, 1964, 1968

First there are plans
then reports
This is the language
we know how to communicate in
Everything must be foreseen
Everything must be
confirmed later
What really happens
doesn't attract anyone's attention
    Adam Zagajewski *Plans, Reports*

They ask so little of us; only to say that we respect what we despise,
    that we hate what we love.
    Boris Pasternak *Dr. Zhivago*

You, censor, are not so terrible
Not the Kazamaty,* nor drops of salt water
that trickle down stone walls,
Nor the crack of a whip or bloody curses
Only sunlight in the curtains,
A whistling kettle, the homely smell of coffee.
Lounging in the corners and the high-pitched
Ripples of laughter of a familiar official
Holding in her hand a pair of ordinary scissors.
    Adam Zagajewski *A Little Song About the Censor*

Who will bear witness to these times?
Who will record them? Certainly none of us:
We've lived here too long, we've soaked the epoch
up too well, we're too loyal to it to tell the truth
about it. . . .

. . . it can't be done:
survive and stay pure. . . .
    Bronisław Maj

* A Tsarist prison

MARY AND I passed through Warsaw in 1960, she to meet some of the people and see the city that had made such an impact upon me in 1957. To cross the Oder from the German Democratic Republic (there was a name!) and reach the Polish border station with its team of chatty, cheerful, khaki-uniformed young women, a little radio playing a pop tune, was to arrive in Freedomland. These officials were human beings, a fact not at all obvious among the hyenas and jackals on the other side of the Odra.

A night in Poznań and the next afternoon in Warsaw, guaranteed as always to make any first-time visitor regret his decision to come. We paid our social call upon the Grocholscy, Mary alert to how much the Colonel's aristocratic grace depended upon the practicality of Madame, whose worn hands and kind, exhausted smile stayed in her mind. I introduced my wife to Anna, who had recently returned from her year in Paris. No business deal in France can be consummated legally. When you re-sell a house, for example, after two years at a tangible profit, you can exchange back into dollars only the amount that has been notarized. The buyer, however, refuses to state the actual price on his notarized statement since that will mean a higher tax assessment, in fact will threaten the existing assessments of every house on the street. Accordingly, 8 to 12% of the payment will be in cash under the table, non-convertible.

"You can buy some nice antiques."

I had been so moved by Anna's hunger for an education, her longing to break out of this hermetic box, that I had put those guilt-flavored francs into an account in her name at American Express. The franc was devalued a couple of times before she could touch the account, but it was still a considerable amount of money by Polish standards.

Passports were not issued by the Ministry of Foreign Affairs, which sheltered too many unreliable liberals, but by the Ministry of the Interior—the police. The only reason, obviously, that an American would bankroll such a grant for a young woman was to use her as a prostitute or as an agent of the CIA. Accordingly, it took a year of police interrogation (think of being paid to have a long talk with a woman like Anna every week) before the passport was reluctantly handed over.

The money was well spent. A year in Paris after a lifetime of Warsaw is a joy to imagine: you accompany this young pilgrim walking along the Seine towards Notre Dame beneath the great sweep of sky that the river brings with it, visiting Monet's *Water Lilies* at the Orangérie, or simply sitting at a café with a new friend, to absorb every quality of beauty and pleasure, every detail fresh, nothing taken for granted, that Paris offered. To escape History. "Of my four grandparents," she once remarked years later, "three died in Siberia, the fourth of exhaustion after he'd been freed from Dachau." Or as a friend remarked, one reason Anna never married was that too many of the men among whom she might have found a husband had been slaughtered as boys in the Powstanie. Paris had evaded History: surrendering without a shot in 1940, left behind when the Germans fled in 1944 to offer the world its revolutionary motto: Security, Property, Comfort.

Upon return, however, every traveler had to undergo more interviews, with two officers. Her original interrogator asked the questions: "What Poles did you meet? What did you talk about? What books did you read? Write down your budget for each month. Where did those 10,000 francs come from?" The other kept his eyes on her face: "Why did you blink your eyes? What did you mean by that smile?"

I had my own experience within the state security apparatus when I served as sergeant typist for a team interrogating Italian and German civilian internees at prison camps in Modena, Livorno, Florence during the summer of 1945. Were they genuine security risks or simply unfortunates (90%) who might be released? To be questioned by the police is frightening, but it also means that someone is very interested in what you do, in what you most intimately think. To leave that world for New York or Paris where you can do anything and no one cares—that can be lonely. It was in the Modena camp that I was handed a French-speaking roughneck picked up in our haphazard dragnet.

"How have you served France in her years of suffering?"

He muttered on at top speed, but one word I caught: 'Milice.' I responded with a friendly smile:

"The Milice were a fine group of men. You served with them?"

The brutal face brightened.

"Oui, Monsieur."

"Darnand, mon vieux, was a courageous French Patriot," I purred silkily, reaching for the form which would put this guy away for eight more months. The Milice of Joseph Darnand, hanged a few months later as a traitor, were an ugly crowd that did a lot of the Nazis' dirty work in southern France, a fact that a Harvard-trained mind would pick up and remember.

"Oui, Monsieur, how right you are!"

We shook hands warmly.

In search of topics to talk about with this charming young woman, the first policeman had told her about his family, his little boy interested in many, many things. So, when she returned from Paris Anna had brought back a toy fire engine. The cop was speechless. Lots of people had offered him bribes, no one had ever given him a present. Anna shared her father's relaxed attitude towards the police.

"They know what I think of them. I don't break any laws. If they want to arrest me, that's up to them."

Jacek Woźniakowski's wife Maja in Kraków bitterly regretted the thousands of hours taken from her children, standing in line, for what were to Anna quiet hours when she could read or pray. She had a spirit at peace with itself, free from fear, I felt, and she had found interesting, useful work, painting the ceilings, on her back like Michelangelo, high on the scaffolding of rebuilt churches, carving three doves within a doorway lintel of the Old Town, a detail of beauty for the eye.

The Colonel asked Mary and me to drive him and Madame to the estate outside Warsaw that they had once owned. He was anxious to show us the little cottages and their gardens that he had deeded to his employees before the war.

"If only enough people of our class had done that! Women will never choose Communism if they have a home and a garden."

A conclusion shared by Stalin, for different policies.

We met with one of the young men I had encountered selling that magazine on American literature. Jerzy felt we should expose ourselves to some of the gaiety for which his city was—at times—famous and suggested a nightclub in the basement of the Palace of Science and Culture. This was Warsaw's skyscraper, similar to Chicago's Wrigley Building, only bigger, a 'gift from the Soviet People,' in Moscow Monumental—'small but in Perfect Taste.' A group of Hungarian ladies in diaphanous scarves of violet, orange, and turquoise were dancing *Lady of Spain I Adore You*, followed by a jazz orchestra with *You Take the A Train* and *Muskrat Ramble*. Reassuring: old tunes, old performers never die, they go to Warsaw.

I returned in 1964 with daughter Amy, seventeen, and son Bruce, fifteen,—my old friend Barton's namesake—on our way to a village way up in the Baltic potato fields where the Woźniakowski family had rented a cottage, and where we would leave Bruce for a maturing adventure. In Science and Culture's giant auditorium we heard a program of Revolutionary Songs of Freedom put on by a famous company from East Berlin. The star was a massive Freedom Fighter from New York whose parade started by our seats in the upper balcony. What had brought him and his Freedom Songs to Berlin? "Please, sir, tell me the story of your life." He didn't have the time. Booming out the *Battle Hymn of the Republic*, he strode down the steps banging his guitar. On stage this turned, of course, into *We Shall Overcome*, with which the audience could sort of follow along. ("And who, sir, is *We?* Define *overcome. Whom?*"—always the academic.) He knew at least ten words of Polish, for which the natives are always touchingly appreciative, and he shouted the names of Castro and Kennedy, which received equal applause. It was an archaic, almost Habsburg, performance.

A digression: Miłosz had mentioned once that despite the abysmal housing conditions, Poles, even if their home was a bed and a couple of suitcases cut off by a blanket hanging from the ceiling, married very young. The other person's body kept out the cold, and to whisper together in the dark supplied a fierce privacy. By the 1960s I heard of ways how that story played out. Times were better now, but in Warsaw women aged, in spirit as well as body, faster than men. Younger, prettier, more optimistic women willing to look for some greater security with an older man, made themselves available, and the loyal companions of those terrible years often found themselves discarded. Time, however, except on the final page of romantic novels, does not stop, and the confident, charming older man also ages, gains weight, acquires varicosities, and having backed the wrong superior is transferred to Przemysl, and it is the ambitious second wife who finds herself staring at the ceiling at 3 A.M.

1968

My skills and accomplishments . . .
My East European expertise in how to remain silent while
arrested or how to fool the censor.
My repeated championship of my housing project in standing
in line,
My hometown record for accepting fate (both in the short
and long runs), my certified diploma in waiting for a bus . . .
Stanisław Barańczak *Curriculum Vitae*

It was night. A heavy leather blanket hung over the entrance of the *Bristol* to keep out the winter. I ran into the street catching soft March snowflakes in my face, absurdly glad to be here, putting behind me the school and Boston and the sense of being confined in LBJ's madhouse, where every statement or thought had to be bounced off his tortured view of the world and of human nature, as if we lived in Bulgaria.

I stopped a gentleman.

"Prosze pana, gdzie głowny urżad pocztowy?"

(Please, sir, where is the main post office?)

"Najpierw na prawo; potem na lewo."

(First to the right and then left.)

"Dziękuję bardzo."

A block further on I asked the same question. To be in Poland again, to have ordered a small cherry brandy, (wisniówka), accurately, at the *Bristol's* bar, to express myself fluently in this beautiful language, this is what I had hoped for, prepared myself for again and again on these trips to *My* Europe. Here was a sign of my own life thirty years ago, when I had been a witness to what this world had been before the deluge, to the children playing in their ghetto park, to the cavalrymen on their beautiful horses.

I had come again when the rubble was being turned back into buildings and when people once again made ironic jokes and talked about God and the purpose of Art. From that experience I had gained, in a way, the sense of meaning that led me to start my own school, which might become a small center of goodwill and reason.

I was walking rapidly along the Krakowskie Przedmiescie towards the Stare Miasto to go beyond this monumental part of the city to the Old Town's scale, narrow streets and human details, like Anna's doves, in lamp light and black shadow, which had been rubble like everything else back in 1945 but had been rebuilt with determination and sensitivity.

I had left Prague for Boston less than a week before to conduct the memorial service at school for our colleague, Seymour Alden, as I had promised his widow, Louise. It had been a proper ceremony, one of his students reading from *Psalm 139*—

If I ascend up into Heaven, thou art there:
If I make my bed in Hell, behold, thou art there.
If I take the wings of the morning,
And dwell in the uttermost parts of the sea;
Even there shall thy hand lead me,
And thy right hand shall hold me

The students sang *Come, O Come, Emmanuel,* his favorite. Seymour, always the teacher, would have respected a good ceremony like this as a model for showing each one of them, when the time came, how to lead a similar service. And to help free his widow and their three daughters from memories of a long slow death at home from cancer—"nothing is so bad it can't get worse."

How would Seymour have fitted into life in Warsaw? Hard to say. At one level satisfactorily enough. He was a resourceful man able to make do with little. As a medieval historian he would have been fascinated by ways in which the city had dropped out of the twentieth century and turned itself into a federation of feudal baronies, a forest crisscrossed by barbarian tribes. I don't think he would have survived the German occupation, however. As a man of honor he would have been less able to learn the tricks necessary to stay alive. If he lived on into the Communist years, it would not have been belonging to the losing side that would have burdened him too much. History is the story of losers. He would have been disheartened by the slovenliness of Communist management and more than that, by its contempt for the truth. Even to live in Boston, to keep on teaching at Commonwealth during the 1970s, would have been painful for him as the school's sense of purpose and mutual trust eroded. Opposition to the Vietnam War, where we—students and faculty—stood pretty much together, would grow into a cynical rejection of any established principle and institution of American life, including, of course, our school.

⁂

I have not only the right
but, also the duty to display all the
human weaknesses: no one, for example, compels me
to be a hero, i.e. to speak the truth,
not to inform, to refrain from the very human
need to kick a man when he's down, nothing
that's human is alien to me . . .
  Stanisław Barańczak *The Humane Conditions*

When I reached the gate to the university area in which stood the Grocholski apartment (though the Colonel had died some years back), a guard with a steel helmet and a sub-machine gun slung over his shoulder demanded my passport.

At the apartment, Anna (now a professional art historian) and cousins and friends gave me details. The classics are safe, and people go to performances of Shakespeare and Chekhov, Moliére and *The Crucible* or *Death of a Salesman*,* at low, government-subsidized ticket prices, to be exposed to a richness and complexity of character and also to language they do not find in current work. That is perfectly all right, Socialism stands for culture. Adam Mickiewicz is the national poet, what for Americans might be the combination of Whitman, Longfellow, and Frost. *Pan Tadeusz*, a closed book to any non-Polish reader in its episodic wandering around the Lithuanian gentry estates of Napoleon's time, is the national epic, which school children must memorize by the hundreds of lines so they can recite it to themselves in prison. *Dziady* (Forefathers' Eve) is a romantic classic in many acts. But then students—dumb kids—have to spoil everything by clapping and cheering at the lines where some foolish idealist condemns the dishonest old men who take bribes and fawn upon the Russians.

⁊

The theatre is closed. The irresponsible students keep on making noise and outside on the sidewalk wave signs in the air. This means a response from the security police, who are apt to be men who grew up in orphan asylums and have a sense of loyalty only to the government that pays them and gives them orders and some rather nice privileges in food and housing. They have vestigial emotional relations with other people, none at all with the spoiled brats who go to the university and think they're better than anyone else.

Police action precipitates another level of student response, though of course the police carry clubs, and guns too, which have not yet been used. It is hard to measure violence precisely, but it is true that even if the police enjoy hitting students, they enjoy hitting girl students even more.

The American police, too, could lose themselves in violence. In April 1969 radical students took over Harvard's administration center in protest against the Vietnam War. One reason for revolutionary action is to allow young people to feel that they belong to their times, and Harvard had produced too

* From Warsaw to Beijing, Arthur Miller was the first American playwright introduced on the Communist stage: his contempt for bourgeois hypocrisy satisfying the censors, his contempt for all corrupt authority, which they missed, rewarding his audiences. The censors also missed—a classic is a classic—the dangers of Chekhov and Shakespeare. The self-delusions, the sheer random suffering that humans endure all their lives have not ceased to exist just because Communist writers are forbidden to discuss them. Shakespeare's smiling villains, his conflicts between loyalty and betrayal do not need a classroom teacher to point out similarities. Richard III was too extreme to fit into Warsaw (Bucharest perhaps), but Claudius, who wanted to befriend, know better, set limits to, and eventually kill Hamlet, suited Polish politics perfectly.

many of the Best and the Brightest who believed that Vietnam could be remade in the image of American society, or at least that their personal careers could be aided in the process. So the Students for a Democratic Society seized University Hall, passed hand to hand down the stairs a large black dean as if he were a sack of cornmeal, and my then son-in-law sat at the desk of Dean Ford, smoking his cigars and reading his mail. President Pusey asked the city police to clear out the strikers, as was his right. But he was not present when the police did attack at 5 A.M., did not see the fear on the faces of police and students terrified at the harm they were wreaking upon each other, hear the screams, shouts, wails; witness the uncontrolled weeping of men and women, police and students, at the end.*

Polish riot police were better trained and more experienced.†

The 1960s. Nostalgia—"Those were the times of youthful idealism." Perhaps. The Vietnam War had a quality of hopelessness and despair, and bottomless cruelty, that rivaled that of the Powstanie of 1944—and now *we* were playing the role of the Germans. (The visits to Hanoi organized by the authorities for Polish, Czech, Bulgarian intellectuals were shocking experiences. Instinctively they loathed anything sponsored by the Communists and instinctively admired the Americans, but the savagery of American bombing was impossible to deny.) The Vietnam years lasted longer than the Powstanie. And here in Harvard Yard, later on at Columbia University, and over and over elsewhere, were young men and women trying to turn their country's policy around and force the Johnson administration and their fellow citizens, basically terrified of taking any stand that might have them labeled unpatriotic, to face the pointless cruelty of that war and to do something about it. As other young men and women had challenged the police and democratic public opinion in Mississippi and Alabama to change the rules and basic assumptions of racial inequality. Europeans, at least Western Europeans, despised Americans as naive, ignorant, protected from reality, and yet those wordy, duffle-coated radicals around their smoky café tables were quite safe. It was Americans who were serving as infantry.

Youthful idealists enjoyed the romance of marijuana, ignoring parents and teachers, trusting the smiling stranger on Harvard Square. To envious young people ten, twenty years later, rock, hair, sex, angering and frightening parents seemed fresh and brave. May 1945 in the Po Valley our trucks passed the

---

* The account of Theodore Sizer, Dean of the School of Education, then an eyewitness.

† Joke: Who are the best educated police in the world? The Polish, silly, they're always at the university.

same young men who had picked up rifles and tied red cloths around their arms, instant Partigiani—Viva il Communismo: Libertá!—whom we envied for their freedom.

The idealists of 1968 were also middle class. LBJ did not want to jeopardize his war by alienating the people who mattered by taxing their incomes and killing their sons, so it was easy to obtain student deferments. Private school headmasters wrote letters supporting Jonathan's request for status as a Conscientious Objector—eventually I became ashamed of the job. It wasn't my sons, my nephews, even my students (except for one black) who were shipped to Vietnam. It was Irish, Poles, Italians, Hispanics, blacks from the cities, dumb small-town boys whose names eventually got engraved on that marble wall in Washington.

∽

One of my reasons, or excuses, for the trip had been to arrange an exchange of student pictures with an art school in Warsaw. I found my way there and admired the pastels, gouaches, watercolors, brighter and more fanciful than what our youngsters usually turned out. The director liked the idea of swapping pictures with an American school, but with times as tense as they were then she was afraid to take any initiative unless I obtained a clear go-ahead from a certain official at some office in the Ministry of Education.

So, off I went, unafraid of Polish bureaucracy, proud not to be like other Americans, threading my way through doormen, security guards, secretaries. No, the official was not there. Where? When? The woman on duty wasn't interested in making herself clearer. Yes, she did give me the number of another office. No, no one there cared to explore gently the card-castle of my linguistic knowledge. "I am an important American." Indeed. Beaten, I trudged back to the *Bristol* and ordered a small wiśniówka.

At Commonwealth I used to get angry at the irresponsible black students who would be found, after I had warned them of the academic trouble they were in and had set out priorities and guidelines and practical ways of managing their time, half an hour later shooting baskets in the gym. They were at my school on large scholarships to prepare themselves for an improvement in class status and a career of social leadership. Well, shooting baskets was one thing that they knew how to do well. I knew how to order a cherry vodka. (The next academic year we did arrange a small, nice quality swap of student art.)

I took the train down to Kraków, across a landscape of snow still in the furrows of the fields, bare trees laden with flocks of jackdaws, to call upon the Woźniakowski family whose son was in the same precarious status as the students back in Warsaw and where the thug-like Workers' Militia had cordoned off the statue of Mickiewicz, the poet of trouble-makers.

Back in Warsaw from Poznań* and Gdańsk, I was eating in the breakfast room at the *Bristol*, filled by a large delegation of Asians—Mongolians?—wearing round knitted caps, giving orders to the harried waitresses in bad Russian. I didn't find the scene exotic any more, nor the police in the streets. How quickly could I leave? I was due in Paris in two days to meet Mary, with David and Paul, our two youngest, on our way to my brother's house in Athens. Where could I go, right now?

I was registered at a hotel in Copenhagen by sundown. Who could have imagined a more perfect antidote? I passed courteous, handsome policemen, well-built houses and churches, clean streets, children with laughing mothers, shop windows designed by artists: books, toys, trips to Africa, soup plates and crystal goblets, tasteful linens, cameras, oriental rugs, pornography, operas, neckties and gleaming shoes. Everything was gleaming and clean and well made.

Suddenly, in a little over an hour, I'd had enough. What did all of this stand for, except for pleasing oneself by spending money? (I get fed up with this dreary moralizing that fastens itself on me. Remember how desperately important it seemed to run as far away from Poland as possible?) It would be nice to live in Copenhagen, but nothing that happened there was of any significance. The struggle to hold to some sort of integrity, at a high price, in gray, discouraged Warsaw, that meant something.

> *They will probably come just after the New Year.*
> *As usual, early in the morning.*
> *The forceps of the doorbell will pull you out by the head*
> *from under the bedclothes; dazed as a newborn baby,*
> *you'll open the door. The star of an ID*
> *will flash before your eyes.*
> . . . .
> Stanisław Barańczak *The Three Magi*

---

* Police state etiquette: Somehow I had been invited for drinks at the home of the young, knowledgeable American consul in Poznań. Present were his wife, a child, a couple of other Americans, two Poles. As we were making our goodbyes, the Poles spoke together privately. "When we are questioned by the police as to who was here and what was talked about, we want to have the same story. We talked about the Negro problem and Vietnam—simple."

9

Warsaw 1978, 1985

Nothing has changed.
The body is a reservoir of pain,
it has to eat and breathe the air, and sleep,
it's got skin and the blood is just beneath it,
it's got a good supply of teeth and fingernails,
its bones can be broken, its joints can be stretched.
In tortures, all this is considered.

. . . .

tortures are just what they were, only the earth has shrunk
and whatever goes on sounds as it's just a room away.

. . . .

   Wisława Szymborska *Tortures*

It's the twentieth century, so
I go to bed with the newspaper,
my glasses, pills, and wristwatch
are within reach;
I don't know if I'll fall asleep,
I don't know if I'll wake up,
that's all.
   Ryszard Krynicki *Almost All*

BETWEEN 1968 AND 1985 I made, with Mary, only one brief stop in Warsaw, in March 1978. I remember particularly our visit to *Wedel's*, an old-fashioned café on Nowy Swiąt, where ladies out shopping would stop for a revivifying cup of coffee or chocolate and a piece of pastry. The hats would have been different in 1938, but the atmosphere would have been the same, and times were so bad that a pleasant cup of coffee was an absolute necessity—although not for Jews, the Wedel firm was notoriously anti-Semitic. How close those ladies, dressed like my mother, were to the end of their world. Back to 1908 and different hats again, this time on the heads of Russian officers' wives, and History is waiting for them too.

We were clients of First Secretary Edward Gierek, who had borrowed billions of dollars from foreign banks,* ostensibly to modernize and expand Poland's export industry (freighters, golf carts, enameled kitchen ware), but in actuality to please consumers enough through subsidized prices to preserve social peace and send visitors like ourselves back home with reports that Warsaw was just like any other European city, only cheaper.

In 1970 Gierek, the boss of Silesia, had replaced poor old angry Gomułka, who could not grant higher wages to shipyard workers and coal miners because he could not reorganize the worn-out, badly run Polish economic system, and could not do that without reorganizing the corrupt Communist management system. Gomułka's response to workers' demands for a more realistic and democratic administration had been to call in the police. His, and Brezhnev's, invasion of Czechoslovakia had done just that in 1968 to get rid of Dubček and his reform Communism.

Gierek was said to be intelligent. He had grown up in Belgium, the child of a miner's family, and therefore could talk face to face with Giscard d'Estaing without the need of an interpreter, a detail pleasing to Polish self-esteem. Madame Gierek, rumor went, used an air force plane to fly once a week to Paris to go shopping and have her hair done.

Not all of Gierek's frustrations could be blamed on himself.† The 1973 Yom Kippur War between Israel and the Arabs boosted world-wide oil prices, which hurt Poland directly and also helped bring about a world-wide economic downturn that depressed its export markets.

The workers at the Lenin Shipyards in Gdańsk were beginning to demand not only higher wages and lower food prices, the cause of the bloody 1970 strike, but also free trade unions. In a capitalist country the unions protect the workers against their selfish employers, but in a socialist country where the workers' own state is the employer, worker and employer cannot logically be in confrontation with each other. The union's job is to administer health services and pensions, vacation benefits, and cultural activities, nice things indeed, but not very important.

The spokesman for the shipyard workers, the twenty-seven-year-old electrician, Lech Wałęsa (an electrician, moving around the plant to deal with breakdowns, was in the perfect occupation to listen to and know other

---

* Not unlike Ronald Reagan. Poland's foreign debt, $2.5 billion in 1973, had risen to $25 billion by 1982. Lawrence Weschler, *The Passion of Poland*, Pantheon Books, N.Y., 1984, pp. 216–221.

† This background material on the 1970s, the Solidarity period, and on Jaruzelski's seizure of power comes partly from Weschler's *The Passion of Poland*, originally a series of articles in *The New Yorker*.

workers), disagreed. The working conditions at a factory in socialist Poland, not only in wages but hours, safety measures, the right to speak freely to management, were as bad as in any horror-story capitalist plant anywhere.

In turn the Communists could not deal honestly with such complaints. They could not admit what everybody knew, the self-serving corruption of its leaders, the Nomenklatura. As in the Soviet Union, this group, perhaps a hundred thousand in number, was the closed circle from which middle management was drawn and which enjoyed good salaries, perquisites, and job security. A member fired because he mismanaged the Kraków streetcar system was sent to run a dairy co-op outside Bialystok. When he fouled that up, off he was posted to mismanage a hospital in Wrocław.

Gierek lacked the freedom to make any serious changes. If he allowed Polish workers to reject the Communist way of doing things, the habit could spread too quickly. That, after all, was the reason that the Hungarian reform movement of 1956 and that of the Czechs of 1968 had had to be suppressed. If rejection of Leninist Communism was just a code term for rejecting the hegemony of the Soviet Union, then Brezhnev could not conceivably tolerate the existence of a hostile Poland on Russia's border—as the United States could not tolerate a hostile Nicaragua or El Salvador.

An unexpected complication would appear in the election in 1978 of Karol Wojtyła, the archbishop of Kraków, as Pope John Paul II. He was not the liberal that American Catholics hoped. He restrained the Latin American movement of liberation theology, which demanded that the Church's message should insist upon a preferential option for the poor. He condemned sexism, but was not interested in changing the role of women within the Church. He did, however, possess the force of character to stand up to Communist pressure and threats and to speak to and for his people in times of their greatest suffering.

As the authority of Gierek weakened, that of General Wojciech Jaruzelski, Minister of Defense, strengthened. Solidarity now had ten million dues-paying members. At the same time, the chaos within Poland, with endless lines in front of near empty stores, no force in society enjoying the authority to accomplish anything, with even Solidarity—sometimes brilliantly, sometimes confusedly led by Wałęsa and his colleagues and rivals—unable to function clearly, and with the increasingly menacing threats from Russia,* meant a nation on the edge of hysteria.

---

* The Americans played an unclear role. Because the Carter administration was tied up in the Iranian hostage crisis, the Russians were freed for their Afghan adventure. That in turn limited their freedom of action in Poland. The State Department warned the Russians against intervention, but a Russian invasion would have so damaged their prestige around the world that a certain type of State apparatchik in Washington would have been very pleased.

On the night of Saturday, December 12, 1981, the army acted. At 6 A.M. General Jaruzelski proclaimed 'a state of war.' Thousands of activists were interned, all Solidarity offices were seized, the country's frontiers were sealed, all public gatherings banned, all schools closed, all mail and phone service closed down. The army, which almost all Poles trusted, was held in abeyance, and the dirty work was done by the 25,000 to 30,000 member Internal Security Forces, the Zomos, one factory at a time.

"A gang of thugs attacked an insane asylum," was a wise-crack that Lawrence Weschler quotes, but despite the Polish reputation for inefficiency, the seizure of power under Jaruzelski was brilliant in its secrecy and execution, even more expertly carried out than Pinochet's coup in Chile back in 1973.

Now what? To cheer people up, large quantities of food appeared in the stores. Within a week the government reported that most of the country had been normalized. The heroism of those days was the steadfastness of several thousand miners holed up in the occupation of two Silesian coal mines, enduring dark, hunger, total isolation, sustained by the faith that the rest of Polish workers were as resolute, which they weren't. Jaruzelski announced that martial law is better than civil war or, as he said years later, a Russian invasion.

There was not the sadistic cruelty of Pinochet's police, but the internment camps were harsh enough. Some demonstrations and underground resistance broke out, by now as symbols, and were cruelly repressed, and then came releases and amnesties and random concessions.

There were moments of elation: the Pope's second visit in June of 1983, Wałęsa's receiving the Nobel Peace Prize (as with Miłosz's Nobel Prize in 1980), but what seemed to come was the silence of internal emigration. The country's economic collapse and gutted gray shell of a cultural life would just go on and on. One unexpected result was a baby boom. From June 1982 through June 1983 Poland had the highest rate of population growth of any major country in Europe, not the boom of joy and expectations that had immediately preceded the upsurge of Solidarity, but one of spiritual deflation—the only way to still find the slightest meaning for one's life.*

> *If china, then only the kind*
> *you wouldn't miss under the movers' shoes or the treads of a tank;*
> *if a chair, then one that's not too comfortable, or you'll regret getting*
>   *up and leaving;*

---

* Weschler, *Op. cit.*, pp. 186–187.

if clothes, then only what will fit in one suitcase;
if books, then those you know by heart;
if plans, then the ones you can give up
when it comes time for the next move,
to another street, another continent or epoch
or world.
    Stanisław Barańczak *If China*

1978's ephemeral call on my usual towns—Prague, Olomouc, Kraków, Warsaw—did not offer anywhere near the rewards of a longer trip to Brazil two years previously. The diversity of Brazil fascinated me, and the possibility of involving the Merrill Foundation in some modest proposals became the excuse for a visit. The foundation's trustees claimed to be uninterested in philanthropy abroad except for Canada (where Merrill Lynch and Safeway Stores had sizable investments) and England (all nice Americans feel a grateful warmth toward its cathedrals and gardens), but one trustee who had served under Kennedy and Johnson as ambassador to Chile felt a strong commitment to Latin American needs. As an Establishment liberal, he was compelled to present these needs under the rubric of stopping Communism, but if that argument could fund the Marshall Plan or some useful grants by our grade B foundation, so be it.

I was interested in a Cambridge-based economic development agency named Acción that was committed to fighting the Latin American disease of unemployment by encouraging small-scale entrepreneurial activity rather than overcentralized, overadministered government projects. Our foundation had already financed Acción enterprises in Mexico and Peru, and might do the same now in the coastal cities of Bahia and Recife.

Just as it was possible to walk along the old-fashioned streets of Kraków and Prague with little awareness of the up-to-date dictatorships that oppressed them, it was easy in the middle of *O Milagro Brasileiro* to ignore the murderous military rule in the background. A lot of policemen armed with heavy pistols were hanging around, but that is true in every Latin American city. Nevertheless, the brand new highways and electrical power pylons, the nationally manufactured Fokker airplanes and Olivetti typewriters, the skyscraper cliffs of Rio and São Paulo seemed proof that Brazil was a partner of the American system. And in Bahia and Recife when I inspected the micro-empresas (a sandal-making workshop, a printing press, a shop making beer mugs out of old bottles) that Acción was backing, with help in accounting, tax management, banking procedure so that the business could obtain commercial loans at 18% rather than 40% interest, and with such aid allow 200 mini-capitalists to go from two employees to four, which meant

400 new jobs—more jobs, with a minuscule investment of capital, than from a Volkswagen assembly plant—here was an undramatic capitalism where everyone benefited. Exactly what was needed in Poland if those dumb Marxists freed themselves from the handcuffs of ideology.

Nevertheless, not in the first conversation with a new acquaintance but in the third or fourth, the visitor began to pick up a chilling set of details. A brilliant, American-educated economist, Delfim Nieto, supplied the brains of *O Milagro* and had raised up a new ruling class of MBAs who were leading Brazil out of its stagnant traditions. They preferred a clean military dictatorship to the chaotic populist regimes that had preceded it, but as graduates of Harvard and the London School of Economics, assumed that the colonels would be kept in their place. They were mistaken.

If one of these bright young men made the wrong remark—"Let's face it, we have a shitty government"—to the wrong friend, he might have representatives of any one of three security police forces pounding on his door at 4 A.M., be taken to any one of three prisons, with no notice of where he was, what was the charge, how long he would be kept, or how he would be treated, whether with an old-fashioned rubber hose or modern electrical shocks. No fooling around with habeas corpus—his lawyer was as useless as his beautiful bilingual secretary.

If he had received a serious Christian education he might reflect on the transitoriness of earthly delights and sing sad Protestant hymns to himself: *Abide With Me, Fast Falls the Eventide* "when other comforts fail and helpers flee, help of the helpless. . . ."

In Recife I had the privilege of speaking with Dom Helder Camara, who in Brazil occupied much the same role as Cardinal Stefan Wyszynski, who during the 1950s and 1960s supplied the force of the Polish church. It was the ancient privilege of the primate of Poland to stand for the people before the king, and both old men, by their status, force of mind and character, and almost universal respect, held a position where they could speak Truth to Power. Cardinal Camara was hated and feared by the military, who attacked him as a Communist. Passing police cars shot up his palace: "They're afraid, though, to murder him—French intellectuals would protest." The next step was to pretend he did not exist. No media organ was permitted to mention his name. This did not hinder his courage in saying obvious things and in dealing with the poorest people, such as trying to organize house servants for minimum rights. And hiring lawyers to supply papers for squatters in the interior, who were being pushed out by the great land corporations like Volkswagen. Without papers they were given $200, enough to get drunk on; with papers they received $2000, capital for a new life.

The following could have come word for word from Eastern Europe: a teacher at a private school in Recife asked her little girls to write down which Brazilian they respected the most. "For me it's Dom Helder," one child answered, "because he's such a good man and tries so hard to help the poor." The teacher showed the paper to her headmistress, who showed it to her favorite police officer, who summoned the girl's father to his office. "What sort of Communist lies do you talk about in front of your kids? You be careful, or they won't be having their father around for quite a while!"

The relevance of this digression on Brazil to a book centered on Poland and Czechoslovakia is to compare left-wing and right-wing repression and, to go further, the role of torture, and then the role of the United States. In Poland the repressive forces were Communist. In Latin America, the *repressed*, according to Senator Jesse Helms *et al.*, could be dismissed as Communist, and therefore military repression in Brazil, Guatemala, El Salvador could be ignored. During the 1960s and 1970s there seemed no limit to what ingenuity could produce within the military dictatorships of Brazil, Uruguay, Argentina, and Chile, against individuals considered revolutionaries or traitors. There was Christ's Crown in which a metal band is squeezed tighter and tighter around the victim's forehead till it cracks; the parrot's perch, whereby an iron bar is wedged behind the victim's knees, to which his wrists are tied, the bar placed between two tables, and the victim hung upside down; burning the genitals with cigarettes; an electric needle placed under the fingernails of a pianist; a cockroach introduced into the anus.*

In 1957 I met a student in Warsaw who described an interrogation by Bierut's police in the early years during which the prisoner, naked, stood in front of an open window in February while police threw buckets of water on him. Gottwald, in the early years of Czech Communism, gave special attention to breaking the kulaks—peasants of any property and spirit— which included having a number beaten to death. The Czechs, however, relied on sending political prisoners to work in the uranium mines along the northern borders where after a few years they died from cancer.

⤜∾⤛

Brutality there was aplenty but there does not seem to be such examples of perverse torture—pretty much ignored by American presidents except Jimmy Carter—as in Latin America, or in the prison cells of NATO allies

---

* This material on South America comes mainly from Lawrence Weschler's *A Miracle A Universe—Settling Accounts with Torturers*, Pantheon Books, N.Y., 1990, whose writings on Solidarity/Martial Law and on post-Communist Prague I have also drawn from.

like Greece under the colonels or Turkey. In Czechoslovakia, where the opposition came mainly out of the intelligentsia, the most effective punishment seemed to be turning the architect into a garbage collector.

The leaders of Brazil were mainly graduates of the Escola Superior de Guerra, launched in 1949 by veterans of the Brazilian Expeditionary Force who had fought under American command in Italy. At American war colleges, like Warsaw-pact officers in Moscow, they traded shop-talk and listened to lectures that strengthening the nation against external attack was in fact less important than shoring up its institutions against the internal enemy and learning how to recognize that enemy behind his many masks of charitable priest, idealistic teacher, inquisitive journalist, and Christian housewife.

So, if you believe that World War III has already started and that the protection of our children and our gardens is intertwined with the protection of our foreign investments, military prestige, standard of living, and the respect owed to People Like Us, then the system that accepted the bombing of Dresden can accept the discomfiture of a few insolent young men. In June 1982 the Secretary of Defense Caspar Weinberger stated that the United States must be prepared to fight and *win* a sustained nuclear war. No one phoned for men in white coats to come and take him away.

⁂

I return to Warsaw in late October of 1985 to call on friends, to collect pictures for an exhibition of Czech and Polish graphics at a Boston gallery, to visit Lublin for a pilgrimage to the Majdanek death camp and the gem-like Renaissance square of Zamość, to walk along the streets, listen to the language. A Jewish friend has given me $50 to hand to a photographer who can buy Finnish printing paper only with hard currency. "I have money for you," a simple sentence.

When he arrives at the hotel he is both angry and frightened. I shouldn't have used the word. If the phone was bugged, *They* would question him: how much, from whom, for what, had he paid the tax on it? Did the Security Police have the resources to bug every phone in Poland and the patience to listen to every conversation? He didn't want to talk business in my room. The bar was noisier and safer.

"He was that nervous because he was a Jew," explained a friend at Krakowskie Przedmiescie 30.

The people at the apartment are irritated by the tantrums and lies of martial law, tired of standing longer and longer in lines for less and less, sad for the friends who have been hurt worse, but perhaps immunized by never having expected much. That lack of expectation—a less emotional word than *hope* —makes them seem more predictable, less bothersome to the authorities, and they endure the ups and downs of this police state, it seems, without apprehension.

What do I think of President Reagan? The only people I associate with at home hold the same views, so I relish being able to say aloud what I usually repeat to myself. Reagan is interested only in the welfare of the wealthy, benefited by his tax laws, but he sells a paint job of patriotism and wholesomeness to the simple. He tells lies that are not really lies because he registers no relation between what he says on Thursday with what he had said on Monday. The lack of any rational thought process. . . . They are not interested. What a relief to have an American president standing up so resolutely to the Russians, who understand only simple words backed by guns. He is smart enough to see, as liberals are not, that Ortega and his Sandinistas are on their way to establish exactly the total control that Castro did.

I nod politely.

A large gypsy family in flowered skirts is begging at the corner. Gypsies were slaughtered so thoroughly by the Germans that one should be courteous, but I have heard too many stories about the woman who engages you in conversation while the children's little hands race through your pockets. I give 50 złoty to the grandmother and hasten away.

Knowing that I am interested in art, Elzbieta, Anna's younger sister, takes me to the atelier of one of her friends. "Here is someone who has the courage to paint in his own style. He isn't afraid to disagree with the Communists." That's nice, but the geometric abstracts aren't very good.

Elzbieta drives me to the church that belonged to Father Popiełuszko, murdered a year ago by the Security Police. For the anniversary a photo exhibit of his life is hung inside the building: his work with youngsters and pensioners, his courage in asking questions. The grounds outside are a storm of flowers, from little private bouquets to a great wreath from the Bus Drivers' Union. A row of stones is painted with the names of Poland's terrible camps: Sobibor, Treblinka, Majdanek, Oświęcm, Birkenau, and now Katyn. "The Communists were not allowing that the last time I was here," Elzbieta remarks. They still force themselves to insist what everyone, including themselves, know is a lie: the Polish officers in the forest were murdered by the Germans and not by Stalin's security police. The Sunday pilgrimage with its flowers and visitors puts Elzbieta in a sour mood.

"Tourists who are tired of long rum drinks on the beaches of the West Indies want something new. We sell them spiritual experiences. It's a way to earn hard currency."

In a room where people unanimously maintain a conspiracy of silence, one word of truth sounds like a pistol shot.
Czesław Miłosz *Nobel Prize Lecture, 1980*

10

Warsaw 1989, 1990, 1991

I arrive.
A hundred people, two hundred eyes.
Watching. Waiting.
I know what for.
  I am to tell them
  why they were born,
  why the horror called life
  goes on and on.
  Anna Swirszczynska *Poetry Reading*

I used to believe that justice would be done.
So I did not cry when my hair was pulled,
I suffered silently the unjust slap in the face,
slander both visible and invisible,
lost belongings, my burned doll,
the war which came instead of youth. . . .
  Anna Kamienska *Heaven*

I prefer not to ask how much longer and when.
  Wisława Szymborska *Options*

Another couple of months in the West and, while tying your shoelace in
  the street,
you realize that you're actually doing it just to tie your shoelace,
and not in order to routinely check
if you're not followed.
  Stanisław Barańczak *A Second Nature*

Forty years of socialism and still no toilet paper!
  Proverb

MY TRIPS NOW START or end in Oxford, where my son David and his family live, and after a city that beautiful, on so human a scale, so at one with the passage of time—perhaps that's not true: perhaps the story of the twentieth century is the revolt of those who were not invited to walk across the court-yards or share the after-dinner port in Oxford's common rooms—it is harder to force myself to insist that what happens in Warsaw is more important. Around the corner from the *Randolph* to the bus for Heathrow is an open market with a sumptuous congress of fruits and vegetables, lorded over by a pile of eggplant, that I will remember all during my days in Poland. I buy a bunch of bananas as a hostess present.

A couple of years before, Janet, my son Bruce's wife, who ran the music program at Commonwealth, had invited a choral group from Yaroslavl, an industrial city on the Volga about 150 miles north of Moscow, to give a concert in our gym. She had already led three trips of singers, mainly suburban housewives, to the Soviet Union, from Riga to Irkutsk, from Leningrad to Tblisi, Yaroslavl gradually becoming their home base. These summer tours turned into the supreme mission of her life as she established friendships with Russian musicians, learned the language, went from conducting Russians in one song, Americans in another, to the same song sung by both groups, then with Russians and Americans shoulder to shoulder like teeth of a comb.

Forty singers from Yaroslavl's rubber factory had made a return visit, staying in homes, singing in churches and schools. None had ever been outside the Soviet Union, only a couple knew a few words of English. Their offerings—Tchaikovsky, liturgical and folk music, a song from *My Fair Lady*—were unadventurous but professional. Then our school chorus, with teachers as well as students, sang a Haydn *Gloria*, something from *Porgy and Bess*, two rowdy choruses from Bernstein's *West Side Story*.

Everyone had a good time. I found myself close to tears. This is what I had dreamed of, that some day my school would play a part in the reconciliation of our two peoples. A prayer of thanks to Mr. Gorbachev. As I walked away from school with the chairman of our board of trustees, a lawyer who had lost his leg to a German shell burst, he said, "You know, this is the first generation of American kids to grow up without thinking that a nuclear war is inevitable."

And a few years later the first conversations are beginning about World War III, exploding along the great half-circle from Korea and Japan to Pakistan, Iran and Syria, nuclear warheads for everybody.

1989

On the plane to Warsaw I read an interesting magazine article on the Polish economy. How would it be possible to rebuild this Third World country to any level of competitive capitalism when there was no valid infrastructure: long distance telephones that work, bank credit, insurance, accurate and honest accountants?

I distrust jazzy systems managed by well-groomed wiseguys. Profits will be skimmed off by the sharpies, and the natives will be billed for fancy machinery that shortly breaks down. My faith stays at the micro level: the peasant woman from Lomza who comes every so often on a tourist visa to Boston to visit her sister, where she is passed from hand to hand within a Polish and Jewish network, cleaning houses for $50 a day cash. After a month she returns to Lomza with $1500 in ten and twenty dollar bills concealed upon her person to help her husband buy a tractor. That is what keeps Poland going.

The airport is shabby, dreary, chaotic—how tired I am of using those words. A contract is being negotiated with an American firm, I am told, to build a new facility, but the Americans insist on employing their own workmen and the Poles resent being treated like Africans.

Warsaw's new-model Palace of Science and Culture is the *Marriott Hotel*, expressing itself in glossy pictures of its state-of-the-art conference rooms and, of course, its casino with Beautiful People in tuxedos and low-cut evening gowns gathered laughing around the roulette wheel.

By three it is already into a November evening when I arrive at the Grocholski apartment at Krakowskie Przedmiescie 30, the kitchen crowded as always with relatives and friends, presided over patiently by Jacek's younger daughter, Anna, whom I knew 25 years ago as a little girl, with her noisy boys and her silent husband, Colonel Grocholski's youngest son, who now runs the institute for the blind at Laski. Americans are cool, preferring neither to receive nor to give too much, but I must play the role of Pan Karol the Good, respond to the ceremonies of welcome and accept gratefully the heavy, far-too-expensive coffee-table picture books. Old family movies are being shown, centered inevitably around the Colonel and summer days on the estate in Podolia. Aunts in hats, men in cavalry uniforms, a world where the horses were more beautiful than the subdued women in long white dresses, and for a moralizing historian like myself, a world of caste, religion, and death.

There has been democratic changing at the top, with a rumor that Jacek Woźniakowski, now 70, will be the next mayor of Kraków. His son Henryk, around 40, is working himself to death as Prime Minister Mazowiecki's deputy minister for press relations. After all the slovenly louts who have tried to run this unhappy country, isn't this a cause for rejoicing? But even if the Communists shuffle off the stage, won't they be waiting in the wings? Like the Nazis in 1945, they were the people who knew how to get things done. The new people are amateurs.

Anecdote: A would-be entrepreneur broods about how to get started. An idea! He goes to Sweden, commits a non-dangerous crime, is put in prison (fed better than at home), on release is given a sum of money by these kindly Swedes with which to make a New Life. He races to Stockholm, buys every electronic gadget in sight, returns to Warsaw, and peddles his booty for dollars. Capital!

Suggestion: With recent amnesties there is space in Polish jails. How about sending an experienced deal-maker to Governor Cuomo, whose prisoners in New York cost $30,000 per year. For $5000 apiece, paid in advance, the Poles will take ten thousand. Polish jails aren't nice, but less violent and drug ridden than American. Everyone benefits!

At midmorning I am picked up by Jacek Zielinski, one of the artists I recruited for the show of Polish and Czech graphics in Boston. He drives me to his apartment in Ursinow, a new housing district south of the city. Jacek Zielinski and his artist wife, Anna Mizeracka, had waited ten years for an apartment anywhere after having lived all their married life in one room. I have never seen a more inhuman area: haphazard sprawl of shoeboxes without a shop or a restaurant, its only trees the television aerials. Pan Zielinski is a sad, thin man, whose inflamed eyes become worse each year; his wife is crippled by multiple sclerosis. Inside their rooms they have created a home of some dignity, centered around two massive carved pieces, an armoire, and a table that came from some family property, plus a very professional steel press.

Although Pani Anna has made a few consciously Polish works—a loaf of bread, hands in prayer—you could not live with their pictures of death and futility. The little figures are jammed together in prison cells or totally alone on a staircase that ends in a blank wall or shut one by one in isolated chambers, these latter images dating from the atomization of life during the first winter of martial law. We talk for almost four hours, mostly about art, in a careful mix of Polish and English. Pani Anna speaks very clearly; I can almost understand the words that go past me. I have bought a fair number of their lithographs and etchings for college libraries and art centers so that American students can gain some hint of the historical world these emerge from, and so that these two over-burdened people can support themselves and fight to create their witness of this world beyond the wasteland of

Ursinow. The awareness of art is perhaps like the awareness of God, a door opened for the briefest moment.

May 1990

Warsaw is the last stop in this year's trip that began in Budapest. With its flowers and green leaves and girls in pretty frocks, May is a hypocritical month. Come to Warsaw in March when the streets are damp, cold, dark, muddy. On the flight north from Kraków we flew over fields parceled out in the narrow strips that cramp Polish agriculture and send their young men away from these thin farms to look for jobs in the cities. In the spring-green forests are many brownish trees—the same Waldsterben (death of the forest) of Germany and Czechoslovakia? To the west looms an impenetrable surf of smog from the Silesian coal fields.

Poles complain about the constant rise in prices, but for a foreigner the slumping złoty keeps them low. Back in 1985 I was fined a thousand złoty for driving without a seat belt—$9. Today a thousand is worth nine cents. Figure how your savings for a house, your children's education, your whole view of the world come out with that sort of change. The five dollar bill is the unit of currency.

I have budgeted only one night in Warsaw before going on to Oxford and then home, one call upon Krakowskie Przedmiescie 30. Henryk and Stefan are bigger and more civilized now: one boy scrapes away on the cello for Pan Karol, his brother plays a piano piece. We trade family news. I try to remember how many grandchildren I have accumulated. The youngest Woźniakowski, Jan, is studying at Harvard Divinity School, bemused that the primary topics of discussion for American seminarians are abortion and homosexuality. Jacek is still trapped as mayor of Kraków. This shows his city's respect for a man of honor, but he was not prepared for the daily: "Prosze, boss, the bus drivers are out on strike, the sewage plant has broken down, the level of sulfur dioxide has just gone 500% over the international maximum—what'll we do?"

The political system in both Poland and Russia is in disarray. Mazowiecki, the liberal Catholic intellectual who speaks for my friends' class, seems unable to strike a balance between inflation and unemployment, beleaguered not only by lack of discipline and deepening distrust of the democratic process, but by lack of interest. A lot of political parties have mushroomed— one for beer drinkers—but the Polish cynicism towards authority, even their love of ironic jokes, which helped keep the Communist rule a bit less inhuman (I'll hear the same complaint in Czechoslovakia), stops them from any positive habits of citizenship. Gorbachev, who once offered the hope of civilizing the Russian monster, has lost control. What will happen to Poland if that system explodes or implodes? Yes, he has admitted that the Russians were the murderers at Katyn, but why did it take him so long?

I cannot present much evidence of America's superiority. George Bush, helped along by Saddam Hussein's arrogance, distracted Americans from other matters that he could not manage effectively by bringing his people into and out of a well-run little war, but I am tired of comparing my countrymen with the Germans who cheered on Hitler when he was beating Poland and all the other easy countries. In 1939 the Germans lost one man killed for every—how many?—twenty, thirty Poles. In 1990 the Quakers estimate that the Americans lost one man for every thousand Iraqis, including children dead from disease and hunger. That's pretty good. Bush took care that Americans saw no close-up pictures of Iraqi dead, as Hitler took care that Germans saw no pictures of the corpses at Auschwitz.

My holiday treat is a morning walk to the Stare Miasto. The eye refreshes itself with the small scale, the craftsmanship, ignored or forgotten elsewhere. Once again I come across the lintel with Anna Grocholska's three doves, carved in her early days at restoration. In 1945 everything here was rubble as it was everywhere else, but eventually these 'old' buildings became inhabited by Party members with impeccable connections. Are they kept in such good shape in order to attract Swedes and Germans? It doesn't matter. Many of the buildings around the Rynek have been newly repainted. There are display boards for drawings and watercolors of façades, horses, nudes, aged mountaineers, peasant girls. Some are nice enough for Christmas presents, others schlock, but a way, again, to earn hard currency.

Passing by a church on my way back, I see some new things. On the steps a young woman holds two little children and a sign, "I have no place to live." Next to her sits a man with no legs and a sign that he had fought in the Powstanie. At the edge of the steps, another young woman, head down, a large cardboard in Polish and English against her knees: "I have AIDS. I have lost my job. My family have pushed me out of my apartment and taken my child. I don't know what to do. Please help me."

One is caught short. You poor woman. You poor, poor woman. What else, besides some money? Even that is confused: a note for 10,000 złoty, which ought to be significant, is worth less than a dollar.

Poland, even under Bierut, never suffered Stalin's terrible purges of the mid-thirties and the last years before his death. A Moscow intellectual frequents the café where he used to meet X and Y. One day they don't show up.

There is no need to ask why. Arresting the innocent was a neat way to keep everyone terrified. AIDS has become something like that. (And, given the poor hygienic standards of Polish hospitals and the new interest in drugs, it is going to spread fast.) Another comparison: the police state's metaphor is the 4 A.M. knock on the door. It is done loudly so that every person in the entire building hears. In America, during this stage of the business cycle, our equivalent is the pink slip, without warning, in the weekly pay envelope. The man or woman who receives this is totally alone. It might be catching, like attention by the police.

November 1991

This time by Swissair through Zurich, two hours at the airport, with no time to walk along the Limmat, look at the swans and visit the Herrenmunster, its carved Bible scenes on the front door with Mrs. Potiphar making a pass at Joseph. The souvenir shops are too expensive for anything more than chocolate bars for Anna's boys and her brother Henryk's girls.

"Polish shops are full now. All you need is money."

Warsaw has become famous as one of Europe's crime centers. Because I don't believe in credit cards, my raincoat has a lining of $5 bills and I hold it close to me as I walk along the black waste of Krakowskie Przedmiescie. A block away from the *Europejski* is the new Mercedes boutique. For 500,000,000 złoty (about $45,000) you can buy an upscale model. Correct Americans despise any man driving such a car: he needs therapy to free himself from such ego-enhancement dependency. In Poland it is only an embezzler, smuggler, gangster, or totally dishonest cabinet minister who flaunts his wealth this way. How many weeks will he drive it before some idealist throws a brick through the windshield?

At a corner of the window is an even more provocative display: a bright red mini-Mercedes, behind it the picture of a nine-year-old in a tuxedo opening the door for his girlfriend in evening dress, an ermine wrap carelessly thrown around her shoulders. Together they will safely tool around the estate.

Next door is a bookstore I always visit. Even in the strictest times, the bookstores of Warsaw and Prague were colorful. A new fashion is military history, in the Communist days as off limits as pornography: undressed females and cavalry charges, the rewards of freedom. Polish history is an archipelago of battles, and it is always possible to dig up an uncle who fought against the Turks or the Swedes, a scythe-carrying peasant under Kosciuszko who fell upon the Russians at Raclawice in 1794, or rode with Colonel Grocholski to the gates of Kiev in 1920, all the way back to Grünwald in 1410 when we beat the Teutonic Knights. Our soldiers always fight courageously, but as the war winds down usually seem to be on the losing side. The battles exist as if they are fought for their own sake.

On the Italian front the capture of Monte Cassino (May 1944) was probably the bravest episode of that whole campaign, but with the Americans and British moving north from Anzio, the Germans would have been forced to abandon the monastery ruins anyway. The Polish assault and its terrible losses were not really necessary.

Napoleon made a practice of using Polish soldiers as cannon fodder in Italy, Germany, Spain and Russia. (It was in Lombardy in 1797, that the legionaries under General Dąbrowski first sang 'Jeszcze Polska nie zginęła, poki my zyjemy' (Poland is not yet lost while we still live), which, with its poignant adverbs, became the national anthem. Doing Napoleon's chores went so far as serving in Haiti, 1802-1803, to put down rebellion of the blacks, in the course of which most of the Poles died of yellow fever and dysentery.

I used to teach the *Iliad* in my tenth grade Bible class. Homer was a prisoner too of this lethal esthetic, the well-made spear, the rattling chariots—but his realism stops all foolishness: the dead are of more interest to the vultures than to their gentle wives.

"The brutal rock shattered the sinews and bones of his leg and the Trojan ran up and struck him by the navel with his spear. His entrails poured out on the ground and he dropped to his knees with a scream."

The current situation is too confused and directionless, filled with spite and betrayal, to talk about much at the apartment. Mazowiecki has been replaced by someone with even less authority. Who knows what set of values Lech Wałęsa believes in as president? (Who knows what values George Bush believes in?) Karl Marx shares part of the blame. He had such contempt for anyone who disagreed with him that Lenin and Stalin and the rest of the gang felt justified in not tolerating any form of opposition. Anyone who held a different point of view was either an idiot or an agent of the CIA. This removed any legitimate way of choosing new leadership so that by the 1980s Communism—world-wide—was managed by a brittle, irritable, luxury-loving gerontocracy.

Polish authorities have taken the gamble of making the złoty freely convertible, which leads to this year's anecdote. A Russian worker is hired by the state to replace Silesian miners on strike. He is paid two-thirds of the Polish wage—not very much—but Russians, shiftless at home, make excellent workers abroad. Eventually he ends up in Warsaw, exchanges his złoty, minus a hefty fee, into dollars that he takes back to Minsk and resells at 1000% profit. Have your Economics 101 class write an essay on who pays the bill.

Better, of course, than the medieval commerce of a truckload of Russian eggs swapped for a truckload of Polish cosmetics.

"Can you imagine what a truckload of eggs would be like after going over Russian roads in winter?"

"Well, our cosmetics aren't very good either."

My Boston travel bureau's voucher for Kraków does not look convincing so I trudge over to the main railway station (dworzec centralny) to verify it. This takes me past the gross conceit of the Palace of Science and Culture, still there, but the vast empty space in front has been turned into a scrub forest of shacks and stands, rather like the Mercado Oriental in Managua, selling every sort of tacky merchandise, a memorial park for socialism. The sellers, I am told, are mainly Romanians and gypsies, who have come to Poland as a sort of bargain-basement land of opportunity.

The Polish railways are well run, but is this flimsy piece of paper valid? I ask a clerk, who yells at me. When I show that I don't understand she yells louder. The underclass at the station are thin, worn Romanian women with baskets of trinkets and dry rolls. A little boy holds up a hand-lettered cardboard: "We are hungry. Please give me złoty so my mother can buy bread." I am so rattled by the ticket clerk that I bark at him, for which I am immediately sorry.

"We Poles are not heartless," someone explains later. "There are places run by the church or the city where these people can find a place to sleep, take a shower, get a hot meal, but after Ceaușescu the Romanians are so terrified of any form of authority that they prefer to sleep in a corner of the station and beg. And no gypsy man will ever take on any sort of work. They drink and play cards."

The women and children offer an even sharper measurement on the Mercedes boutique. Freedom = capitalism or, you might say, capitalism = freedom.

A former student of mine writes from Paris that she met a black Peace Corps volunteer who said that all blacks in the Corps have been removed from Poland after one of them had been beaten up by a gang of skinheads. In the town where he taught, old women crossed themselves when they passed him. Black people are children of the Devil.

On a building near the railway station is a small stencil of a cross superimposed upon a star of David, above a message: Christ was also a Jew. It is worth being reminded.

Lublin 1960, 1985

"Whither the battle?"—and the young men arm.
The women pray, "God is Napoleon's shield,
Napoleon ours," as to the outcome calm.
Spring well remembered! Happy who saw thee then
Spring of the war, spring of the mighty yield,
That promised corn but ripened into men!
Phantom of dreams where still you stand revealed,
In slavery born and weaned to chains, I see,
And shall in life, no spring to equal thee.
Adam Mickiewicz *The Year 1812*

You were the peacock and the parrot of nations.
Juliusz Slowacki

LUBLIN WAS A FRONTIER town. To its west, no matter the lack of any order in Polish society, the irresponsible egoism of its nobility, the desperate poverty of its peasants, existed a flavor of Europe. Towns, however weak, were marked by the towers of church and ratusz. To its east stretched the featureless plains of the Ukraine—no boundaries, no limits. Armies mounted on horses were fueled by the grass under their hooves. Not all the invaders were as self-sufficient as the thirteenth-century Mongols, who nourished themselves by opening their horses' veins and drinking their blood, but the plains would lead to the obsession of going farther and farther, without rational limit. Lublin was a goal for the Cossack armies of Chmielnicki in 1647 and the Turks in 1680, and from the opposite direction for the Swedes in 1655 and 1709. Napoleon's army of 1812, with its Polish soldiers, marched east out of Lithuania, way to the north, but the Germans in 1917 and 1941 saw Lublin as a gateway to the Ukraine, with its wheat fields and oil fields that would make Germany independent of history. Piłsudski's cavalry (with Colonel Grocholski) in 1920 claimed that Kiev was a Polish city and for a moment became addicts again of Destiny, which promised them the lands from the Baltic to the Black Sea, from Wilno to Odessa, a sphere of influence, indeed, from Finland to the Caucasus.* The Soviets had launched that war in 1919 to pursue their own fantasy: to break through a boneless Poland and join up with a revolutionary Germany in order to form the Communist nucleus that would dominate Europe. Stalin never forgave the Poles, of any political flavor, for having frustrated this.

When Rokossovski's army was rapidly moving West in the summer of 1944, Lublin became the site of the first 'independent' Polish 'government,' under the Soviets, rival to the exile government in London.

The lack of limits reminds one of the Vikings whose ships ranged from Greenland to Constantinople. Or the great plains of North America for the farmers and railroad builders. In Ole Rolvaag's tragic story of Norwegian settlers in Minnesota, *Giants in the Earth*, the heroine goes mad because nothing in that emptiness conforms to the order, the limits of fences and village and church tower with which she was raised.

Those deadly plains were caught by Henryk Sienkiewicz in his trilogy written in the 1880s, books of war against the rebellious Cossacks (*Fire and Sword*), heretical Swedes aided by the treacherous Radziwills (*The Deluge*), and cruel Turks (*Pan Michael*), though his vision was colored by memories from train trips across the American prairies. The trilogy was an epic of romantic violence, treachery, loyalty, devotion, love and death, read by every Polish schoolboy who wanted to become like wild, brainless Pan Kmicic with his turned-up moustaches 'who killed whomsoever he was ordered to kill and cared for naught else.' Boys liked to speak a secret language in the peculiar seventeenth-century Polish that Sienkiewicz's characters employed. Even the fighters of the Home Army during the German years used pseudonyms from Sienkiewicz, who eventually founded a socialist, orange-

---

* The most interesting details raised by Professor Richard Pipes out of his research in the recently opened Central Party archives in Moscow concern Piłsudski's odd pro-Bolshevik neutrality during the Russian Civil War in 1919. The leading White general, Anton Denikin, refused to recognize the frontiers of an independent republic beyond those of 1815–1830 Congress Poland, that is, the lands around Warsaw. Accordingly, even as unofficial skirmishing between Poles and Bolsheviks was sharpening in the fall of 1919, Piłsudski denied the Whites all military assistance and insisted that Denikin be crushed so that he could deal with a weak and isolated Bolshevik Russia. The Bolsheviks in turn were willing to grant the Poles just about any territorial concessions they wanted since it was—in the words of Julian Marchlewski, a Polish Communist who served as intermediary between Warsaw and Moscow—only a matter of a relatively short amount of time before all Poland became Communist. (Richard Pipes, *Russia Under the Bolshevik Regime*, Alfred A. Knopf, N. Y., 1993, p. 90)

growing colony at Anaheim, one day to become the site of Disneyland. Today Sienkiewicz's reputation is finished in his homeland. His novels are not for girls and few boys in Poland read anything now.

Lublin became wealthy in the sixteenth century, a sort of Dodge City or Omaha, as a transshipment center for the horse-drawn wheat from the Ukraine loaded onto rafts floating down the Vistula past Warsaw to Danzig and thence across the Baltic to Western Europe. It was less a town of the *Szlachta*, however, (but which included pennilesss, proud hidalgos, forefathers of the peasants who had saved a wounded Jacek Woźniakowski from being captured and tortured to death by Ukrainians) the land-owning gentry who were Poland's ruling class, than of the magnates who owned vast estates to the East administered from their fortress-like manor houses. One sees a likeness to the ranches of Texas or northern Mexico, also fortresses with thick adobe walls against Comanches, Apaches, Yaquis, bandidos, marauding revolutionary armies ready to kill the Chinese storekeepers just as the Cossacks killed Jews. The manor-house garrisons were officered by the gentry who had lost their own property through any combination of drink, gambling, mismanagement, or misfortune, a warrior caste similar to the samurai of feudal Japan.

Each manor house also had a Jesuit priest. During the sixteenth century, when the rest of Europe was butchering itself in religious hatred, Poland had a reputation for tolerance, but the Counter-Reformation, led by the Jesuits, had introduced a new rigidity. The enemies whom gentry and Magnates fought from one end of Poland to the other belonged to other religions: Lutherans, Orthodox, Moslems, in the Ukraine Uniates—Russian Orthodox, more or less, in liturgy, but accepting, more or less, the authority of the pope in Rome. The Jesuits tried to enforce a more formal Polish Catholicism (one is reminded of the later straight-from-Moscow Commissars who tried to discipline their own parishioners), whose pressure for religious correctness helped provoke the great Cossack revolt of Chmielnicki in 1648.

This mixed ruling class of Szlachta and magnates that dominated Lublin formed the irrational republic (*Rzeszpospolita*) of Poland. It might be termed the most democratic state of Europe because that class was so large and unchecked, most of the time, by the monarch, whom it elected. With its rule of unanimity for every law passed and even for its very duration, the parliament (*Sejm*) stressed the sacred freedom and equality of each member. The lack of royal authority left real authority in the hands of the great magnate families, and the desire of its foreign neighbors to keep Poland weak encouraged them to bribe gentry members—not difficult—to disrupt any decision. As a result, democracy came to equal self-indulgent, aristocratic anarchy and an increasingly paralyzed government to be divided among Russia, Prussia and Austria in the partitions of 1772, 1792 and 1795, when the Polish state disappeared entirely until November 11, 1918, to reappear under Piłsudski.

Jean-Jacques Rousseau was intrigued by the democratic imaginativeness of Polish political assumptions, and since he was a major figure in Jefferson's thinking, it was possible for Szlachta intellectuals, unfettered by Protestant pettiness about facts, to claim that the American constitution was based on Polish models.

In the summer of 1960 my wife and I drove to Lublin from Warsaw, glad to be free, and in 'real' Poland, through villages each with its own duck pond. No pigs. What had happened to the national animal? (Rationalized by the Communists into factories, fed by conveyor belts, the methane from their manure powering some giant steelworks?) We made a picnic lunch on a willow-shaded embankment of the Vistula. A barefoot girl with a small herd of geese, straight out of a hundred nineteenth century paintings or poems composed by exiles in Siberia, came by to stare at us.

In Lublin, we stayed in the modern part of town, at a graceless hotel that one might imagine duplicated all across the Ukraine to the Urals, and from which I went to make a call on the rector of the Catholic University. KUL* was just about the only autonomous educational institution in the Communist imperium, a politic concession to the Church. Although its facilities were poorer than those at the Marie Sklodowska Curie University on the other side of town, its integrity made it a critical part of Poland's limited independence. Even if an intellectual like Jacek Woźniakowski could not be trusted to teach real history, he was permitted to teach art history, carefully, at KUL, in a way quite alien to Communist style.

～∞～

The Merrill Foundation, whose capital had been provided under the terms of my father's will and of which I was chairman, had made a grant of $25,000 to KUL in 1959 through Catholic Relief Services. The money supplied hard currency for student and faculty study in the West and for the purchase of books and scientific equipment. The Ford Foundation had exploited the momentary thaw in Communist control during the early Gomułka years to fund a generous program of fellowships in Western Europe and the United States. Although afraid of heretical ideas, the Polish government needed non-Soviet training in medicine, science and technology. Ford agreed on

* Katolicki Uniwersytet Lubelski

condition that for every two fellowships granted in those fields, a third should be in the humanities. The long-range vision of this program made it one of the finest examples of American philanthropy.

Our foundation possessed a tiny fraction of Ford's resources, and its priorities were safe institutions like Amherst College and Southampton Hospital. Nevertheless, small grants could be imaginatively targeted. My formal reason for this trip to Lublin was to obtain enough factuality to make a second grant saleable to other trustees and thereby ensure the intellectual survival of Poland.

I found the main gate and the porter's office. The rector wasn't there. Nor was the porter at all interested in helping a stupid foreigner who didn't understand anything even when it was shouted.

That ended my responsibilities. By chance Mary and I found ourselves in Złota Ulica, walking past the Renaissance elegance of its townhouses. These were the homes of merchants, or a townhouse for the landowners, as a cotton planter might build a summer house for himself in Savannah or Charleston.

The peripatetic Italian opens his book of designs.

"This is all the rage in Padova."

"Very nice, but Kieniewicz has a tower like that. I want one twice as high. And the façade painted red."

"Signor, you won't find anything like that anywhere in the Veneto!"

"And who's paying?"

What sort of people had lived there? What did they talk about? The price of grain, clouds on the horizon from Turks or Russians, impudence from Jews, from Cossacks, originally peasants who had run away from their masters and the constraints of church and village but on the lawless prairies of the Ukraine had become a separate people. Gossip from the court in Warsaw? Duels and feuds. For a few months I served in Algeria and Italy with a Texas National Guard regiment, and my colleagues enjoyed some of the same good-ole-boy gladhandedness that in a moment could turn into lethal rage. Love of extravagance and ceremony, pickled cucumbers and shouting. In 1683 nobles like these had ridden across the Carpathians under King Jan Sobieski to rescue Vienna from the Turks and returned home with oriental carpets, tastes for coffee and shaven heads, infatuation with profitless military adventure.

What did a woman do? Prayers, embroidery, giving orders to the servants, playing the lute, attending mass? Suppose she was burdened with intelligence?

From this Renaissance street we wandered into the old town of winding alleys that had grown in vegetative style since medieval times. In 1952 we had lived in a somewhat similar city, Graz, the most southeastern German-speaking city of the Austrian empire. Hungary lay to the East, the Slovene and Croat plains to the South. I was a Fulbright exchange teacher at the local gymnasium in a city known for its National Socialist sympathizers threatened by those lesser peoples. Our own home was a cardboard apartment house beyond Conrad von Hötzendorfstrasse hardly superior to Polish models, and the narrow streets wandering around the Hauptplatz held smells—cabbage, drains, underwear, beer, tobacco—close to those of Lublin. One can sense the claustrophobia that must have made those sunless streets prison corridors, the sound of coughing and children with bandages over their running ears.

Lublin, of course, had sheltered an intense Jewish life possessed by no German-speaking city. The dailiness of that God-covenanted culture, the unscholarly piety of its humble people are memorialized by Isaac Bashevis Singer: 'chicken soup with noodles and tiny circlets of fat like golden ducats' as if even soup can enter holiness, and the imps and devils, ghosts and spirits that seemed to arise out of the bottomless studies of Yeshiva.*

Messiah did not come for the Jews so the Jews went to Messiah.
Isaac Bashevis Singer *The Last Demon*

It wasn't until 1985 that I returned. Lublin was an adventurous distance from the two cities that I always visited, Warsaw and Kraków, at the eastern border to which no one cared to travel, where no inhabitant spoke a word of any foreign language besides Russian. If you were fascinated by the idiosyncrasies of Poland, as I was, they existed there, undiluted.

Poland doesn't motivate Significant People to make the journey. The phones don't work. There are greasy thumbprints on the spoons. Horrid fantasies keep the timid away: rumors about the toilets, being expected to say *przystrzyc* upon entering a barber shop, being robbed by gypsies, arrested by the secret police, assaulted by drunks. But if you don't expect too much, don't insist on plastic interchangeability with the total society managed on contract by Holiday Inns, then things function well enough. You are rewarded by courtesy, a straightforward unpretentiousness, a humorous realism in facing up to life's disappointments.

* Cynthia Ozick, *Art and Order*, E.P. Dutton, N.Y., 1984, p. 221.

In Warsaw you can move along an archipelago where English is used (add on German if you know it; French is spoken by middle-aged ladies), by most young people with any claims to education or ambition, by anyone acquainted with the mechanics of survival in the late twentieth century. Or the foreigner can try to build some structure of his own in the language.

Before each visit I try to make, *this time*, a solid effort to learn the language, moderately successful at my desk in Boston, less so in Warsaw where the edifice is smashed by a confrontation with a railway clerk or erodes from fatigue. Like a chair put together by an unskilled carpenter, not very pretty or well made, it can be sat on, and it is his own. A faithful set of nouns and adjectives, some expressions, have stood by me, led by a few verbs, though the latter are apt to desert under pressure. Unreliable little prepositions come and go. 'Twelve' and 'twenty' play games with each other. Scraps of Russian and Czech amuse children and either amplify a dialogue or confuse it.

In Warsaw this time I'd been lodging, for some reason, at the *Viktoria* rather than the *Europejski*, where Bruce Barton and I had stayed in 1939. It was new, classy, expensive, with shiny marble floors, a Tuzex store for foreign luxuries in dollars, fax machines, elegant prostitutes with long lynx scarves.

A phone call awakened me at 1 A.M. Panic.

"I am so sorry if I have disturbed you at this hour," said a silky, not-too-young voice. "Would you care for any feminine companionship?"

"Hell no!"

"You prefer boys, handsome young men?" asked the now less silky voice. I slammed down the receiver.

Always the Bostonian, I complained next morning to the concierge.

"We are so terribly sorry, sir. You must know that such adventuresses unfortunately exist."

"Nonsense," said the friends on Krakowskie Przedmiescie. "They hand out the names of all English and German-speaking guests to those women, then take a cut. They're quite expensive. One of our exports."

I drove my Avis car across the river through the marketplace suburb of Praga, where General Suvorov massacred the inhabitants in 1795 and where the Red Army camped as spectators during the liquidation of the Powstanie in 1944, where I took the road southeast. It was the day after All Hallow's Eve, and the cemeteries were still washed by flickering waves of light from candles in their glass lanterns. The road bordered the Vistula, past poplars and willows hung with mistletoe, past signs recounting where the Red Army had heroically forced a crossing despite intense fire from the Hitlerite Fascists. A stop at Kazimierż Dolny, a gem of Mannerist architecture from the seventeenth century, carved reliefs of saints and fantastic animals, cardinals and flowers as if squeezed out of a pastry tube, now visited by an aimless group of French-speaking Africans.

Then into Lublin where I found an adequate hotel with a large number of tall dark young men in blue uniforms speaking Arabic, who turned out to be Iraqi air cadets. The next morning a return to Złota Ulica. In just 25 years, however, its Renaissance elegance had turned shabby and decayed. Scaffolding lined the row of façades, but on a Monday morning not a workman in sight.

"Easy," Jacek explained later in Kraków, "the contractor has good Party connections. He receives an allotment of tools, plaster, timber, nails from the state and sells them on the black market. Nothing can be done till he receives his next allotment, which, if someone keeps checking on him, he'll use just enough in actual construction so that he isn't put in jail."

I took off for Zamość, one of my formal goals, maybe 30 miles southeast of Lublin where a Texan personality named Jan Zamoyski had stamped his foot on the ground in 1578 and commanded a city to be built here, now, and named after him. He hired an architect and town planner, Bernardo Morando from Padua. Kraków, Lublin, Lwów attracted many Italian and Italian-trained architects. The anarchic formlessness of those plains made me treasure even more the harmony of the square and its arcaded houses, the graceful ratusz with its tower and double staircase.

"Zamość was the first town in Poland and one of the first of a rare few in Europe which was planned and laid out not only in terms of function but as a work of art. It gave shape to the ideas formulated in the Italian Renaissance, among them the theoretical concept of the 'ideal town.' . . . Zamoyski was a man of great enterprise, energy and culture as well as a profound knowledge of the humanities gained in Italy. The town was to be not only the principal center of his latifundia, but the capital of an area that he regarded as his personal kingdom: a hub of commerce, a mighty fortress against the invaders from the East, a cultural and religious center, and the great man's seat and residence."[*]

Zamoyski founded an academy for the training of citizen nobles. Unlike the Jesuits' rigidly uniform program, it offered both classic and contemporary education, more secular and patriotic, which attracted the sons of prominent families, from a variety of ethnic and even religious backgrounds.[†]

[*] Michael Pratt and Gerhard Trumler, *Great Country Houses of Central Europe*, Abbeville Press, N. Y., 1991, pp. 223–224.

[†] Frank Sysyn, *Between Poland and the Ukraine*, Harvard University Press, Cambridge, 1985, pp. 47–49.

The city stood on the stylistic borderline between Renaissance and Baroque. Plans for a synagogue, library, arsenal, public baths, sophisticated sewage construction system were worked over all during the seventeenth century, but as the Counter-Reformation tightened, society became less tolerant under Jesuit pressure and thought ossified.

Until 1939 a Count Jan Zamoyski still owned 60,000 hectares (150,000 acres) of land around Zamość, confiscated by the Communists in 1946. In 1993 he is a senator and a leading member of the Society of Industrialists, who demand the restoration of their property and indemnities for their losses.

On the façade of a modest house in one corner of the rynek is a marker stating that it was the birthplace of Rosa Luxemburg in 1870. She was the revolutionary who with her partner Karl Liebknecht refused, unlike all the other timid German socialists, to support the Kaiser's war, was imprisoned, and then in 1919 murdered by army officers. Having lived in a house with such a view across the square to that beautiful town hall, she should have been glad to remain there as a contented housewife?

Big History washed over Zamość late in August 1914 as the Russian and Austrian armies collided with each other, and there was heavy, disconnected cavalry fighting in the woods and fields southeast of the town.*

Zamość was always an important Jewish center, the first settlers coming from Lwów in the 1580s, followed by other Sephardim from Turkey, Italy, and Holland. In 1939, 45% of the population was Jewish; under the Germans the city was briefly renamed Himmlerstadt.

My next stop was even further south and east, to the village of Tyszowce, only a few kilometers from the Russian border. The grandparents of one of my school's Jewish students had come from this village. Perhaps it might be placed into my great album of Polish memories. There were old, white-washed wooden houses with thatched roofs and progressive ones of brick with tile roofs. The main street was tied up in a traffic jam where a dugout-shaped horse-drawn manure cart blocked a tractor pulling a trailer of sugar beets.

---

* World War I material on Zamość and Przemysl comes from Winston Churchill's *The Unknown War, the Eastern Front*, Thornton Butterworth, London, 1931. This history, one of Churchill's earliest, shows his ability to control a vastly complicated subject while giving a sense of the chaotic drama as well as the intellect and character of the figures who were trying to accomplish something. Note: more men were killed in the first six weeks of war in 1914 than in the almost twenty-two months, 1939–1941, from the German invasion of Poland until their invasion of Russia.

In the villages on the other side of the Soviet border, Polish until the whole country was shoved westward in 1945, the churches had been torn down to make room for parking lots or converted into warehouses, leaving an emptiness that ached like a missing limb. On Sundays when the wind blew from the West, the villagers could hear the faint sound of church bells from Poland.

⟨∞⟩

Here was an older Poland, of long fields, with willow and oak trees, a clean spare landscape as I drive south to the Beskids, the eastern end of the Tatry, now across the old Austrian border into eastern Galicia, the scene of chaotic fighting in 1914 and 1915 around the great fortress city of Przemysl, base and depot of all Austrian armies. Churchill has a high respect for the Austrian commander-in-chief, Conrad von Hötzendorf, who made Przemysl his headquarters. He was a brilliant strategist but demanded more from his hodgepodge army than its confused, poorly equipped and poorly officered, exhausted, demoralized men could deliver. The fortress itself ran out of supplies and surrendered to the Russians in March 1915 with the loss of 100,000 prisoners and 1000 guns. Had it served a purpose in slowing down the enemy offensives or had its protection cost the Austrians far more than it was ever worth?

I spend the night at a hostel, perhaps church owned, beside the great ruined castle of Krasiczyn. How wealthy were those great magnates like Marcin Krasicki who could construct such piles, how weak the king, what low wages could be paid the workmen!

I stop for lunch at Biecz. It possesses a powerful fifteenth-century church and an imposing ratusz, but the sole kawiarnia is run by an unconcerned girl who offers crackers and hot water with tea bags.

In search of some monument suggested by Jacek I trudge across Tarnow through swarms of children bursting out of school. A noisy crocodile of dwarfs stumbles by, each of them wearing bright-colored caps and mittens knitted by grandmother. A seven-year-old, wrapped up in her monologue of schoolyard politics, holds onto mother's hand. There appears a galaxy of adolescents, three girls arm in arm for security, three boys revolving about them like fighter planes or wolves (I am unsure of the analogy), vivaciously charming as the girls are obliquely responsive, with the clatter, plumage, gestures of a courtship ballet of grouse or cranes. It is, at times, a sweet land.

But beside the pleasures of wandering through southeastern Poland the serious purpose of that second visit to Lublin was to see Majdanek, as in 1993 I felt compelled to see Auschwitz. The twentieth century stands for skyscrapers, movies and television, mass bombing, the destruction of forests, concentration camps. There are new people, ignorant or cold-bloodedly evil, who deny their existence. The camps are a Jewish slander, a Zionist myth. It is worth while to make a personal visit, every ten or twenty years, to one of those camps to remind oneself that they existed.

At war's end I was typist for an interrogation team of the 88th Division at a prison camp outside Modena, in the Po Valley. We were billeted at the Palazzo Ducale along with one or two thousand survivors of Dachau, Buchenwald, Auschwitz, Mauthausen, most of them liberated by the Americans but trucked down to Italy by soldiers of the Jewish Brigade (originally of the British 8th Army) who had hoped to get them onto ships bound for Haifa or Tel Aviv before the British established a blockade of Palestine. Modena was as far south as they reached.

One of the boys who ran out from the palace to carry our bags in return for chocolate was a thirteen-year-old Hungarian named Bernat. I was impressed by his spirit, we became friends, and in the evenings (I saved food from my supper rations) we used to walk around Modena and in our poor German talk about his life and mine.

Bernat and his family (his father a carpenter and a wholesale nuts-and-honey dealer, his mother the daughter of a rabbi) lived in a village named Tab, just east of Lake Balaton. The Jews and Hungarians got along badly, and each afternoon as he ran home from school Bernat was involved in a fight. Nevertheless, though an ally of Germany, Hungary was proud to be an independent nation. It might mistreat these Jews but it also protected them, the only country on the continent of Europe besides Switzerland and Bulgaria that did, until the day in March 1944 when the SS took control.

The Jews of Tab were marched from their homes to the railroad station, their Hungarian neighbors closing their shutters so they would not have to see them. ("You can never trust a gentile.") Bernat's mother tried to comfort her two frightened boys: "We'll make it. We're not afraid of hard work. We'll stick together. We'll get through OK." The train moved slowly, picking up other cars from the stations it passed on the way to Budapest. There they waited for 24 hours in the railroad yards for a locomotive to take them across Slovakia to Poland. Can you imagine what an August day would be like in one of those freight cars?

What struck Bernat when the train finally halted at Auschwitz were the crowds of men running back and forth in black-and-white striped suits, like pyjamas. Wearing pyjamas at mid-day? Then the old prisoners and the new-comers got all mixed up, and he never saw his parents or his brother again.

"How old are you, kid?" a Polish boy asked in Yiddish.

"Twelve."

"They'll put you to death if they know that. Tell 'em you're 16. A lot of people here are undersized."

Bernat was put to work sorting nuts and bolts from wrecked Messer-schmidts into the proper containers. He learned about the German labor classification system: One line of newcomers was Arbeitsfähig, the other Nichtfähig. The latter—too old, too young, too sickly—were sent straight to the gas chambers, the former not for a while. A mother had screamed and fought when a guard tried to take her baby away to be carried off in that second line. The guard grabbed the baby and smashed its head against the wall.

"Now will you act rationally?"

Men and boys occupied the same barracks, under Ukrainian Kapos, who were hated more than Germans. Rich people died soon, adolescents who had grown too fast, French and Spaniards. Poles and Hungarians were tough. Then, as the Russians rolled across Poland, the Germans evacuated Auschwitz, and by train and truck shipped the prisoners to western Austria, to Mauthausen, a few kilometers west of Linz.

Years later, when Bernat had gone from living with our family in Missouri to Cornell University, and had become a lieutenant in the United States Army on his way to Harvard Law School, he showed my wife and myself around Mauthausen. Here were the barracks, over there the gas chamber and the terrible stairs up which prisoners carried heavy stones. Sometimes German guards at the top would knock over the prisoners and laugh to see them tumble down the stairs. Around the camp grounds were monuments to Soviet citizens, Yugoslavs, Poles, French, even Americans and Australians, who had perished here, but not a word about Jews. For the Communists they did not exist.

What was peculiar about Majdanek was not simply the source of its prisoners, humble Jews from Grodno, Kishinev, Czernowitz, Lwów, Košice. Nor its statistics: in one week in October 1943, 45,000 survivors of the Warsaw ghetto were murdered there, shot by machine guns, 18,000 in a single day. It was not isolated in the countryside like Mauthausen and Treblinka but rather was at the edge of a major city. The burghers of Złota Ulica could have climbed onto the roofs of their Renaissance houses and seen its guard towers. When the wind blew from the west they must have smelled the burning flesh. Did they talk about it over the dinner table?

I needed only a few minutes to drive to the camp from my hotel. A huge, deliberately hideous slab of cement—a spread of broken teeth—marked the gate. In the icy twilight I walked down a lane between two double walls of barbed wire, fixed to their posts on porcelain knobs to show they had been electrified. A few dark brown wooden barracks were still standing. At the end of the lane was a muffin-shaped concrete structure where the gas chambers or crematoria,* I forget which, had stood. Again there were tablets to the Polish, Romanian, Soviet victims, no mention of the forbidden word.

What to say? Gypsies protest that the Jews never mention those who died wearing a black triangle with Z (Zigeuner) on it. There are no monuments to homosexuals. A militant like Malcolm X made a point of insisting that more Africans died on the slave ships than Jews did in these camps.

There was a marriage between Jews and Poles that lasted 600 years, not a very happy one, but one where both parties absorbed far more from the other than either cared to admit. Then, after about six years, almost nothing remained. In 1939 the Jewish population had been about three million, about 10% of prewar Poland. That is just about the percentage of blacks in our country. Now it is less than 0.1%—most of them over 60, though there are voices pointing to a new revival among young people.

In a hotel room at night, a smoke of thought drifts by. The Japanese conquer America—our high school products are too poorly educated and undisciplined to make good soldiers. The victors want space for their settlers and so start rounding up blacks and sending them off to relocation centers in Montana and Idaho—a few empty camps from 1942 recycled. These 'relocatees' are street-corner idlers, rap musicians, addicts, convicts, welfare mothers and will be taught—the new authorities promise—computer technology and wholesome calisthenics. They will soon return to their communities much improved in body and mind, but let nobody be deluded by Japanese courtesy: anyone who interferes with the process will be shot. After a while, when other people are occupied with other things, the prisoners are put to death. The camps refill with new groups.

* Paul Celan, "from which the victims are given a grave in the air."

How violent would the protests be? The Japanese have taken many hostages and possess a monopoly of weapons. It would be harder to shelter a black child than a Jewish child with brown hair whose name was changed from Sarah to Olga. Harlem, Detroit, South Central Los Angeles are being rebuilt with attractive new housing and sushi restaurants. Tchula, Mississippi, is bulldozed to leave foundations for a high-tech optics factory. Less crime, better schools, lower welfare costs. At cocktail parties, someone is almost always sure to start off: "You've got to hand it to the Japs—"

But it isn't only the music, and the faces you remember. It was the way they walked, and dressed, their laughter, the rhythms and vitality of their voices, the smells of their food. Even the explosions of anger gave intensity and some extra sharpness to life. There is less flavor to the days. People aren't happier or less afraid.

Enough of that.

∾

I was looking through a large picture book of the Holocaust wondering whether to purchase it for our school library; I found a horrible photograph of a column of naked women being marched to a gas chamber somewhere. Worse to me, however, was the picture of a group of middle-class Dutch Jews at a railroad station in Amsterdam waiting for a train to take them to some collection point for transferral to another train that would transport them, although they did not know it yet, to Poland. In their travel tweeds, with their solid suitcases, the middle-aged women looked like my mother, waiting for her train to Long Island or Palm Beach. The horror, worse than that of the naked women marching through the mud who knew that they were at the edge of death, that if God existed they would find out within ten minutes, was the ignorance. After all, Germany was a proper country they had visited many times.

What secret delight for the guards who could savor, bit by bit, revealing the truth: demanding a watch or a necklace, snickering when someone asked about lunch, a quick paw at the chest of a younger woman; the changing of expression, the cries, the begging for mercy when each person realized they were heading to some place where there might not be even soap or toilet paper. What was left of that tweed-clad self-respect when the train arrived in Poland?

> The children cried 'Mummy!'
> But I have been good!
> It's dark in here! Dark!
> Tadeusz Różewicz *Massacre of the Boys*

She's got a wardrobe from which
the dresses managed to escape
they would have gone out of style anyway
   an armchair from which
   somebody once got up
   just for a moment
   that lasted the rest of his life
pots and pans full of hunger
but handy when
you want to eat your fill
   portrait of a murdered girl
   in living color
she could also have gotten a black table
good condition
but she didn't like its looks
   sad somehow.
   Jerzy Ficowski *Ex-Jewish Things*

Ignorance about those who have disappeared undermines the reality of
   the world.
   Zbigniew Herbert *Mr. Cogito on the Need for Precision*

12

Kraków 1939, 1960, 1964, 1968, 1978

In your eyes, Europe, we are history's reservation
with our dated ideals
with our dusted-off treasure box
with the songs we sing
We give up our best
for the dragon of force and violence to devour
the young boys the beautiful girls
the best minds the most auspicious talents
. . . .
    Julia Hartwig *In Your Eyes*

It is more difficult to live honestly through one day than to write a book.
    Adam Mickiewicz

THE GERMANS MOVED EAST so rapidly in 1939, west so rapidly in 1945 that Kraków escaped the fighting that devastated so many Polish cities. Its most painful loss fitted its intellectual distinction. As told by Waclaw Lednicki, who taught me Pushkin at Harvard in 1941 (though the poet he really wanted to discuss was Mickiewicz, the Russian's moral superior), after the city had fallen to the Wehrmacht that first week in September, the military governor announced that even if the Polish state had vanished, the nation remained. Germans and Poles might still understand and respect each other. A sign of this would be the reopening of Jagiellon University, the oldest in Central Europe, now under German protection and encouragement. The faculty, which had scattered in all directions, would be invited back, students again enrolled, and the university would take its rightful place in the construction of a new Poland.

Most of the faculty did return later that fall and gathered in the great lecture hall to hear the welcoming address by the new chancellor. Then the doors opened to admit German soldiers who rounded up the disoriented academics, and loaded them onto trucks that took them to a camp, perhaps Sachsenhausen, where most of them died in the course of the winter.

When Germans insisted that Poles had no culture, sooner or later they were proved right.

⟨∞⟩

Who were the Germans, the people, for a while, who were at the center of our every thought? In Italy, American soldiers—too many for my taste—were apt to respect them more than they did the British, certainly the Italians, for their discipline, tenacity, manliness, and as a nose-thumb at military authority.

Nevertheless.

In mid-summer 1945 I served with the 88th Division around Verona in processing the repatriation of prisoners—farmers and construction workers as first priority—plus a half-hearted effort to uncover possible war criminals. Our unit was billeted in a farmhouse which had been occupied earlier by German soldiers. Across one wall of the kitchen an artist had painted a nostalgic landscape of *die Heimat*—fields and wild flowers, a stream, cows, village rooftops, mountains—what he and his comrades were trying to protect against Asiatic Communists and against Us with our tanks and bombing planes, our Negroes and Jews.

In a corner of the kitchen stood a well-made whip: a carved wooden stock two feet long, four or five leather thongs the same length, knotted. It hadn't been made for animals. A strong man could have torn apart the back of anyone—who?—he was whipping with those knotted leather thongs. The whip with the pretty landscape, side by side, was not bearable, and we broke it up and threw the pieces outside.

And, in a later war, who were the Americans? On March 16, 1968, a company of soldiers belonging to the Americal Division landed by helicopter at the village of My Lai in Quang Nai province, with orders, one man later stated at a court martial, to kill everything that breathed, and over a period of four hours shot chickens, dogs, cattle, and perhaps 350 Vietnamese men, women and children. Only a handful of soldiers faced any legal proceedings on this. Lieutenant William Calley, who had personally killed 22 civilians, was sentenced to life imprisonment, shortened to four and a half months. He became something of a popular hero to patriotic Americans and had a jukebox tune dedicated to him, a faithful soldier.

The author of this story in the May 2, 1994 *New York Times Sunday Magazine*, Tim O'Brien, also a Vietnam veteran, concludes that evil has no place in our national mythology. A military judicial system treats murderers and common soldiers as pretty much one and the same. America declares itself innocent—it is no big deal.

When Bruce and I headed south from Warsaw, in the last days of July, 1939, I gave up my earlier plan of visiting Łódź, the great Jewish textile city I had read about in Israel Singer's epic *Brothers Ashkenazi*. We did stop at Częstochowa, to make a pilgrimage to the great fortress-monastery of Jasna Gora and its shrine of the Black Madonna. The heroic defense against the Swedes in 1655 formed the climax of Sienkiewicz's *Deluge*, which I had read the previous summer as a 35-cents-an-hour grocery clerk in Bozeman, Montana. With generations of young Poles, I stood upon the battlements shouting defiance at the brutal invaders and their treacherous running dogs, the Radziwills.*

We stayed at the *Francuski*, the most elegant hotel of Austrian Poland in 1907, across from the medieval walls of the barbican. I know we walked around the main square and paid a visit to St. Mary's church and listened to the trumpeter whose call each hour from its tower ends on a half note because a Tatar arrow pierced his throat in 1241. We were moving across Europe so fast, however, that only a couple of pictures remain. One is of a picket of cavalrymen, white and red pennons on their lances, escorting an anti-tank gun the size of a sewing machine. The other is of the crowded streets in the Jewish quarter of Kasimierz, the boys our age with earlocks and the middle-aged housewives with red wigs.

The smoke of Nowa Huta floats over the town like the flags of victory.
  1950s slogan

With Mary I visited Kraków again in 1960, when we called upon the Woźniakowski apartment on ulica Wyspianskiego. The tired post-war look of household things reminded her of our stay in Vienna and Graz in 1951–1952 when that past had been so close.

Jacek and Maja and their family were essentially my Kraków, and seeing their children grow up, and then the grandchildren, within the irregular frames of my visits, was my way of measuring time.

One could accept Warsaw, like Berlin, as the capital of a police state. Its spirit-dimming public buildings of underwear-gray, like Moscow's, had been erected to ensure total control, with the jerry-built apartment houses designed for secret microphones. As with Prague, however, it was hard to envision Kraków as part of that system.

* On a stay at Harvard as a Niemann Fellow in 1957, Jacek Woźniakowski warned me that Jack Kennedy would be our next president. A Radziwill had married into the family, and the Radziwills always picked the winning side.

Like Prague also it was a sort of architectural palimpsest, with Renaissance structures added on to Gothic, later flavored with monuments of the Baroque and the nineteenth century. The great Wawel complex, castle and cathedral, at the edge of the city, dated back to St. Stanisław, slain before the altar by King Boleslaw in 1079. The castle was built around a courtyard whose arcaded porches were obviously designed by a Florentine. On one of Kraków's November days, one can imagine a homesick Italian princess, shivering despite her sable jacket, listening to the rain's long tedious lecture, wondering whether the sun will ever shine again. The Wawel and Kraków itself decayed in an eighteenth century dominated by the Church and the rural gentry, the burgher class less and less important. After 1846 the castle became an Austrian barracks and military hospital. Bored and drunken soldiers would break this or that. A surprise that anything is left.

My favorite backdrop of the Kraków stage are the dirty gray apartment houses, destroyed in Warsaw, put up from the 1870s and 1880s until 1914, part of the middle-class domination of the world, from Chicago and Buenos Aires to Manchester, Brussels, Hamburg, and Kraków, supported by cigars and Oriental rugs, faithful servants, newspapers, soap, roast animal for Sunday, sewer pipes and street lights, railways, heart attacks (replacing smallpox), brown velvet curtains, noisy arguments between father and son, opera, street cars, corsets, politicians, policemen, German and business for the men, French and refinement for their wives.

After the collapse in 1864 of the last uprising against the Russians, there came a strong movement in favor of middle-class values, within all three separate parts of Poland, against a religious, almost mystic political romanticism of heroic conspiracy. The new railway that linked Warsaw to Vienna and Moscow was a respectable alternative to a cavalry charge. On the one hand was the threat of Polish being replaced by Russian in the schools and law courts, on the other, opportunity in the rapid industrialization of central Poland best seen in the surging textile city of Łódż. In Prussian Poland, opportunity was employment in the great coal and iron works of Silesia, threat was Bismarck's Kulturkampf against Polish Catholicism, and the heavy-handed Germanization of the agricultural lands around Poznań—a policy also followed by Hitler after 1939. Bismarck, however, was constrained by certain limits of how far he could punish opposition, and the vast sums at his disposal for buying up peasant properties provoked a stubborn Polish counter movement. When, in 1901, in the village of Wrzesnia near Poznań, a Prussian teacher beat a Polish child for refusing to say the Lord's Prayer in German, it provoked across Europe not only anger but ridicule. (Similar to teachers at Protestant mission schools in Arizona who beat Navajo children when they used their own language.)

In Galicia, where the Poles enjoyed the greatest political and cultural freedom and the worst economic backwardness, the conflict was not so much between Austrian and Pole as between landlord and peasant. The wild jacquerie of 1846, burning down manor houses and murdering gentry families, is not a topic that fits the Polish myth.

This economic development, based on the rapid extension of the railroad networks, absorbed the Poles into Russian, German, and Austrian economic life. Divided as they were among three imperial masters, how was it possible for them to maintain the sense of belonging to one nation? When war came in 1914 Poles fought, often against each other, as soldiers within the three armies, and when peace came in 1918, the new republic proclaimed on November 11 had to fit together a viable nation out of three entirely different states.*

To return, however, to walking along the streets at dusk in November or March, feet already cold and wet, the first zigzagging drunk avoided, lights of security and comfort glimmering behind the curtains, what middle-class resident could imagine the secret police? For the workers in the railroad yards, for students and artists, yes, but not for *Us*.

Jacek's job was to deal with that police state in a typically Polish manner. He was an editor of *Tygodnik Powszechny* (Universal Weekly), the voice of the semi-tolerated Catholic liberal opposition whose independence was based on a careful estimate of the possible and Jacek's weekly interviews with the censor. The magazine appeared on Friday. On Thursday, therefore, before it went to the printer, censor and editor would go over every article. The first reaction of each new official was an automatic *no* to almost every piece. Jacek's duty was to point out the essential harmlessness of the material, its obvious loyalty to the ideals of socialism, its harmony with the basic tradition of Polish history, its factual accuracy (caution—policemen don't like facts). Of course, the editors might be mistaken: this article should be scrubbed, that paragraph could be rewritten.

After a while the censor looked forward to his Thursday meeting with a cultured, patriotic, and interesting man like Dr. Woźniakowski as the high point of his week. Jacek and his colleagues had to make sure that there was enough (not too much) offensive material to be indignantly rejected for the censor to

---

* This material comes mainly from Stefan Kieniewicz et al., *History of Poland*, Polish Scientific Publishers, Warsaw, 1979, an impressively objective book put out during the relatively liberal years at the end of Gierek's administration.

know he was doing his duty, but the system could be bent as it could not in East Berlin or Prague. Eventually, however, some higher up would read through a copy of *Tygodnik*, be scandalized at what was being printed, fire the contaminated censor, and Jacek must start all over again with a new troglodyte.

> *The languid demons*
> *of torture cells in provincial*
> *cities, small communists with stiff little hearts*
> Adam Zagajewski *The Gothic Canvas*

The American equivalent of Communist censorship is ignorance and lack of interest. On the other hand Poles have exactly the same attitude for anything Czech, and vice versa.

Years later I read *Lost in Translation* by Eva Hoffman, the autobiography of a Jewish schoolgirl whose family had survived the occupation and lived in Kraków until they emigrated to Vancouver. One might imagine that the Canadian city would be the longed-for refuge of comfort and freedom for any Polish Jewish family. The author's message, however, was that despite post-war meagerness and Communist repression, Kraków enjoyed a paradoxical intellectual and emotional freedom that Vancouver could not approach. There was theatre (Shakespeare and Chekhov with subsidized tickets) and music and dance to share and to argue about vehemently with one's friends. There were stimulating intellectuals one sometimes encountered, like Jacek Woźniakowski, who had not been liquidated by the Germans or Russians, who still existed even if in humble positions (Jacek's first job had been as a translator for an English newspaper), and who had lived during the war with an intensity that no one on the safe side of the Atlantic could comprehend. There was the exciting, however dangerous, game of changing one's face between what was shown the outer world and that shown one's family and closest friends. To have survived, to still survive, required wit as well as tenacity.

In contrast, Vancouver was not only bland and dull, it offered far less freedom to this spirited immigrant girl. The demand for total conformity came not from the police but from her high-school classmates. The rules, dangerous to disobey, were to speak act dress laugh just like everyone else. A heretic who violated them was a traitor and to be shoved outside society.

Since my retirement in 1981 from Commonwealth School, I keep busy by hunting down brief teaching invitations at a scattering of colleges from Atlanta to Maine. My favorite topic is totalitarianism as the dogma of our century, the ways by which it is enforced, its essence of lies and fear, and the role of its messiah, V.I. Lenin. I start with a slogan scrawled on a wall between Naples and Rome that I saw in 1937: Nothing against the State, Nothing above the State, Nothing outside the State. Lenin would have substituted the Communist Party for lo Stato. Hitler would have put, what? The Will of das Volk? Mussolini was mistaken in setting Italian Fascism and its state and nation as a paradigm for totalitarianism. There were just too many conflicting loyalties—to your hometown and its customs, to the church, to Mamma—and too much simple grit in the machinery, like inefficiency and graft, to fulfill his ideal. The definition, however, was accurate. For an American college student in the 1990s, not able to travel to North Korea or Cuba, the nearest example of totalitarianism will be his dormitory.

One reason why I remained fascinated by Poland was to witness how a man like Jacek Woźniakowski—and admittedly he would not have survived in East Germany or in Czechoslovakia—was able to stand up against Mussolini's definition. What strengths did he possess, did his society possess?

In his guided tour of the city that summer of 1960, Jacek took Mary and me to Kasimierż, which Bruce Barton and I had seen about twenty years earlier. We visited the synagogue and its surroundings, Esther Street named after King Casimir's Jewish mistress. The buildings remained, but no Jews. The impact was even more disheartening than in Warsaw where every physical sign had been destroyed. Here in Kraków there were houses, street signs, a cemetery where vandals had broken the gravestones, but beyond a few aged folk, no Jews. In the camp memorials, no mention. In the picture books of Polish art, landscape, history that I was given by my hosts, hardly a word. It is a painful subject still for Poles. Jacek edited a carefully researched history of the wartime heroism of those who protected and sheltered Jews. In Yad Vashem, Jerusalem's great memorial to the Holocaust, there are many trees planted in honor of righteous gentiles with Polish names.

Kraków had always had a liberal tradition. There were far more mixed marriages, particularly among the intelligentsia, than the stereotypes recognize. In Sholom Aleichem's tales of Kasrilevke, as presented in *Fiddler on the Roof*, when the daughter of Tevye the milkman runs away with a gentile, forcing her heart-broken father to say a kaddish for the dead upon her name, the handsome young Pole says they'll go to Kraków. There's a town where they can make a life together.

Jacek's heart, however, was in the family home of Zakopane, built in over-sized peasant Gothic in the custom of the 1890s, when the gentry tried to share the painter Wyspianski's infatuation with peasant life. It rambled irrationally with many out-of-the-way bedrooms where lived obscure and silent relatives: a German aunt who wove, an aged uncle who was writing a never-finished epic about the mountaineers. The house looked up to mountains and forests, and down to the lavish pink villa and its guards belonging to the Prime Minister.

One morning Jacek took Mary and me climbing into the high Tatry along the Czech border, to show us the famous lake—Eye of the Sea—rimmed by rocky peaks, totally hidden that day by fog. We did reach the border, a high grassy ridge, through forests of fir trees, and we could walk along it, a foot in each country. Just on the other side, eating and drinking, sat a large party of Them, with shapeless suits, gross faces, vulgar manners.

"Czechs!"

On the way back to the city we stopped at a village named Dębno, for oak trees, where there was a famous dark little wooden church with painted interior like the ones of northern Norway, and a famous wood-carver. I bought a large plaque of a crowned and suffering Christ brooding upon the sufferings of the world, a bird (ptak) perched on his shoulder, a design the old artist was proud of. His carvings brought him more money from city folk than he knew what to do with, and it was too easy for him to dispose of it in drink.

Next to the church lived a woman who wove exquisitely clean and simple linen, even growing her own flax. Mary, who loved every detail of women's weaving, wanted to buy a couple of meters for embroidery. The woman was hard to persuade. She enjoyed, she said, simply to unfold the bolt and run its cloth through her hands. And of course the złoty we were trying to give her were simply pieces of paper.

❦

I took the train down from Warsaw in March 1968. The student disturbances that had crowded the university area around the Grocholski apartment with steel-helmeted security police had spread to Kraków, and I found the same tense atmosphere. The center of all danger was, of course, the monument to Mickiewicz in the rynek, facsimile of an original destroyed by the Nazis. It was sealed off against symbolic gestures by a gang of thugs in black over-coats with clubs and red armbands and the inspirational name of 'activist workers.' (Where would Frost's or Yeats' monument in the English-speaking world inspire such fervor and fear?) There was a serious, excited spirit in

Jacek's apartment. The phone, of course, was bugged, and the treacherous implement had been wrapped in blankets. Henryk, a university student, spoke earnestly about the demonstration his comrades were planning: they acknowledged the education given them by the socialist state, they were not acting like spoiled children, as the party paper claimed, but had a right to protest against the irresponsible violence shown by the security police, especially against girls. After the younger children had eaten, Jacek, Maja, and I sat around the supper table, under the lamp in that darkened room, listening to Henryk. It was a scene from Gorki or Conrad.

"They are so weak," Jacek said. "The police are so strong."

Maja left to hear the children's prayers.

I was witnessing a scene out of Polish history, the mother reassuring her children in a time of danger. Their family, their faith had lasted from generation to generation, invisible but strong enough to hold the nation together. Their language in which the prayers had been said. Even a final prayer for Party Secretary Władislaw Gomułka that he might come to look at his suffering land more reasonably.

Afterwards we listened to the much heralded two-hour television address by Gomułka to the party faithful. The drama was not entirely black and white. Gomułka had stood up against the hard-liners in 1951 and paid for it with three years of prison, he had shown a forcefulness, and tact, with Khrushchev in 1956 that preserved Poland's independence against Soviet tanks. He maintained a modest standard of living wherein his (Jewish) wife queued at an ordinary shop for family provisions, unlike the Byzantine luxury of Tito and his peers. In a way Gomułka had represented a path from an intolerable Stalinism to a socialism where decent men could lead decent, happy lives. His stubborn courage in the mid-50s, however, had turned into age-hardened arrogance, and by September he would become one of Brezhnev's firmest allies in the invasion of Dubček's Czechoslovakia.

That speech by Gomułka pretty well ended the Jewish history of Poland, eliminating the remaining one per cent of 1939's three million. He was not anti-Semitic (only Fascists were anti-Semites), but he was anti-Zionist. When the Nazis were finally expelled, many alienated Jews had sided with the Communists, and, given their tragic memories and the ever-green traditions of Polish anti-Semitism, only Jews strongly sympathetic to Communism had remained there. A figure given by Nicholas Bethell—and hotly disputed—in *Gomułka—His Poland, His Communism** is that half of the UB (*Urzad Bezpieczewstwa*—the security police), at least in its early years, were

* Holt Rinehart and Winston, New York, 1969, pp. 254–262.

Jews. When the war broke out between Arabs and Israelis in June 1967, the entire Soviet bloc sided with the Arabs and branded the Israelis as aggressors, which encouraged, of course, a sentimental philo-Semitism from anti-Communists. Nevertheless, the stereotype of Jews as Communists was convenient for the government, which could placate protests by blaming the usual scapegoat. Most non-Communist Jews had already emigrated to America, Australia, Canada, and Israel. After 1968 grandparents remained.

The evening at ulica Wyspiańskiego left me with a poignant mix of reflections. The fragile and yet tenacious integrity of the family with its roots in history had stood against Russian, Prussian, Austrian authority, sometimes in suicidal cavalry charges, sometimes by a mother listening to the prayers of her children. And this expression of up-to-date totalitarianism was expressed both by chanting party members shaped like rusty pieces of iron and by clever wordmongers eliminating Revisionists one year, Dogmatists the next, cosmopolitan formalists and petty bourgeois nationalists the year after.

❦

Where did you get that leaflet, sir, what is your reason
for being out on the streets at this hour,
what gives you the right to wear that black armband, quiet,
we're asking the questions and being polite about it too
as you can see and we expect that politeness back, sir, who
gave you the right to these rites,
whom does your Poland belong to, where
is the Mother of God hiding, contacts, names,
addresses, quiet, we're out here working
late at night and listen to you is that how they taught you
to talk polite at the university
on the state's money, who taught you
those expressions, who instigated
that expression on your face, quiet,
we inflict suffering, you must realize
what times are like
and where you are living, dates,
names, facts, just you be civil
        Stanisław Barańczak *The Weight of the Body*

My visit gave Jacek an exuse to leave the city for twenty-four hours, drive south past the late-winter fields to his beloved mountains.

We stopped for lunch at *Poraj*, Zakopane's one private restaurant, which served good food at reasonable prices. Poraj's recent offer to show the ministry of tourism how to upgrade the slovenly state restaurants had panicked everyone in authority. It was easy to imagine the public's conclusions if such capitalist advice made the mechanism too quickly better.

Under Polish custom, in a crowded restaurant a newcomer sits down at any empty place, and a young woman asked permission to share our table. When she removed her jacket we saw the pin stating, in English, *I am a Virgin*. A Pandora's box of questions: Was she? More important, *why?* Where had she found it? Purchased? A gift from her dying mother? An expression of religious or political beliefs, from what point of view? What response was she hoping to elicit? Sober approval? A flaming challenge to any self-respecting male? We finished our lunch in silence.

It was ten years before Mary and I, on our way to a conference on rural development in Istanbul, were in Kraków again. By 1978, year of that visit, Edward Gierek, who had replaced a discredited Gomułka in 1970, was enjoying the last fragile year of Polish 'prosperity.' Despite the rise in oil prices, 1978 was still a boom year throughout Europe. Orders for Polish ships and golf carts were plentiful and credit was easy. Spain had become a new trading partner, and Henryk and I conversed in Spanish instead of French. Rioja had replaced Hungarian and Romanian wine.

By late 1970s the police were no longer trying to uncover the 'flying universities,' study groups in private homes trying to learn what exactly *was* Polish history since 1939. In *1984* George Orwell stated that Big Brother held total power not simply out of fear of his police but because no one knew the facts to prove him wrong. History was whatever the Party, at that moment, said it was. Róża and Anna Woźniakowska and their friends were challenging Orwell's conclusion. No one knew the complete truth, but piecing together bits of it, as with a jigsaw puzzle, out of books from abroad, out of parents', and even grandparents' memories, they constructed a version of reality.

At the same time, the censors were losing confidence. It was easier to import books. The rise of Solidarity at the Lenin Shipyards in Gdańsk, a labor movement that believed in speaking for the workers, not for the state, gave a sense of movement, of hope, in which the students, again, could play a part.

There's nothing more debauched than thinking
this sort of wantonness runs wild like a wind-borne weed
on a plot laid out for daisies.
. . . .

They prefer the fruits
from the forbidden tree of knowledge
to the pink buttocks found in glossy magazines—
all that ultimately simplehearted smut.
The books they relish have no pictures.
What variety they have lies in certain phrases
marked with a thumbnail or a crayon.
. . . .

Wisława Szymborska *An Opinion on the Question of Pornography*

13

Kraków 1985, 1989, 1990, 1991

A tyrant's proclamations (in whatever era)
Are merely words

Someone else must translate them into a manhunt
Someone with a knack
Someone who likes his work

Someone adept at getting the right people
To the right place at the right time
To pound on the door with a crowbar or a fist

Someone who draws up the timetables for raids
As if they were crosswords in the Sunday paper

Someone who doesn't bother with whatever's coming next
It's no longer his affair
He's not responsible
Hell's humble servant
An exemplary employee an adroit technician
    Artur Międzyrzecki *Someone Else*

1985

THE IMPOSITION OF MARTIAL LAW by General Wojciech Jaruzelski in 1981
turned the clock back 30 years. Dealing with the police, the courts, the censors, ceased to be a game. Few people were actually killed but many were
beaten and the jails were real enough.

At that time I was in the middle of a major change in my own life, giving
up my job as head of Commonwealth School. I also felt it was not right to
witness as a tourist these new ordeals and dangers in my friends' lives, and I
did not see Kraków again until 1985.

"*Charlie*—the sexy young fragrance for livin' in the fast lane"—an adver-
tisement in a lobby display case at the *Francuski*. Jaruzelski could not totally
suppress Freedom.

A purpose for this visit was to collect graphics on consignment for a show at a Boston gallery. It is important that Americans see Poland as other than a welfare case. Each print sold meant keeping an artist alive, meant keeping art alive. The Czech part of the job had been easy, selecting samples at a state agency at prices shamefully low. The Polish artists had to be dealt with individually, each with his own method of payment: to a cousin in Montreal, a girlfriend's brother in Edinburgh, out of sight of tax collector or policeman. Some pictures were marvellous in force, imagination, technique. Some were too dreary even for a Cambridge intellectual. Back in Boston it would be a matter of dealing with the gallery owner, of making up myself the difference between the 35% commission I thought correct and the 50% she thought. No good deed goes unpunished.

What were the changes? Jacek took me to the headquarters of a mushroom magnate. Pan Antek was allowed to keep the family mansion with sabres (used against Turks, Swedes, Russians *et al.*) and shaven-headed, moustached ancestors on the wall because of 24-hour-a-day industrial production at a pair of greenhouses in the back yard. The skill and energy required, the desperate need for more food, more exports, more well-trained workers, persuade the government to leave such an entrepreneur alone.

Jacek was angry, however, over the case of a cripple who, on his motorized tricycle, bought bread at one side of town and then resold it at a few złoty markup to workers leaving their factory at the other. He had been arrested as a speculator.

"When every high official steals millions in one racket after another!"

On some errand I wandered into the small Kleparski Rynek beyond the *Francuski*, a market square selling fish and mushrooms (pieczarki), tired apples, flowers (kwiatki), poultry. At one side stood a small line of expressionless, middle-aged folk in dark overcoats which they opened as each potential buyer walked by. Dollars, pornography, drugs, guns?

Women's underwear.

Karl Marx's years of faithful study in the library of the British Museum, the heroic Communists who gave their lives resisting Piłsudski's police, Franco's Moors, Hitler's tanks—

"Nu, panie, wanna buy a hot bra?"

In the main rynek that I would walk around and around, circling the medieval cloth hall (Sukiennice) with its little Christmas stalls, past the statue to Mickiewicz, I always sat for a while in St. Mary's church. I tried to slow down, silence the noise in my head, share the silence and dark, the candles, the prayers of the people, mainly middle-aged women, who took refuge for a while. General Jaruzelski held no authority here, nor did the queues for meat or children's socks. It is easy to become sentimental, but if the 'Free West' has freedom of religious expression, political action, intellectual inquiry, what use does it make of them?

Noise again. At Fort Knox there had been a young Jewish soldier in our barracks. "Poles! I came from a town way in the southeast. The teacher whipped me on my legs and called me a dirty zhid."

One event that had occurred that year was a bar mitzvah at the temple in Kazimierż. Only grandparents, almost, were left, but some thirteen year old had been brought from Philadelphia. Jews in their 60s, 70s came from towns all around and packed the temple, most in tears. Poland had been the oldest, the greatest center of Jewish life in Europe, and here, now, with this American boy was the last bar mitzvah.

My second day was sunny, fairly warm. I returned to the Sukiennice hoping to find Christmas presents for my grandchildren like Kraków's patron, Saint George with his red horse and dragon. (As I grow older I identify with the dragon.) Painted eggs. Carvings of the Holy Family. Walking sticks. Axes with small steel heads used by the mountaineers around Zakopane, the cause of death at the end of three-day weddings.

Music brought me outside. Three or four violins, accordion and clarinet, bass fiddle were playing tangos, polkas, waltzes. Teenagers—mainly girls with girls—were dancing self-consciously. Little girls were jumping up and down in excitement, the circle of spectators was smiling at this merriment. Then a handsome student bowed to one of the little girls, and at her mother's nod, picked her up in his arms and waltzed elegantly around the square, returned her to Mother, and bent over to kiss her hand. The spectators cheered.

I described to Jacek his city of spontaneous gaiety.

"It's all organized by the police," he replied sourly. "Any Pole with brains isn't fooled, but gullible tourists come away with all sorts of silly conclusions."

The little girl a dwarf cop in drag?

My last evening I had dinner at Henryk's apartment, although he was away, perhaps in Colombia, in Pope John Paul's party as editor of *Znak* (The Sign), for 30 years the monthly of the liberal establishment. Barbara teaches mathematical logic (a Polish strength) at the university. They have a lovely eight year old Justyna, who a year or so ago had informed her parents: "I'm lonely. I'd like to have either a puppy or a baby sister." So, they talked it over and here was Urszulka, whom everyone smiled at, and Justyna the age of Jacek's Róża and Anna when I had met them in the 1960s.

"Will your children have a better life than you?"

It's a question I feel compelled to ask, starting with my last parents' meeting at Commonwealth when I suggested that for the first time in American history the answer might be no.

"I don't think so," Barbara answered. "I was born in 1952. Life was very hard then but we had hope. I am not sure now if we still do. The land is poisoned. The wind coming from the West carries fumes that are killing our forests. Our own factories poison our air, our rivers, the food we eat, the land itself. It isn't what happens to our economy, it's what happens to our life. What do our children grow up into?"

Justyna, waiting impatiently while her mother speaks in English, starts to whisper.

"Tak—Justyna asks if you will listen to her play the piano?"

The girl arranges her music on the respectable upright, sits herself very straight upon the bench, and, with her hands raised in the correct way all piano teachers insist upon, plays three arrangements from Schumann.

"Very nice. My seven-year-old (what is the word for granddaughter?) plays the piano also. When I come back you will play Chopin? All Polish girls play Chopin."

This well-beloved, thoughtful girl, following the cultured Polish love of music gives us hope for the future and her reality answers the sad pessimism of her mother.

⌘

1989

I returned in 1989, again in November (listopad), the dark, disheartening month, and with the *Francuski* closed for modernization, a paralyzed process, stayed at the *Cracovia*. A featureless Orbis hotel, but because it stood at the edge of town, I was forced to walk back and forth through the city, early morning, at dusk when the street lights were lit, at night, and Kraków became my worn, old, beautiful Europe.

The system was coming to an end. How long would General Jaruzelski stay on? Would he be replaced by Lech Wałęsa? How much of an improvement would that be? How much was Wałęsa modeling himself now on Piłsudski—the noble primitive: authority, force, moustache? Jacek had been nominated for the Senate but had refused. An honorable and trusted man, perhaps he might be chosen as mayor. Censorship had ended. *Znak*, the monthly, had a newly remodeled office building, dating from the eighteenth century, but would it land the funds to stay afloat?

At the rynek, looking for Christmas presents again at the Sukiennice, at whose kawiarnia I order a coffee and a cherry brandy. The clientele is mostly housewives out shopping rather than intellectuals arguing about Gorbachev, but in any café with its clouds of cigarette smoke, smell of coffee, back and forth of Polish conversation, I remember my first call upon Czesław Miłosz outside Paris, over thirty years ago. For him these details were *his* Poland, what he missed the most in exile, and which he feared he would never find again.

Walking there I'd passed the sad little pyramids of apples brought in by farmers. How many hours would a man stand behind his pile of ten or twelve apples? The Polish government, like Gorbachev's, was trying to restore social discipline by cutting back on the production of vodka. As a result demoralized men were drinking anti-freeze and brake fluid.

"You'll find yourselves as in our inner cities: no men, and society held together by women."

"That's a Polish tradition," Jacek replied. "In the nineteenth century so many men spent so many years in prison or exiled in Siberia that it was the women who had to run everything."

Not a totally exact comparison.

For Maja the good news was a movement to start a loose grouping of little private schools, organized by parents and teachers, as alternative to the brutal state schools. People were working together to accomplish something, not just complaining.

I had supper again at Henryk's apartment in the dark, unfriendly building on Siemiradzkiego, across the streetcar tracks, past the bars. Justyna was thirteen now, and Urszulka stood by the piano while she carefully played Scott Joplin, as close to Chopin as any American ever came.

⁓

1990

I was at the *Pollera*, a small, worn hotel, which, after 40 years of nationalization, had been returned to its original owners. Next door was advertised a weekly amateur striptease competition—*Konkuracja Striptyzowych*. The shops were full, no more lines—at a price. I bought Honduran pineapples as hostess presents. Jacek was mayor, too exhausted to speak.

I had promised Maja that I would raise money for the private schools started up the previous September, so my visit became a sausage sliced ever more finely. One school, of middling size, was in the city; smaller, even more fragile ones were scattered around the suburbs. All progressive schools are

149

alike: teachers and children, blackboards and wall decorations. I might as well be in Cambridge. Likewise all sit-still-and-don't-speak-till-I-tell-you, forty-children-in-a-room schools are alike.

For months I had been receiving letters about conflicts between parents and teachers ("Just because they pay tuition, they think they can say what the curriculum should be"), heating problems, accreditation disputes, fees for dance and swimming, but here was a half moon of fifteen or so little children absorbed in what the young teacher was saying, bursting into laughter, unconcerned about the intruder.

If you want to build a new Poland, this is where you begin. If children are taught not to be afraid, it is easier to teach them not to hate. That seems obvious, doesn't it?

One school was out near Nowa Huta, the famous steel works that supplies Kraków its sulfur dioxide (both Woźniakowska girls had had serious chest trouble over the winter) and a miserable quality steel that only the state will buy. At a distance the towers and gleaming domes, chimneys and curving pipes become a Mongol palace.

If, Western experts insist, the Polish government showed the slightest discipline, Nowa Huta would be shut down immediately. "What do we do with 30,000 workers for whom there is no unemployment insurance, no retraining programs, no housing available should they seek jobs elsewhere?"

The experts wave their hands impatiently.*

And yet this caricature of a steel mill, constructed out of postwar devastation, was a monument not only of Communist but of Polish achievement. We are not beaten. We will build a modern industrial nation.

These claims were true and not true. Poets and Western experts pointed out the lies that wrapped Nowa Huta as sulfur dioxide wrapped its smokestacks. Pollution was a scourge of capitalist nations. If you described dead forests and children dying of lung diseases you might be subjectively correct, but objectively you were describing something that could not exist in socialist Poland, and therefore it was correct for the state to punish you for slander.

---

* Suggestion: a Communist theme park. Rootless radicals from Berkeley and Paris, freedom fighters from Frankfort would pay hard currency to be interrogated by unemployed security police, slip under barbed wire, print illegal poems, sing revolutionary songs in various languages, go to a specially refrigerated Vorkutaland where they chop wood and eat bean soup with imitation weevils, cut sugar cane. What a challenge for some no-longer-needed Stalinist agronomist to raise sugar cane outside Kraków.

Production problems, as in *1984*, are solved by statistics: national shoe production has soared by x% even if there are no shoes for your child's feet. The maintenance of worker morale by petty theft, and of executive morale by gross perquisites. To protest harsh shop discipline is either infantile leftism or the effects of CIA bribery.

⟨◦⟩

Nevertheless, I do not think that Americans who have tolerated the perversion of their own industrial system have the right to throw stones. Our factories are run not by engineers but by financiers who turn prosperity into paper, who skim off quick profits and shrug off closed plants. The only solution is low labor costs, shifting from North Carolina to Poland, if the Poles promise not to cause trouble, more probably to Central America, the home of workers who accept fifty-six cents an hour.

Nowa Huta is also the home of the great modern church, dedicated to Mary Queen of Poland, erected after a 20-year confrontation with the Communists, primarily through the leadership of Archbishop Karol Wojtyła before he became Pope John Paul. Here was defiance, a kilometer away from its showpiece, to Communist authority—a great No, a great Yes. Standing up against the Nazis and the Communists, the church had paid a high price for the authority behind its defiance. It spoke as always for the women who raised their families in Catholic tradition, and I remembered back in 1968 listening to Maja Woźniakowska hear her children's bedtime prayers. The men who attended this church with their wives and children worked in that hideous mill and voted, perhaps not unwillingly, as the Communists wished, but retained some innermost No to any total allegiance.

The building itself lacked the resources for the architecture and glass of a Coventry cathedral, the noblest of all postwar churches, and its murals of Calvary are confusing. What better background for the Crucifixion than a Polish industrial landscape, but the ugly, grim-faced men in Nowa Huta clothing who are forcing Jesus to the Cross look no different from the suffering bystanders.

I must visit, however, the little school at the edge of town. The children have been prepared: "Goot mornink, Meester Merrll." The directress shows me the desks sent by friends in Sweden. A large package of used clothing from Vienna will raise cash at a jumble sale. There doesn't seem to be much overall management for the different schools, however. If I did raise money (2500 letters brought in $10,000), how would it be divided, for what priorities, monitored by whom? How do teachers keep from starving to death?

There were parents who argued that members of such a noble profession should not preoccupy themselves with money. And, of course, this nice little private school for a few lucky children denies, as did Commonwealth in Boston, the democratic assumption that all children have the right to receive a good education—and don't.

"Well, we are not yet into detailed formalization."

Of course. I must attend a working breakfast tomorrow where everything will be explained. In a way, yes. Tired as I am, I understand less Polish than the day I arrived. Suddenly I am no longer able to stomach this role of wise old educator from across the sea, so anxious to help. Who was I kidding? "Przepraszam, panstwa!" and irresponsibly I run down the stairs, through the rynek, past Mickiewicz and the flower ladies, past the great conglomerate of the Wawel, with no need to speak to anyone. I find myself in the old Jewish quarter of Kazimierz. Saturday, but no one is in sight. I stand in front of a little grimy padlocked synagogue.

1991

By train from Warsaw—Polish trains are fast and comfortable, with few customers, cheap. A few years ago a ticket between Warsaw and Kraków cost the price of one black-market grapefruit. This year's hotel, the city's oldest, where Franz Liszt and Balzac stayed, is *Pod Różą*, 'under the rose.' In a pretentious world, Kraków keeps, on the whole, to a human size. There is a gross, glossy *Forum*, out beyond the Wawel, but one doesn't have to stay there. The rynek is a half block away so I throw down my bag and hasten outside to touch each of my favorite objects: Mickiewicz, the flower ladies, St. Mary's, in this city as beautiful as Prague and Venice and the walk along the Limmat in Zurich. I am near enough the cathedral tower to hear the trumpeter every hour till 11, starting anew at 4, so many details crowding upon me that I cannot sleep. The chill means children to and from school in tasseled caps knitted by grandmother, the supreme Polish art form. And in front of the Sukiennice is an odd orchestra of Peruvian Indians, plus a few Poles, singing in Quechua and Spanish, puffing into their pan pipes, bobbing up and down to their drums. (A year later it began to appear that those colorful musicians were often fundraisers for the murderous Sendero Luminoso in Peru, and their cassettes paid for explosives and machine guns.)

Before I set foot outside *Pod Różą*,* my calendar was full. There were too many people, and too many projects to deal with, such as locating resources for a center of Latin American studies in Warsaw. This is a new field of serious interest in both Poland and Czechoslovakia, but no hard currency exists for travel or even book purchases. Any American academic must know a dozen contacts with surplus volumes he'd like to mail. (No, fewer generous bibliophiles than I had expected). An interview with a possible translator for a novel I had recently published: the story of a heroic seventeen-year-old Polish-American girl (Emily Morawski) in a down-beat industrial town of western Massachusetts who rescues a baby from the bottom of a well and then must deal with the problems of becoming an instant celebrity. The book took seriously the culture and problems of Polonia, discussed them in realistic but positive ways, and would be wholesome reading for adolescents. An American investment to balance the smothering weight of Grossdeutschland? The ensuing problems from unrelenting inflation, administrative amateurishness, resource bottlenecks (paper from Turkey), unreliable partners (a wholesaler in Kielce claimed to have sold 800 copies but had gone bankrupt: how about payment from his overstock?) would make an amusing case study for a grade B business school.

The one public establishment out of the group I had backed, a large school in the distant industrial suburb of Podgorze, was putting on a program of Krakowiak song and dance for the generous American. Southwestern Poland, especially in the mountains, has a rich folk tradition in music and costume (tight bodices and swirling flowered skirts, white embroidered woolen suits with peacock feathers in the square-topped caps, as worn by the cavalrymen of 1939), wild and graceful. After refreshments I must pay a formal call upon each classroom, where one feels expected to say "Fraternal greetings from the People's Republic of North Korea."

A capable new directress is looking for money to buy a modern electric stove for the kitchen. The old coal-burning one is impossible by now, and because times are bad the school lunches may be for many children the only hot meal of the day. Sound familiar?

---

* Yes, the *Francuski* at last had reopened, more elegant even than in 1907, waiting, glistening, for 'beautiful people.' As I entered that evening to share this witness to a new Poland, a large, smiling headwaiter put his arm around my shoulder and courteously pushed me back out the front door. Someone as shabby as myself, born in New Jersey, did not suit their self-image. Despite some subjective emotions, I was proud that the Poland I had helped rebuild had outgrown the need for American patronage.

But when I pay my calls upon old friends, I am disturbed by their low morale. Nothing seems to be working. The Communist structure has been broken, but the Communists themselves seem as important as before, even if they call themselves different names. The rules put in to protect non-Communist teachers are being used to make it impossible to get rid of the dragons who are teaching in the same old way. There is freedom, and every single cultural enterprise, Poland's pride, is on the verge of bankruptcy. The musician, the writer, the professor, even the scientist have no prestige, only the Person of Money, no matter how he got it. Old friendships are shredding away (what I will hear in Olomouc) as people become frightened and selfish.

The glum underwear salesman on Kleparski Square, the persecuted cripple selling bread from his tricycle are honored now as the combat infantry of new free-market Poland. What happened before was just a bad dream. I think of the State Department's donations of tens of thousands of anti-personnel mines to the contras in Nicaragua and the government forces in El Salvador, which defended our country against Communism by blowing off the feet of anyone who stepped on them. Then a few years later generous Americans and Germans donated thousands of prosthetic devices so that the crippled children could move around again.

There ought to be neater ways of helping people.

∽∾

Jacek, no longer mayor, is heartsick. The recent parliamentary elections, the dream of decades of oppression saw less than half the electorate voting. Of 67 parties that competed, 29 won seats in the Sejm. The liberal Catholic prime minister whom he supported, Tadeusz Mazowiecki, had been pushed out of office (no one could run Poland today) not only by the ex-Communists, but by former allies in Solidarity and the church establishment. It was the stubborn integrity of a united church that had kept Poland from being like Czechoslovakia, and now the hierarchy is attacking the liberals as Jews and Free Masons who want to force a Western-style Catholicism upon their country. What a waste.

A letter from Jacek Zielinski, the etcher I know in Warsaw, a few months later is made even more poignant by his battle with English: "In the summer time we was as usual at the lakes and we came back with the distress of the changes that happened in mentality of persons which we considered as our friends from many years. Urgent impetus to the possession possibility of obtainment the ground and the houses by the person's which spend the holidays in the same place with us—breaks hitherto solidarity. I'd call it childish disease of the property full of antipathy to others and greed of ownership. And that greed tramples each who stands on their way like animals fighting of territory's extension. . . . It's new phenomenon and in private relations it is very nasty. Perhaps it's first sign of Polish way to real capitalism?"

I am not convinced that a free-market economy is the absolute foundation of democratic reform. I am still imprisoned by a nineteenth-century belief in progress learned at high school. As workers gained the suffrage, built unions, elected deputies to parliament, they fought for better pay, shorter hours, decent working conditions, education for their children, pensions and health care. They were exposed to at least the ideal that all workers are brothers and sisters and not locked into permanent hostility by symbols and traditions that benefit only their masters. These ideals were corrupted by the Communists and the Nazis, Stalin and Hitler. In contrast, naked greed is clean?

About 20 years ago I found myself in Hong Kong, walking along the streets of Kowloon with a former student who was studying Cantonese in order to reinforce a career as social worker in Boston. We passed an open workshop where an obese toad, cartoon figure of rapacious capitalist, squeezed into an armchair, was staring at the passersby with little angry swollen eyes, while behind him three or four young women were frantically stitching garments together on their sewing machines. *Frantic* is the only word for their efforts. He had set their tasks. If they didn't meet them each day, each hour, he would fire them and hire new thin frightened young women.

Hong Kong is the role model for Polish competition-disciplined capitalism, as a few years ago Americans were encouraged by conservative theoreticians to accept the pragmatic authoritarianism of Singapore.

Sell tickets to Mother's autopsy.

Some American states have already started to privatize their prison system. Private companies can run them more effectively, at lower cost, and still make a profit. Public schools. Corporate sponsorship of military units: Merrill Lynch's marine battalion, with the company logo on shoulder patches, cash bonuses and generous stock options for bravery.

Arthur Miller has suggested contracting out executions. Americans love executions: in a ball park at night with lights and cheerleaders, priests and rabbis, marches and hymns. An old man like Miller, though, has perhaps lost touch with today's preference to watch reality through television: the Justice

Hour, Thursdays at 9:00 (younger children are in bed) each week from a different prison. The murderer describes his unhappy boyhood, affirms his faith in God, asks forgiveness. Weeping widow or tight-lipped mother stresses some mix of anger and mercy. The warden hosts a tour of the execution room, and as the criminal is strapped into the electric chair or has his arm prepared for the injection, explains how the procedures are designed to spare unnecessary stress. Though always with good taste, the camera briefly close-ups the murderer's face, then shifts to the governor in his office, who reports how the state's homicide rates are tangibly falling. The hour closes with a message from the sponsor, whose fees help pay for further prison construction and inner-city sports facilities. The seriousness of the program encourages useful discussion among parents and adolescents about morality and social responsibility.

Is Poland, like New Guinea, an example of a cargo-cult phenomenon? When a society is screwed up, like Melanesia when disrupted by Westerners in World War II, revitalization movements explode that are both fundamentalist—"Gimme that ole time religion!"—and magical: building jeeps and airplanes out of bamboo, setting them on hilltops and waiting for them to be filled with cameras, machine guns, radios, wristwatches, chocolate bars. The West says, "If you adopt a market economy you'll get these things." To make this happen the natives destroy everything of value that they possess. The ancestors are propitiated by the choice of a shaman (a 'real' Pole—Lech Wałęsa), and unquestioning obedience to ritual (Mary Queen of Poland).

"I hate to say so but what Poland needs is a man like Pinochet who's not afraid to stop printing money and paying out all those social benefits, who'll close down the plants that aren't profitable and lay off the workers who aren't needed, who doesn't care if children go hungry, and who'll just lock up the union leaders and journalists who make too much noise. Then we'd eventually get an economy like Chile's, which is the only one in the Third World that works. And we'd give him a nice pension so he could buy a villa on the Mediterranean, or we'd have him shot as a fascist."

PART III

~

THE HABSBURG LANDS

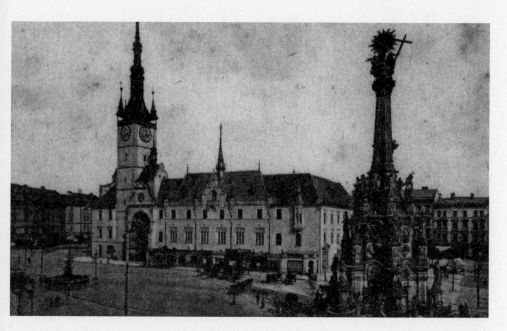

Habsburg Olmütz, city hall (radnice) and main square, 1913.

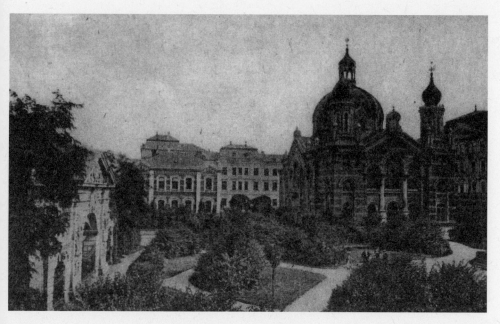

Olmütz, the synagogue, 1909, destroyed in 1939.

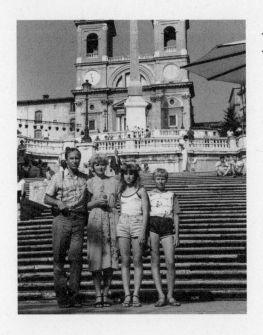

Jiři and Vera Kořinek with Jana and Jirka, on vacation in Rome.

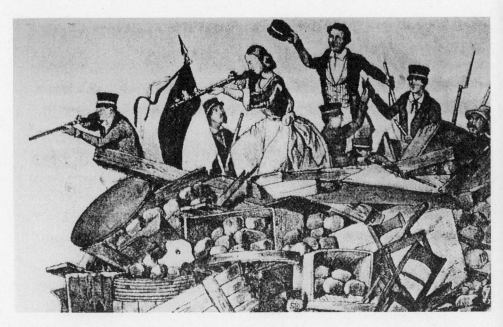

Prague 1848. The first few glorious days, so close to those of 1989, of the uprising against Austrian oppression. From some unnamed Czech history.

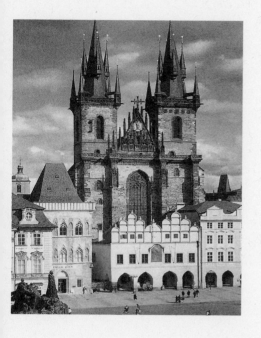

Old Town Square with façade of Tyn church, monument to Jan Hus in lower left quarter.

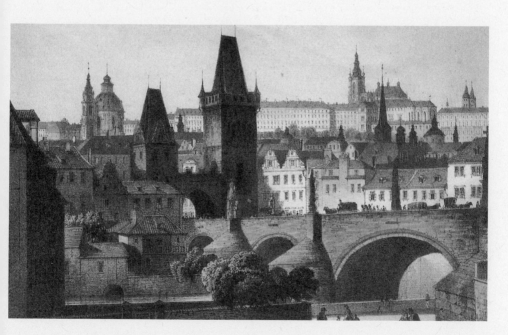

Prague, Charles Bridge and up to the Hradčany castle and the tower of St. Vitus cathedral around 1840, By F.X. Sandmann.

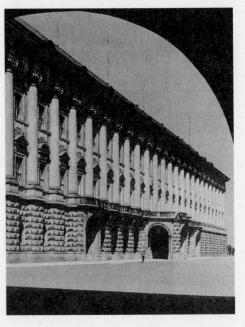

The Černin Palace, on the Hradčany hill, was built in mid-18th century for Count Černin, Austrian ambassador to Rome, Venice, and Istanbul, an illustration of the wealth and power of the upper nobility. It was later used by the Ministry of Foreign Affairs under the empire, Masaryk's republic, the Communists, and Havel, as well as being the German headquarters during the war. The Habsburg empire had humane qualities, but this monstrosity represents the Staatsmacht upon which the superstructure rested. Photograph by Eugen Wykowski in Praha Objektivem Mistru, 1983.

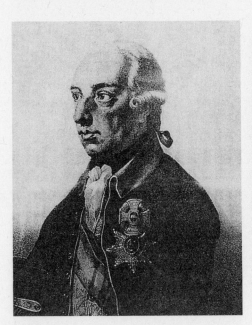

Josef II, 1741–1790. Became emperor in 1765—the mentor of all authoritarian rationalists.

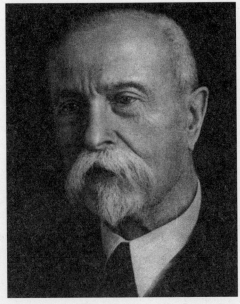

Tomaš Masaryk, 1850–1937, president 1918-1935—for a while Europe's philosopher king.

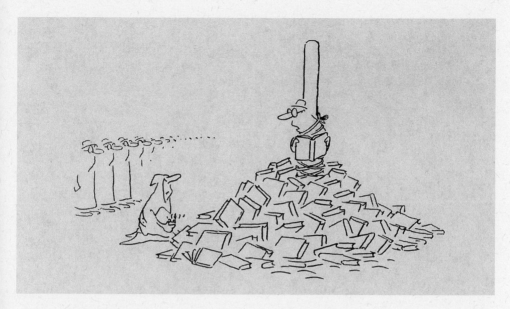

"Wait. I'll just finish this page…"

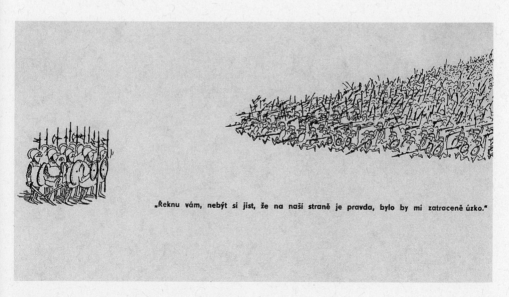

„Řeknu vám, nebýt si jist, že na naši straně je pravda, bylo by mi zatraceně úzko."

"Listen, If I didn't know that Truth was on our side,
I'd be scared to death!"

Censored Laughter. Cartoons from 1969 after the Warsaw Pact invasion of
Czechoslovakia.

14

K.u.K.

The State is the march of God through the universe.
  Hegel

. . . there's always the billowing edge of the fair
  For booths that please
the most curious tastes are drumming and bawling
              Especially
worth seeing (for adults only) the breeding of money!
Anatomy made amusing! Money's organs on view!
Nothing concealed! Instructive and guaranteed
to increase fertility!
  Rainer Maria Rilke *Elegy X*

MY CONTRIBUTION to the never-ending argument about the Great American Education Crisis has been a compulsory course in Austro-Hungarian history. This makes sense. In its ambiguities and paradoxes, with so few heroes or total villains, Habsburg history challenges the American weakness for simplistic, good guy/bad guy, happy-end reasoning. In any society, what are the sources of unity or fission? Was the ramshackle K.u.K. (Kaiserlich-imperial-Austrian-und Königlich-royal-Hungarian, the attributes of the monarch according to whether he was in Vienna or Budapest)* accretion of ethnic units the sign of its obsolescence or of a modernity reaching beyond the nationalisms that have caused such suffering in our own century? After eight years of Ronald Reagan Americans have gained a new awareness of Emperor Franz Josef.

Sadly enough, no one, even in my own school, has shown any interest. The universal significance of the lives of Josef II, Metternich, and Franz Josef is ignored.

---

* Since no English-speaking child can take the French seriously when he learns they say 'oui-oui' to each other, just think of the jokes it was impossible not to make with 'ka-ka.'

Josef II (1741-1790) is the earliest and most modern of the three. He was the perfect headmaster, always right, with a fanatical intensity of belief in the power of the State when controlled by reason, and in his authority, unhindered by law or tradition, to speak for such a state. He was the spokesman for all the headmasters of the twentieth century. In our country Woodrow Wilson shared his pedantic self-righteousness. Franklin Roosevelt had Josef's vision of reconstructing society, but was a more adroit politician. One thinks of Nehru, of Kemal Ataturk, and the Shah, who each in turn insisted on modernizing, westernizing, and secularizing his country unconcerned as to whether these reforms were wanted or not. And any number of loyal Communists in the years after 1945 who believed that their authoritarian rationalism would eventually be blessed by the god of History.

Josef, freed by Voltaire from the prejudices of his priest-ridden mother, Maria Theresa, sought to end Catholic limits upon freedom of thought, constraints upon the Jews, the cobwebbed traditions of guilds, cities, provinces, the corporate building blocks of the Empire, and aimed to lift the burdens imposed upon the peasantry by generations of brain-dead nobility. He would promote unity within his polyglot mishmash by insisting upon the use of German—which included closing all Czech libraries—and by settling German colonists in Hungary and the Empire's Slavic lands. Today Josef would re-close Czech libraries for the new language of reason—American. A true Habsburg, he preferred the predictable mediocrity of Salieri to the anarchic genius of Mozart.

Josef's efforts to pound his provinces and social classes into geometric shapes were less and less welcomed, and failure brought increasing isolation to the embittered idealist. The last year of his life he renounced all his efforts: his pupils had failed him.

His legacies were the Oriental agglomeration of the Austrian bureaucracy (what Tolstoy's Russian officers at Austerlitz dubbed the Hofkriegschnappswurstrat), and an even wider scattering of clots of Germans (Volksdeutsch) across the maps of Eastern Europe who eventually became enthusiastic fans of Hitler's Grossdeutschland.

One might even name Mikhail Sergeyevich Gorbachev as Josef's most inspired follower. In his crusade to bring rational reorganization (perestroika) and truth-telling clarity (glasnost) to replace the corruption and paralysis of post-Stalinist Communism, Gorbachev freed his country from dictatorship and the world from the fear of nuclear war. He also wrecked Russia's economy and broke the Soviet Union to pieces.

spies and informers,* on the censors who kept out unwholesome books.†
People's readiness to make decisions declined. Problems were best put off.
Anything new, anything strange was distrusted. Schubert was the musician
of that time and place, and though his greatest work, like Beethoven's, was
created in solitude and pain, there is the charming myth of the evenings of
piano and song in his friends' drawing rooms.

୶ଡ଼ଡ଼ଋ

The role of the State is to protect the rich against the poor.§

When Emperor Franz died in 1835 he was replaced by the openly feeble-
minded Ferdinand whose only remembered statement is "I am the emperor
and I want dumplings!"** There was administration but, somewhat like the
age of George Bush, no government. Metternich was locked into his obsession with maintaining a calm surface and could not face any real problem,
like the rapid growth of a desperately poor industrial proletariat flocking
into Vienna from the villages, except by strengthening the police. When a
revolution in Paris drove Louis Philippe from the throne of France on February 24, 1848, three weeks later Vienna exploded. Metternich's law and
order fell apart and the chancellor fled, like Louis Philippe, to exile in England. The students and their working-class allies were surprised at the System's collapse, the hollowness of authority—one is reminded of Prague,
Berlin, Bucharest in 1989—throughout, and beyond, the empire. In
Budapest, Milan, Venice, Dresden, and Prague, Vienna became a center of
hope rather than the model of repression. The students and workers man-
ning the same barricades followed the bare-breasted goddess of liberty in
proclaiming the brotherhood of all peoples and the defeat of tyranny and
reaction. What a glorious dawn seemed to be appearing! One can almost
envy the heroes who died, certain that they were winning, in those early
months of 1848—and 1990.

---

* The main target was the educated middle class who might be infected with liberal ideas
from France or England. Such a family often hired servants straight from a Moravian village
just so that they could not understand and repeat what was said around the dining table.

† Byron was such a writer, a trouble-maker who disturbed the peace—to be compared with
Elvis Presley at the end of our silent 1950s? Or in Reagan-Bush America, black rap?

§ I have used three books as my major sources for material for nineteenth-century Austrian
history. First is Hugo Hantsch, *Geschichte Österreichs*, Vol. II, Vienna, 1949, which was my
demanding teacher of language and background when we lived in Vienna in 1951. Next is
Edward Crankshaw, *The Fall of the House of Habsburg* (Viking Press, N. Y., 1963, and Penguin Books, 1983). Third is Ilsa Barea, *Vienna* (Alfred Knopf, N. Y., 1966). For a more limited period, Carl Schorske, *Fin-de-Siecle Vienna*, Alfred A. Knopf, N. Y., 1980.

** "I am the president of the United States and I will not eat broccoli!"

The amateur revolutionaries had no leadership, no cohesion or direction. It becomes boring to hang around those barricades—where are the toilet facilities, what's for lunch? The civilian population becomes impatient, supplies are running low, prices are going up. Will the workers go back to where they came from? When, at the end of October, the barricades are finally stormed, the government employs Croat troops, traditionally loyal to the monarchy, traditionally ferocious, and ready to savage the revolutionaries whom they saw as allies of the Hungarians, who from one point of view were heroic freedom-fighters and from another the ruthless oppressors of their Slavic subjects.*

A new eighteen-year-old emperor, Franz Josef—conscientious, diligent, untiring—was crowned in Olomouc, to begin his reign of 68 years. The forces of liberty were defeated in Germany, Bohemia, Italy, and, with the aid of Russian troops and mass hangings, Hungary. The revolution became a heroic memory, a myth. In his twenties Franz Josef already had an old man's mind. He was convinced of the impossibility and impiety of constitutional methods. Instead he dreamed of a brilliant autocracy, Austria as the central authority of Europe, and Vienna as the imperial capital. With those noble convictions, he was less aware that real power was passing to Berlin and St. Petersburg.

With one day's fighting, on July 3, 1866, Austria became a second rate power. The war had broken out over whether Austria or Prussia would be the leader of German-speaking Europe. The Austrians were hamstrung by their practice of stationing in Lombardy a regiment recruited in eastern Galicia, so that no garrison would ever sympathize, or even be able to communicate, with the people around its barracks. Somehow this hodgepodge had to be concentrated to meet the Prussians. The Austrian commander-in-chief, General Benedek, idolized by his soldiers, put those men with antique weapons against the deadly menace of the new Prussian breech-loading rifle. "He knew, none better, the effect on a soldier's morale, when, standing up to reload, pushing in his powder and shot and ramming the charge home, he can be shot five times by a man who, lying down, has only to slip a cartridge into the breech, twist home the bolt and fire."† Moreover, Benedek knew northern Italy, not Moravia, but Italy was to be reserved for a Habsburg archduke to win an easy victory. At the village of Sadova, the Austrian army was destroyed. Bismarck's generals wanted a victory parade through Vienna,

---

* Ilsa Barea, *Op. cit.*, pp. 192–202
† Edward Crankshaw, *Op. cit.*, p. 222.

but the chancellor had pressed the war for limited objectives: recognition of Prussia's leadership of Germany. Austria would be needed as a future ally, and Bismarck insisted upon peace terms that spared the beaten foe's dignity.

⟨∞⟩

Their prestige crippled by this Prussian victory, the Austrians had to accept a new defeat in 1867, the authority of the Hungarians as (the almost) equal partner in management of the Empire. This compromise of the Dual Monarchy precluded the more reasonable division into three parts, with the Slavic provinces of Galicia, Bohemia, Moravia (Slovakia and Croatia too?) as an equal.

From then on, Austrian and Viennese history moves in two directions. One is the creation of the imperial capital (Kaiserstadt) as a city of Prunk (ostentation) and Pracht (magnificence). The old ring of fortifications had been demolished and the horseshoe-shaped Ringstrasse that replaced it would be lined with splendid hotels and apartment buildings and glorious monuments that would fool the passerby into believing show equalled reality. One flamboyant example of eclectic Schmacklosigkeit* paraded after another: The neo-Renaissance of the Opera, the Burgtheater, the Kunsthistorisches Museum, where the work of art most truly celebrated was the glory of the Habsburgs; the neo-Gothic of the Rathaus and Votifkirche (erected by the Emperor in thanks for a failed assassination attempt); the neo-classic parliament. Almost from its opening this last, where deputies shouted at each other in half-a-dozen languages, banging their desk tops and throwing inkwells, was a meaningless structure, observed cynically by an alienated, mordant young provincial, Adolf Hitler, when it was not dismissed and the business of Empire was carried on by the senior bureaucrats.

If this was theatre, however, what a wonderful show! Visiting families from Agram (Zagreb), Brünn (Brno), Lemberg (Lwów) found here the glittering center of their existence. A walk through the gardens surrounding these Prunkgebäude,† doffing their hats to the military parades,§ an operetta by Strauss or Lehar in the evening. For Mutti, coffee and pastry at *Dehmel's*, a moment of prayer at the Stefansdom, a morning of shopping, for Vatti, perhaps a little time with one of those tightly corseted young ladies. No vision of heaven could surpass a day in Vienna.

* Tastelessness. English is too pale a language for late nineteenth century Vienna.

† Buildings of splendor

§ The boyfriend of little Gustav Mahler's nursemaid was a soldier in a Moravian garrison town, and the glorious thump-thump of those regimental marches found its way again and again into his symphonies.

On the other hand is the evasion of reality not too far beyond this circle of monumental Kitsch?* Vienna was also a city of desperate poverty: clerks in the giant state buildings who sliced each kroner into cabbage and shoes for their families, unskilled village-born construction workers who faced unemployment and hunger whenever the business cycle slumped, Jewish pushcart vendors from Galicia and the angry shopkeepers they threatened.

Metternich was gone and, most of the time, so were his secret police, but the upper-middle classes, both Catholic and Jewish, still lacked the status of their counterparts in Manchester and Birmingham. They could make money (often lots of it) on the stock market, in real estate, railroads, manufacturing. They could involve themselves in culture (does Wagner replace Brahms?), in buying Oriental rugs, and then withdraw into family concerns: will Mitzi make a proper marriage? Will Franzl avoid syphilis? Politically, however, they were marginalized. The Imperial authorities did not care to grant honest power to constitutional government. And old-fashioned liberalism, based upon reason, education, and money was being threatened by anti-liberal mass movements.

These included the well-organized nationalism of the Czechs, which seemed able to just about paralyze government in both Prague and Vienna; the anti-clerical, anti-monarchist, anti-semitic Christian Socialism of Karl Lueger, permanent mayor and hero of Vienna's lower middle class (and Adolf Hitler); the more dangerous anti-Semitic Pan Germanism of Georg von Schönerer, who wanted to abandon this ramshackle Habsburg goulash and ally his followers with the Germany of Bismarck. Just about the only people with any genuine loyalty to the Emperor and to political liberalism were the Jews, attacked by every other national group.

The leading actor of this theatre was, of course, Franz Josef. It is intriguing to compare him with Ronald Reagan.† A foolish concept. In character and personality no two men could be more different. The monarch was armored by an impenetrable reserve, whereas the actor's mask was of democratic affability. The Austrian was driven by an exhausting sense of responsibility to his self-appointed duties, the American unconcernedly allowed his subordinates to manage what they would. The former was haunted by a

---

* A homey, chocolate-box version of Schmacklosigkeit.

† "Does Reagan think?" I once demanded of a Republican friend who held a high position in the president's National Security Council. After a pause he replied: "Look at the chipmunk. He knows nothing about Russian literature, nothing about economic theory, and yet in facing the deadlines of chipmunk life, he does pretty well. That's Ronald Reagan." Reassuring, and yet as one drives around New Hampshire's backroads one passes many flattened chipmunks whose instincts had not prepared them for a phenomenon like the automobile.

sense of tragedy, in family and in state life, and an awareness of the coming apocalypse that would destroy dynasty and empire. The latter bet that if you did not look too closely at your troubles, they would go away.

And yet both old men, tall, handsome, confident in the roles they had assumed, allowed themselves to be accepted as father figures. Both rulers were shrewd, callous, even cruel in their ability to cast away loyal servants who were no longer useful to them, and to destroy their own families as well, but if their subjects chose to believe that they were kindly and caring, that image could be made profitable. The ceremonies where they performed as wonder-working icons, in the reception hall at Schönbrunn, in the Rose Garden of the White House, even the photo opportunities of hunting chamois in the Alps, chopping wood at the ranch, gave their subjects a sense of stability. Neither ruler troubled his people with dangerous questions. If the surface was preserved for the moment, that was good enough.

> *It is not necessary for a prince to have good qualities but very necessary to seem to have them*
> Machiavelli *The Prince*

The most interesting proposal for saving the Empire came in 1907 with the introduction of universal male suffrage. The clever conservatives who thought this up reasoned that the forces of nationalism tearing the empire apart were essentially the work of middle-class townspeople: journalists and stationers, artists and students, half-educated agitators and unscrupulous politicians. The real people, the silent majority, were the peasants, miners, artisans of remote villages with a profound loyalty to God and Emperor, whose most stirring experience was service in the imperial armies. They intensely resented the chattering classes who claimed to speak in their name. The poor and uneducated, as Reagan and Franz Josef knew, are profoundly conservative.

It was a neat idea but came too late. The tensions and rival ambitions, the interlocking hatreds and fears of Europe, and the forces of dissolution, pessimism, fatigue within the empire, were too far gone. There was almost a universal sense of relief when war finally came.

15

Olomouc 1960, 1964, 1978, 1983

Cyclopses, olms, informers and the angels
of the Apocalypse have
very small eyes. But a lot of them.
One small eye at every keyhole.
    Miroslav Holub *Brief Reflections on Eyes*

BACK IN 1960, under a pouring rain, Mary and I had left Zakopane in the mountains of Poland on our way to Brno, from there to Bratislava and Vienna. At about half way to the Cieszyn border crossing into Czechoslovakia, we witnessed a sad drama. A gypsy was whipping a pair of horses to pull his wagon across a swollen stream in order to escape a policeman. The latter was burdened, I think, with a motorcycle, of no use on a rain-soaked path. Gypsies are less charming in reality than in Viennese operettas. They have few friends. We had just been assaulted by two women when we stopped at the kawiarnia of a small town on our way. "Hey, you want your fortune told!?" they shouted, grabbing our hands. They pointed angrily at this line and that, our palms not revealing any good news, demanded money. No, it wasn't enough, nor was the next bill I offered. Even so, the dainty yellow wagon with its painted peacocks and flowers and the frantic struggles of its driver believing that if he could get across the stream he would be free of twentieth century state authority, were sad.

The Czech officials at Tešin did not want us to think that crossing the border from one fraternal nation to another would be an easy matter. Unfortunately, our papers seemed in order. They could not find any obvious contraband. We weren't innocent. They simply hadn't been able—as in an old-fashioned New England boarding school—to pin anything on us. The Communist headmasters did not want their pupils to compare notes. Workers' delegations, folk-dance companies, volley-ball teams, yes, an individual asking questions, no.

After our days in Zakopane we entertained fantasies of bourgeois comfort in Brno. The rain only became worse, however, and at Olomouc I persuaded Mary to see if any hotel rooms might be available. The *Palac* offered us the bridal suite (empty—she had changed her mind? His first wife had suddenly turned up?) while the staff hastily cleaned up the debris of a wedding. At least there was the hope of lots of good things to eat and drink. The restaurant was so full, however, that we were seated at a small table with a young couple who had obviously planned a special evening together. Nevertheless, the fact that neither couple knew a word of the other's language guaranteed total privacy. Perhaps without us they might have held hands, but they could have gone on discussing details of how to poison her elderly husband with perfect freedom.

After dinner, the rain having stopped, I wandered through the town, looking at posters for the film festival—a Bavarian Western, a war drama from Hungary, passion from Romania—but returning to the *Palac*, ran across a boy swapping značky with the foreigners who had come to this international cultural capital. I gave him leftover Irish coins and Danish stamps, and we shared a few German words about ourselves, and our addresses.

In the claustrophobia of these hermetic national boxes any foreign contact might be a thin chance for Jiři, this thirteen-year-old Ulysses longing to sail beyond the horizon, to open the door. Back home I sent him stamps, and postcards of Boston and the Grand Canyon, harmless enough for any censor, and we exchanged simple phrases, later switching to English, about what went on at my school and his.

Two years later Commonwealth's Lithuanian-born Russian teacher wanted to organize a trip as far east as Moscow in order to bring alive the country whose language her pupils were studying. For my money Russia is a flat nothing, like Texas with dirty plumbing; the thought-provoking countries are Poland and Czechoslovakia. Reluctantly she agreed, and when a postcard informed Jiři of this trip, he wrote back excitedly that he would organize a party for our students when they arrived in Olomouc.

It was a big affair, with more flowers, beer, wine, and food for our twenty Americans than Jiři and his pals could well afford. Our folk had formed the habit of throwing frisbees or kicking soccer balls in the middle of a city street to strike up acquaintance with the natives. David played country-and-western. A couple of Czechs got out their own guitars. Both sides had songs and pocket dictionaries; they made friends in German, English, and Russian. The dialogue tended to stick at the level of "Your system is better for you and our system is better for us"—but the Twist had just raced across America, and our hosts wanted to learn this *tveest*. Our kids had records with them. Point your toe, swivel your hips—"Here, like this. . . ." These young people had literally never set eyes on a person of their age of that nationality. "Here I am," they thought, "talking with these Czech (American) kids." It was exciting, and with the music and dancing and wine came the sudden conviction from the eyes of the face so close to yours that you both understood so much more than the words in the dictionary.

As the evening drew to a close the mood became darker, and the excitement changed as it came up against the almost erotic tension of knowing that the two countries were supposed to be enemies. Even our light-hearted youngsters had seen the barbed-wire fences and the machine-gun towers as their bus had crossed from West Germany into Czechoslovakia. What could this sudden love among boys and girls bring about? They said good night to each other almost in tears.

Next morning, while the Americans were loading up the bus for the next lap to Kraków, a number of the Czechs, even those who were supposed to be taking a final exam, came by to see them off, bringing gifts of sausage and cheese and more flowers. There were girls on both sides openly weeping. "Come back. We will never forget you!"

In one of Yevtushenko's poems there are the lines: "Finished with lies and crooked ways, one day posterity will burn with shame remembering these peculiar times when honesty was labeled courage."

∽

I myself returned to Czechoslovakia in 1964 with Amy and Bruce, stopping at Banska Bystrica in central Slovakia on the way from Vienna and Budapest to Kraków and Warsaw and eventually to the village of Sominy near the Baltic. The Woźniakowskis had rented a cottage in Sominy for the month of July, and I believed that a couple of weeks with them would improve Bruce's understanding and character. Amy had been on the student trip to Moscow and at the Olomouc party had met a certain Miroslav. He was supposed to be at a forestry school near Banska Bystrica and wasn't, but ten, fifteen of his classmates—the number kept growing—were trying to reassure Amy, who knew some Russian, that that fact made little difference. As the tiresome father, I was being eased further and further away from the center of this conversation. By the time I extricated my beautiful seventeen year old, it was time to look for supper and a hotel.

Banska Bystrica entered history August 29, 1944, as the center of the Slovak national uprising. Unlike the fighters in the Warsaw Powstanie, the Slovak rebels were Communist, as were a large contingent of French war prisoners who joined the battle from somewhere. The uprising began with murderous revenge against Slovak and Hungarian collaborators, but its main purpose was to attack the retreating Wehrmacht units strongly enough from the rear to allow Petrov's 4th Ukrainian Front to make a breakthrough. The

Russians could claim, as they did before Warsaw, that they had outrun supply and that their soldiers were badly battle worn. Nevertheless, in the same way they were willing to sit quietly on the east bank of the Vistula while the Germans wiped out the Polish Home Army, they were tempted not to push too hard in Slovakia. Even if those partisans were Communist, it was wiser to have Eastern Europe liberated by the Red Army alone and avoid the messiness of Yugoslavia where Tito's forces claimed too much of the credit. The revolt was liquidated by late October, with Himmler's SS handling a sadistic pacification.*

Save for those few weeks Banska Bystrica lived an existence painted in simple colors. Austrian oppression had at least led Bohemia and Moravia into German-speaking Europe. The Hungarian oppression of Slovakia led nowhere. Lajos Kossuth, the flaming freedom-fighter for Hungarian rights in 1849, could not understand what the words meant if challenged on Slovak rights. Primary schooling in their wretched language was the most they could expect—and probably a waste of time and money.† Between 1900 and 1914 over 15% of the total Slovak population emigrated to Pittsburgh, Bethlehem, Gary, Cleveland, Chicago. In Masaryk's republic Slovakia was supposedly the equal other half but was treated as New Yorkers would the peasant world of Mississippi, which exacted a high price by the time that Vaclav Havel had become president.

My children and I traveled across the High Tatras and north through Poland to Sominy, some miles southwest of Gdańsk. It sat on a sandy plain, a checkerboard of potato fields and pine forests sheltering deer and boar. Boiled potatoes and eggs with bread were the daily dish, sliced cucumbers in sour cream and a piece of meat on Sunday. Paper in the local privy was from a Polish-Russian grammar. Bruce looked apprehensive as his sister and father prepared to leave, but for the two little Woźniakowska girls it was like having a large teddy bear who made no comprehensible sound but was docile and good natured when pushed or pulled, and whose name of Bruczik could be declined in amusing ways: Bruczkom (with . . .), Bruczku (to . . .).

Amy and I drove southwest to the dark brown Hohenzollern cities of Posen/Poznań and Breslau/Wrocław§ and then back across the border to Olomouc.

---

* John Erickson, *Op. cit.*, pp. 290–307.

† "Teach a Nigruh to read and you spoil a good bean picker"—Deep South proverb.

§ Breslau, with Poles to the north and Czechs to the south, was a strongly German city sympathetic to the Nazis and was smashed to pieces in the terrible fighting between Wehrmacht and Red Army in early 1945. When Poland was shoved westward after Yalta, it was rebuilt as Wrocław. An interesting detail was the large Greek Catholic church for Ukrainian fugitives from Lwow and the other lost lands east of Zamość and Lublin who had always resented the Poles but feared the Russians and who leapfrogged traditional Poland to settle the new German territories.

My visits in that city were to be at the large house in the featureless pre-1914 inner suburbs that Jiři inherited from his father-in-law. The old town is a Central European collage dating back here and there to a tower or a gateway from the eleventh century Přemyslid dynasty, then to the arrogant monuments of High Baroque before settling into the yellow-stuccoed streets of Maria Theresa's time and the comfortable style of provincial Habsburg. When Olomouc's fortifications were razed in the 1880s, parks and gardens, bordered by geraniums and petunias, with ponds in the charge of ducks and swans, were developed for Sunday afternoon promenades and band concerts shaded by horse chestnut trees. Around the main square before the town hall were the bourgeois shops of the nineteenth century. All of this had been absorbed without the slightest visible disharmony into one of the strictest Communist systems in Europe.

Many important individuals have wandered through this neighborhood. Agents of the Austrian Mozart industry print out constant publicity releases about Salzburg and Vienna, though it was Prague where he was really appreciated. Without Olomouc, however, his genius would have been lost forever. In December 1767 eleven-year-old Wolfgang fled there from a smallpox epidemic in Vienna with his father and sister. She caught the disease anyway, which spoiled her complexion forever, but he was saved by the bishop's physician.

Lafayette, Washington's beloved mascot in our Revolution but out of his depth in the French, was held prisoner in the city's fortress (Kazamaty) from 1794 to 1797 by the Austrians. (Lafayette Ulice is a short street, once a gypsy hangout.) It was to Archduke Rudolf Habsburg (also archbishop of Olomouc) that Beethoven dedicated both his great trio and the *Missa Solemnis*. Smetana and Dvořak visited often. Mahler conducted the opera there in 1886, as difficult to get along with as he would be in Vienna. Sigmund Freud, also born in Moravia, served on military maneuvers nearby in the 1880s and during the long afternoons of Austrian army life had the leisure in which to invent the Oedipus Complex.

Masaryk's father, a Slovak, was a coachman at a neighboring royal estate. Perhaps like Emiliano Zapata, another revolutionary who started life as a stableboy, Tomaš realized that the horses were more highly valued than the humans who looked after them. His mother, of German background, came from Brno. Tomaš learned her language and, although he was apprenticed first as a blacksmith, was a brilliant enough student to win a scholarship to an outstanding academic gymnasium in Vienna.* (Habsburg Austria showed more concern for encouraging brilliant poor boys than present-day United States does. Intellectual distinction is undemocratic.) Masaryk went on to study philosophy at the university there, disrupted by nationality conflicts and anti-Semitism, and then at Leipzig. In 1882, at the age of 32, he was appointed professor of philosophy at the newly constituted Czech-language part of Charles University, but, coming from a remote Moravian village, educated outside Bohemia, with an American wife (Charlotte Garrigue from Brooklyn), he was always an outsider in Prague's academic and political circles.

On the stage of Big History, Olomouc escaped the Hussite wars that tore Bohemia apart during the fifteenth century. Religious turbulence and the extermination of the Czech nobility by the Habsburgs and the Counter Reformation after the battle of the White Mountain in 1620 were less bloody in Moravia. On the other hand, the Swedes, whom we think of today as moderate, progressive people who enjoy well-made furniture and soft-core porn, were comparable in the seventeenth century to the Mongols and during the 30 Years' War they sacked Olomouc and burned its university library. In Maria Theresa's time a sophisticated fortification in French style had been built around the city as a protection against any threat to Vienna from the north. Therefore, when the Prussian armies of Frederick the Great, who saw the Austrian empire as a sort of stranded whale to be parceled out at his convenience, besieged it in 1758, they failed.

In 1805, when Napoleon occupied Vienna after his victory at Ulm, the Austrian armies and their Russian allies, including Emperor Franz and Tsar Alexander, withdrew to the safety of Olmütz's† fortress. Tolstoy as his guide, an educated reader follows the armies to Austerlitz, witnesses wounded Prince Andrey's detachment from the irrelevancy of war, measures Tolstoy's conclusion that victory does not go to the army with better leadership but to the first side that cries out, "We've won!" After the battle an arrogant little gang of fifty of Napoleon's soldiers appeared before the fortress gates to demand the surrender of its 10,000 men, but this was too much for the Austrians to swallow.

Then after Metternich's government collapsed in 1848, it was to safe and sober Olmütz that the court machinery transferred itself for the ceremony of replacing helpless Ferdinand the Good with the young Franz Josef. One

* As he remarked to Karel Čapek, the writer and a close friend during his last years, since the Moravian boys had to learn German in order to enter secondary school, they were older than their German and Jewish classmates and therefore stronger in soccer and fights and with more sexual adventures to brag about.

† German spelling

thinks of poor Richard Nixon at the end of his reign, who hoped to find some archetypal elm-shaded college where he could mingle freely and ask the wholesome students how the football season was coming along.

A new monarch could not be allowed to change—could not think of changing—an old Austria, and that Austria's military machine was smashed in 1866 at Sadova, about 25 miles northwest of Olomouc. Von Moltke's Prussians had better training and abler officers, as had been true a century before under Frederick the Great. They also had a beautifully efficient mobilization schedule connected with a rationalized railway system that could concentrate troops from all over Germany to overwhelm Austria, and at Sedan, Louis Napoleon's France. Out of the American Civil War just ended, Von Moltke had learned the importance of the railroad and the telegraph so that from Berlin he could control the three armies that crossed the Austrian borders.

The Habsburg concept of war, archaic armies in handsome uniforms led by princely amateurs, was ended by Von Moltke's clockwork precision. Sadova gave the Prussians the experience and the confidence to defeat the French in 1870. That in turn gave them the confidence, more than that, the hubris of Greek tragedy, to believe they could defeat any enemy—as the American military organization that had beaten the Germans and Japanese knew it could defeat the Vietnamese. Which meant that the most fitting monument for Sadova was the mass graves around Verdun and the Somme, 1916, and the end of traditional Germany. More deadly in the long run, the interlocking gears of Von Moltke's mobilization schedule, copied, as best they could, by the general staff of every other nation, the individual reservist picking up his jacket, his boots, his rifle, his cartridges, the local battalion being fitted into regiment, division, army corps, the time-tables arranged, as the supreme achievement of the Western mind, so that the train carrying the 147th regiment of the 18th Prussian division crossed the Köln railway bridge over the Rhine (the ultimate bottleneck—it would have been infinitely worth while for a French hero to have blown it up) at 2:14 A.M. on the twelfth day after general mobilization, and not four minutes later or earlier—all these gears were so precisely fitted together, disciplined by the perfectly accurate watches that each officer held in his hand, that they could not be interrupted.

At one moment in late July of 1914 a spasm of good sense struck Wilhelm II: might Germany actually lose this coming war, might the possible victory not be worth the probable cost? He raised the topic with another Helmuth von Moltke, the great man's less-than-great nephew, in turn chief of the general staff. The general was reduced to hysteria. *The machinery could not be halted.*

The imperial army would be reduced to chaos. Every general, every officer would resign. Every tradition, every value upon which Imperial Germany was based would collapse. Including, Your Highness, the throne. Wilhelm gave in.

As my career as headmaster was coming to an end, one reason for my skepticism about curriculum came out of my contact with Olomouc. This unexciting provincial city that I had happened upon by accident, that I came to know through one young friend, Jiři Kořinek, was an archetypal Habsburg, Central European city. To know its history thoroughly was to gain a sharper set of lenses for examining any city's crises of ethnic conflict, economic change, and the interrelationships of politics, culture, and morality. In a school some subjects are more important than others, nevertheless, the priority is not the subjects themselves but how well they are taught. To know Olomouc is to know the world.

Most of the time, however, the sociologist is busier than the tragedian.

At the beginning is the village, its feet deep in what Karl Marx saw as the idiocy of rural life. The mother prayed, as in traditional black Mississippi, that her son might not be too clever or her daughter too beautiful so that he did not make trouble with the police or she become the landlord's whore. At one end of the street was the church, at the other the manor house. Perhaps the inn—beer and wine, slivovitz from plums (though not the Russian-Polish curse of vodka), later on the school. Traditional objectives were how to avoid the tax collector and recruiting sergeant, how to keep girls from getting pregnant. A rich tradition of music and dance, though the furiant of Bohemia and Moravia was no protector of chastity, of dress and embroidery and festival (the costumes I remember on the drive from Vienna to Prague in 1939 beyond the truckloads of SS troops). A few Jewish peddlers and gypsies.

Beyond the village, in the fortress town of Olmütz, with its merchants, shopkeepers, artisans, its officials and garrison officers, anyone with any education was German speaking. And as Poles and Hungarians enjoyed repeating, no one fitted into the rhythms of Kakania—love of hierarchy and the properly arranged file cabinet, formality and obedience rewarded by a pension—more loyally than the Czechs.

History, as usual, moved in two directions. One was towards gradual industrialization. Milling and distilling, the first factories for textiles and shoes to replace and eventually destroy village crafts, utilizing the surplus labor of those villages. As those former peasants became factory workers, and as Olmütz itself rapidly expanded, once the barrier ring of fortifications had been torn down in the late 1870s, to incorporate the surrounding villages, then the other question of the city's ethnic identity arose. If Czech families wanted secondary education for their sons (girls could wait), was it available only in German? If a workman got into trouble with the law, were all the procedures in a language foreign to him? And if Czechs were beginning to graduate from their own secondary schools (which came to include Slovak boys whose families could not tolerate the straitjacket of Hungarian education), then there should be better quality jobs awaiting them. (One of the first professions Czechs moved into, as did blacks in Mississippi, was undertaking.)

"Olmütz may be small but must be German!" Which side would control the Rathaus/Radnice? Again we are back in Mississippi, now in the 1970s and 1980s. The introduction of universal manhood suffrage (the Habsburg version of the Civil Rights Act of 1964) in 1907 made it harder than ever for the German minority to hold on to authority. Olmütz's Jewish population grew in size and wealth during the second half of the century, in 1890 built its own synagogue in Moorish style, and, aided by their wealth, Jews were able to enter the town council, where probably they voted with the Germans.*

When war came in 1914, the first goal for German Austrians was to punish the Serbs, and then to discipline all the Slavic minorities of the Austrian and Hungarian lands, and beyond them the Russians—even if this meant accepting Lutheran Prussians as allies. The Czechs obeyed orders in a passive way, but with a common enemy in both Austrian and Prussian Germanism it was possible for them to see the Russians as Slavic brothers. On occasion when Czech troops opposed Russians on the Galician front, whole regiments, banners flying, bands playing, marched across to the other side.

In the provincial museum of Klagenfurt, Carinthia, I remember a painting of Franz Josef on his knees praying for his brave soldiers, while above, in the sky, a dense mass of infantry make a bayonet attack. The peasant soldiers of those bayonet attacks had been slaughtered, or barb-wired in Russian prison camps, at any rate taken from their fields, and the cities were beginning to starve. Now it was the German-speaking Austrians who lapsed into passivity while the Czechs involved themselves in secret societies and street demonstrations.

On November 11, 1918, Olomouc's German town council resigned, and the next week a committee of Czechs took over the Radnice.

---

* The material on Moravia and Olomouc comes mainly from Dr. Jaroslav Peprnik of Palacky University in Olomouc.

How do you create a new nation? There was much to be said for the Empire: a common market from Polish Galicia to the Romanian and Italian borders, a common railway and banking network. Under Austrian management, if you played by the rules, things went pretty well. Now, if any disturbance threatened Central Europe's economy, the new tariff walls were certain to make things worse. For Olomouc, industrial capital of central Moravia, the depression came later but lasted longer, with 3200 unemployed in 1935 out of a total population of about 60,000. In the Sudeten coal, steel, and glass towns on the northern borders, the depression was even worse, and their German inhabitants protested that the authorities in Prague showed little concern.

Out of that misery grew Konrad Henlein's Sudeten Nazi movement, contemptuous of 'this dwarf nation of domestic servants, village musicians, and postal clerks', even if strongly opposed by German-speaking Socialists and Communists. After the loss in October 1938 of the Sudetenland borders and their fortifications (built at tremendous cost, aided by French financing, in the 1920s), there was a sense of demoralization. Beneš was replaced by the weak and ailing Hacha, Slovakia was controlled by the Catholic fascists under Father Tiso, the Germans in Olomouc and nearby villages created the chaos that gave Hitler the excuse of announcing the occupation of the remnants of Bohemia and Moravia on March 14. The country disintegrated. Poles joined the feeding frenzy by occupying the border city of Tešin, Hungarians seized a large strip of southern Slovakia and the mountain valleys of Ruthenia.

Nevertheless, this takeover by Hitler was a deadly mistake. The Sudeten victory in October had given him all the prestige he could want: The Czechs were finished, the demoralized West groveled before his promise that this was his last demand. That March grab shocked Chamberlain into facing the utter hopelessness of appeasement. On March 31 he gave a guarantee to the Poles that should the Germans invade, Britain would fight. War and all that followed became inevitable.*

How did this disintegration of the Czech state and of civil life affect, week by week, the Jewish community? In 1939 the synagogue was destroyed. Under what circumstances? By whom? In what sort of sequence did the Jews become pushed first to the edge, then out of society? Most of the 2000 ended their lives at Auschwitz, 80 miles northwest. Who survived? Were any children sheltered, as in Amsterdam, as even in Warsaw? No Anne Frank wrote a diary. Gentile witnesses kept silent. The Czech world is an ahistorical one, as I have found even in working on this book. In a society where a diary, a collection of letters, an anecdote recalled within hearing of the wrong

* Joseph Rothschild, *Op. cit.*, 1974 p. 134.

person, even evidence of supporting state policy when that policy suddenly changes—we are close to *1984*—reveal more about your actions or opinions 10, 30 years ago than is wise, it is safer to have no contacts with the past. Talk about sports and the weather. Spend your leisure working in the garden.

Yes, there used to be Jews. The Germans sent them to Auschwitz.

On one of my visits Jiři took me around the Jewish graveyard. I have seen Jewish graveyards in Kraków and Lublin, sad because they are the last monuments of poor and forgotten people, they mark the end of a 600-year-old society, and have been vandalized by hooligans. The graveyard at Olomouc was for affluent people. The massive stones, with most of the inscriptions in German, were often of highly polished, expensive black marble. If these people had lived in Boston, their children would have gone to my school. There was no sign of vandalism. The cemetery, though, was completely overgrown. Tall grass, bushes, even small trees grew out of the plots. The two acres are taboo.

Step by step the Czechs, like the Jews, found their city taken away from them. The Gestapo, with cooperation from the local Germans, went into action, registering, constraining, and eventually deporting the Jews while rooting out any possible anti-Nazi opposition as well. Cautious grumbling was the response: "How can I keep my job and stay out of trouble?" The Polish campaign came and went in September 1939. Save for the annihilation of Yugoslavia and Greece, Eastern Europe was carefully quiet until the invasion of Russia June 21, 1941.

Some amateurish resistance appeared briefly, some sabotage—emery dust in the gears, sugar in the gas tank, the cutting of a power line. This was inconvenient, but the prompt arrest, deportation, or execution of bystanders made heroism unpopular.

In Poland this conversion into a slave society had occurred after a short but terrible military defeat: bombing and artillery, ruined bridges and burning towns, dead horses and endless columns of prisoners. There had been a war and Poland had been beaten. In Olomouc and in the whole of Czechoslovakia the change had come without a shot fired. The street signs were replaced by ones in German, but the same policeman might still be directing traffic at the corner. When the Weintraubs' apartment became empty, someone else immediately occupied it. Aloys Schmidt, the butcher, says 'Heil Hitler' when you enter his store, and you take care not to offend him. How do you act?

May 1945. The Red Army arrives from the east. Olomouc is one of the last cities taken on its final advance to Prague. The battle lasts only a few days, pushing out the disheartened Wehrmacht units, the city suffering relatively little damage and few civilian casualties. Russian looting and raping in the villages came mainly, as in Vienna, from second-line troops. Within a year, carrying not much more than the clothes they wear, Aloys Schmidt (if he is still alive) and his family are shoved across the border of Saxony, part of the German Democratic Republic, or into Austria. Does that also happen to Hanna Regler, of a German-speaking family that always voted Socialist, whose husband was arrested by the Gestapo and who died at Buchenwald? That may depend on how influential and how loyal her friends are.

"I fought against the Hitlerite Fascists—here are my scars."

"Yes, but did you fight for bourgeois nationalism or for proletarian solidarity?"

Whatever the mix of state structure and action set up by the Beneš government, it is replaced, step by step, after February 1948 by Gottwald's Communists. But still the surface remains unchanged—the geranium beds in the public garden, the charming little streets from Maria Theresa's time, the beer drinkers in the pubs. Hitlerstrasse. Lenin Ulica.

The difference between surface and reality might lead to a silent madness. I will burn down the church, pull up the geraniums, shoot the swans. Set myself on fire. Turn on the radio and open another beer.

⁓∞⁓

The stage becomes smaller, with homier props, and my picture of hard-line Communism limits itself to monthly letters and visits every so often to the gray stucco house on Žilinska Ulica. Mary and I pay a brief call in 1978 when Jiři and Vera can show off six-year-old Jana and three-year-old Jirka. The house still is in the name of her parents, and we eat intricately arranged salami and sip tiny glasses of slivovitz. It will be an act of hospitality to drive us to Kraków (about three hours) across the Těšin crossing point, but both of them are nervous in Poland and despite our urging refuse to eat a hurried lunch at the *Francuski*. Poland has a reputation for heresy. Is it catching? Will people talk?

Upon Jaruzelski's imposition of martial law in 1981, after the efforts to reach out and share the making of a freer society had been brutally frustrated, Poles retreated into themselves. I had the feeling, however, that despite the cheerful friendliness I always received, Jiři had led his whole life within a silence: the more people you know, the greater chance for trouble. And as Jana and Jirka grew from children into adolescents, reaching out to a wider world and questioning the rules of the family fortress, their father's sense of insecurity increased.

I return in 1983 on a side trip from Prague, with three days for conversation. Jiři has the technical school title of Engineer and started off working for the pump factory, one of Olomouc's export plants. As designer and troubleshooter he had made a couple of trips to Russia, a dour country he disliked. An exciting trip might be one to Nairobi, where cheaper Czech products compete with German and British ones, but it is given to a rival "who doesn't know enough English to find his way to the WC," a Party member. The all too typical corner-cutting, where traditional Czech standards of a job well done are betrayed, angered Jiři, and he resigned and took a lower-paying job teaching industrial drawing at a high school. There is not a Communist or non-Communist way to draw a heating duct. Perhaps he will be left alone.

The big compromises can be tolerated. After all, no one made a conscious decision to put Czechoslovakia in Central Europe with the Germans on one side and the Russians on the other. That is unavoidable, but there is no hiding place from the petty compromises.

Elena appears in class wearing a crucifix. When the period ends, Jiři calls her to his desk. She has the constitutional right to wear a crucifix, but if she does so three or four times that fact will be put on her record card, she will never have a chance to enter the university, and she will finish her days as a factory worker or shop girl.

"Talk this over with your parents." (I have been sending Jiři's children Christmas books set in a small-town English church, where a patient orange cat named Samson is the long-suffering father figure for a crowd of foolish mice—is that religious propaganda, is someone keeping track?) The compulsory weekly classes in Marxist Leninism are led by the school's most boring teacher. While he drones away the students study their physics, write letters, do crossword puzzles, nap. This is no accident. An interesting teacher would encourage questions, and some youngster might ask about the differences between socialist theory and daily practice.

A colleague makes a dumb classroom joke about Lenin. A parent writes an anonymous complaint to the director, described as a decent guy. He calls in the teacher. "I don't like this habit of anonymous complaints. Tell me it's false and I'll tear up the letter and we'll never mention the subject again." Silence. "It was a dumb joke, but I don't tell lies." Twenty-four hours later the teacher is an assistant truck driver. There is no need for terror.

Jiři's Jana has a serious eye problem and needs a major operation. Under universal health insurance, this is free, of course, but who will perform the operation: the department head or a senior resident looking for an educational experience? Jana's grandfather goes to the hospital with a month's salary in a sealed envelope that he gives to the surgeon's secretary. Meanwhile Jirka, 7 now, slices his thumb with a rusty knife. There is no penicillin. A friend tells Jiři to buy a black market bottle of Johnny Walker Red Label, worth $35 (equal to eight jars of Nescafé), and he will give it to the right person. Next day comes a phone call: "Pan Kořinek, we just happen to have found some penicillin. Send your boy right around."

"You could go mad," he says as he forces himself to tell me story after story.

The work discipline in his classroom is nothing to be proud of. At seventeen too many of the students already spend their evenings hanging out, smoking and drinking together in the pubs, listening to Heavy Metal. (No drugs yet—one advantage of a police state.) Nevertheless, final exams come in two weeks. At least now they should put in some effort. "OK, I work hard and I become an engineer like you. I don't work and I drive a garbage truck. Each way I get the same salary. So what?"

Marx and Lenin have freed the proletariat from servitude to the wage system.

The kids who come from the palisades-like housing projects at the edge of the city, where they grow up with no sense of community or responsibility, with both parents always away at work (maybe they'll earn enough together to buy a car someday), can be difficult to fit in.

"What's wrong? You've been looking awfully troubled recently." Stefan is startled. All his life he has been given orders and then bawled out for not obeying them. No one has ever asked him what's wrong.

What sort of a country is this? What can we be proud of? What will the children grow up to have? Our best tennis players are very good. Our best musicians. That shows. The Party cares a lot about the surface. But who teaches kids to tell the truth?

> *Over the house spreads*
> *the eczema of twilight,*
> *the evening news bulletin*
> *creeps across the façades*
> *the beefburger is singing*
>   Miroslav Holub *Evening Idyll with a Protoplasm*

16

Budapest 1937, 1939, 1964, 1990

I no longer believe
what I believed once
But the fact that I have believed . . .
that I compel myself
day by day to recall
And I do not forgive anyone.
      Gyorgy Petri *By an unknown poet from Eastern Europe, 1955*

THE TWO MOST EXHILARATING events of the 1950s were the unanimous decision of Earl Warren's Supreme Court in 1954 to outlaw segregation in the public schools and the 1956 Hungarian uprising. In both cases the entrenched forces of oppression and lies seemed defeated, the forces of reason, decency and courage to have won. It was a hot June afternoon when I heard the news walking down a street in Kirkwood, Missouri, the nearest town to Thomas Jefferson School where I was a teacher, and I remember the smile on my face, my desire to stop strangers and shake their hands and say, "We did it! Aren't you proud to be an American?"

Budapest—in the beginning was the poet. As resentment began to grow against the leaden-footed rule of Matyas Rákosi, Party boss since 1948, university students formed the Petofi Circle, honoring the young poet who had been hanged by the Austrians in 1849 for his fiery defense of Hungarian freedom. (Forget for a moment the Slovaks and Croats.) Like Mickiewicz, he was safely dead.

Nevertheless, when his poems against Austrian tyranny were recited, the listeners made their own additions. Next came the demand for rehabilitation of Laszlo Rajk, a Communist who had fought in Spain (Stalin did not trust 'Spaniards'), and who, though a hard-line Minister of the Interior in the post-war years, had been arrested by Rákosi as a Titoist and hanged in 1949. Khrushchev's sacrifice of the hated Rákosi in June did not slow the acceleration of demands, which widened to liquidation of the secret police and insistence by workers upon their own labor unions (as with Solidarity in the Gdańsk shipyard at the end of the 1970s), until Imre Nagy, the new liberal

Party head, included multiparty democracy and withdrawal from the Warsaw Pact, accompanied by the destruction of Stalin's monster statue on the hills of Buda. Each detail was more than ever could have been expected. *They* could be beaten!

Of course, both sets of hopes were doomed. Eisenhower was not interested in any real change; he kept the assumptions he had grown up with in Abilene. Congress was afraid of public opinion. The administration of *Brown v. Topeka Board of Education* was carried on by the courts, by dogged local boards of education, and by blacks and their white allies who fought to change the country's way of looking at democratic words. Perhaps it was just as well that blacks had to fight for their rights and weren't simply handed them by kindly whites. Perhaps it was a way for some churches to prove that Christianity still had a role to play in American life.

In Hungary it was too much to expect that the Communists could accept such a series of demands. Red Army tank units came back to Budapest, suffered losses from firebombs thrown by boys who had seen too many movies about blowing up German tanks, experienced their hardest fighting against workers in the Csepel auto works, but there was never any doubt.* Nagy took refuge in the Yugoslav embassy, was lured out by a formal promise of safe conduct by Janos Kadar, his successor, handed over to the Russians and more or less passed from hand to hand until given a secret trial and hanged on June 17, 1958.

Thucydides has the Athenians state in his *History of the Peloponnesian War* concerning the protests of the Melian islanders: those with power carry out the measures they will; those without have to endure what they must.

When I came to Budapest in 1964 with Amy and Bruce there were still necklaces of machine gun bullet holes on some of the walls—tourist attractions. In 1937, on my cousin's Grand Tour, I had spent a night at an elegant hotel overlooking the Danube. In 1939 Bruce Barton and I had visited the city twice on our way to and from Bucharest and Sofia. Pest, on the east bank, destroyed again and again by the Turks, and expanded at top speed by commercial and industrial prosperity during the years before 1914 (a district of railroads and stockyards assumed the name of Chicago), is not a beautiful city in comparison with Vienna and Prague. There is the Danube and its bridges, the life of hotels and restaurants (goose livers with paprika), cafés

---

* Alexander Wat, *Op. cit.*, p. 100, quotes Khruschchev's interesting explanation in 1963 for the slaughter he wreaked: "Under Nicholas I Russian troops suppressed a revolution in Budapest in 1848, and we had to wipe that stain from our honor and suppress counter-revolution."

and shops ("the wedding present capital of the world") if you have money and know where to go. (The gypsy fiddler stares deep into the eyes of the German tourist and awakens a lifetime of forbidden emotions.) Within a country that never had a viable democratic tradition, Budapest's most flamboyant edifice is the neo-Gothic parliament.

In 1964 our host was a young orthopedic surgeon, Tamas Farkas, who had thumbed a ride on the bus that two years before was carrying its load of Commonwealth students from Kraków to Warsaw. He had been intrigued by American personality and stayed with the group as it pilgrimaged around the Polish capital. Now he became our guide, which included a trip to Eger, 60 miles east, to a wine cooperative whose director sold bottles for his personal profit to visitors like ourselves. The day had been spent in laughing and cynical conversation, but as we said goodbye Tamas turned serious. "No articles." What? "No articles in any magazine, any!" The Hungarian state, so corrupt, so incompetent, maintained a very effective radar network about any article in any language written about it. When was the author in Budapest, where did he stay, with whom might he have spoken (hotel desk staff kept careful records), and after that it was not too difficult to track down the native who had spoken too freely.

In May 1990 my standard visit to Olomouc and Prague began in Budapest, to provide another line of sight. A third-rate hotel room costs $100, a haircut twenty-five cents. A newsstand carries a Hungarian edition of *Penthouse*, one example of capitalist joint enterprises. I go into a huge delicatessen: a jar of paté will make a luxury present in Warsaw. No clerk speaks either German or English. I strut and hiss like a goose, clutch at my liver, chop it into a paté, pack it into a round can. Just before the phone call is placed for men in white coats, someone catches on. Too expensive. I take my meals—salami, coffee, tokay, chocolate éclairs—at the Café New York, where men at the round marble tables used to wear stiff collars, derby hats, and great turned-up moustaches. In a passageway stands a thin, tired woman offering a not very good piece of red embroidery for sale, a Transylvanian refugee. That style of embroidery helped give the Hungarians under Romanian rule their identity.

I meet up with Dr. Farkas, who guides me around the pretty little Maria Theresa streets of Buda, past the stands of drawings and water colors where one can lay in inexpensive Christmas presents. From the bastion on top of the hill we look across the Danube to Pest. A huge red star still remains on top of one of the ministries. Everyone wants to take it down, but it would be a shame to have something that expensive go to waste. Aren't there still left-wing millionaires in Los Angeles?

Tamas gives me the recipe for success in the old system, two out of the following three: professional skill, Party membership, personal connections. You were out of luck if your surgeon possessed only the latter two, but skill by itself was not enough. The symbol of change had been the ceremonial reburial, June 16, 1989, 31 years after his hanging, of the remains of Imre Nagy, but it is hard sometimes to insist that the rules have really changed. Every single social unit—a hospital section, a factory floor, a ballet school, a soccer team—had its police informer who gave a regular report on every colleague, and these people still go around their daily lives.

On the other hand, during the war Hungary might have been a fascist country, but it had protected as well as oppressed its own Jews. Artists, journalists, intellectuals of Budapest had intermarried quite freely. Many an improvident noble had saved the family estate by encouraging his son to marry the beautiful, dark-haired daughter of a Jewish banker. It was a more mixed society than the Nazis were expecting. When the SS took over the country in 1944 a pattern of camouflage had been established, and though thousands of Jews perished at Auschwitz, more survived in Hungary than in any other Central-European land. Budapest is the only city that retains anything of its old Jewish culture along with a vibrant anti-Semitism.

∽

It is unfair for Americans to criticize Germans, Czechs, Hungarians for their docility. When the circumstances are correct, Americans are just as easy to manage. In 1973 my wife and I took four months off to go on a journey from Manila to Istanbul, associated vaguely with the Harvard School of Public Health, which included time in Dhahran and Teheran. Saudi Arabia did not grant visas to Jews, so my visit began with a letter from the dean of the Divinity School stating that Charles and Mary had enjoyed a traditional Christian upbringing. The Saudi monarchy and its ministers exercised unlimited authority, but the rules were enforced by the Arabian American Oil Company, whose guests, though no one knew exactly why, we were.

The executive staff and their families lived in little Pasadena bungalows, while transients like ourselves stayed in a dormitory flown untouched from the campus of San José State; and in this undemanding environment the mechanism of control was as firm as in Olomouc. Don't mention Israel, on the maps simply a blank space. Don't use alcohol. (From Aramco's many laboratories, of course, there was a cottage industry in distilling 'white' and 'brown' for cocktail parties.) Be careful in the sort of reading material you leave around. The men could wrap themselves in their jobs—I ran across a former student who had learned fluent Arabic—but life was a misery for the wives.

The Holy Quran forbids women to drive automobiles, so if they wanted to take the children to the beach, they had to make arrangements with a Company driver. Shopping in Hofuf and Dammam was interesting but not encouraged (better to stick with the Company's supermarket—even from there really careful housewives washed their lettuce in Clorox), but though the weather in March was still like California, it was forbidden to garden. Saudi women did no physical labor, and it made them nervous to see foreigners of their social class who did, so on lovely spring mornings the wives stayed indoors and watched their Yemeni gardeners tend the flower beds. A few became interested in archaeology and shared adventurous expeditions deep into the desert, a few learned Bedouin weaving and embroidery skills or tried to volunteer in public health service. Anything useful, however, was performed by Egyptians and Palestinians, and for an American woman to want to teach, anything, was resented as lady-bountiful colonialism or as inadmissible criticism of Saudi values. Better to play bridge, invite friends to tea, read novels, beat one's head against the wall. A few years after our visit American women could not leave the Aramco compound unless completely veiled.

There was a primary school for Company children, with Arabs and a few Germans as well as Americans, and pictures of Snoopy and King Feisal on the walls. Probably from deliberate policy there was no secondary school, to eliminate trouble-making teenagers, who were sent to boarding schools at home, in England, or to a progressive school near Hyderabad.

As a historian I was intrigued by the interworking of authority and assumption, and mentioned to one senior American my plan to write an article on this unusual community. Very nice, and it would be easy for me to have it checked by someone at New York headquarters. He was surprised and a bit hurt when I replied that I wouldn't.

Years later I found the correct adjective, used to describe what is done to calm aggressive dogs. It was a castrated society.

The habits lasted. During George Bush's Jihad against Saddam Hussein, the Americans in Saudi Arabia went along with royal policy to spare local sensibilities by permitting only minimal recognition of these infidel mercenaries. It was the Saudi air force and tank columns, infantry too, that broke the Iraqi invaders. The Americans smiled politely.

A bit later, in 1973, Mary and I spent a couple of weeks in Iran. There was not the smothering Saudi-Aramco totalitarianism—"You have a good deal of freedom so long as you don't criticize the Shah"—but the game was more dangerous. One more disciple of the great headmaster, Josef II, the Shah was going to modernize, westernize, secularize Iran, expunge the concept, the very words of humiliation and inferiority from the political dictionary, and together with his beautiful empress create a glorious state.

The oil and cautious conservatism of Saudi Arabia, the oil and dynamic forcefulness of Iran made these two states the cornerstones of American policy in the Middle East. The Shah was the source of fascinating rumors. He had paid *Time* magazine to be chosen as Man of the Year. He had paid $500,000 to the Committee to Re-elect the President in 1972 to have Nixon stop in Teheran on his way back from Beijing and show the world's respect for the nation and its ruler. Every so often a planeload of beautiful young Parisians, of both sexes, would land discretely at his private airport to help him relax. He had a firm understanding of Machiavelli—it is good to be loved, it is better to be feared—and critics who had forgotten how dangerous it was to displease him were invited to dial a certain phone number where they could listen to the screams of wrong-headed people being tortured by his secret police, the Savak.

Even more than the Saudis he saw the need for a crash program of education by which to train a new ruling class. In the early 1970s American academia was not in healthy shape, and there were many not-fully employed professors from even the finest universities who were excited to be offered a post in Iran. Hard work, good pay and eager students, cheap servants, available drugs,* a place in history's forward march, a reinvigorated career. Perhaps a couple of details: be careful what friends you choose, don't ask the wrong questions. If the full machinery of American Staatsmacht did not catch the hollowness of the Shah's power—the corruption, sycophancy, lethal jealousies of his court and its vulgar display, the large sections of the body politic, like the peasantry and the Moslem fundamentalists, ignored— could an associate professor from Cornell be blamed?

Then when the whole system blew up in the faces of the Shah and President Carter, and our country had to confront the dangerous combination of Islamic fervor and a powerful military force armed with American training and equipment, it suddenly seemed wise for the philosopher princes of the State Department to build up a counterweight in Iraq.

---

* Pre-party caution: "Go ahead and smoke marijuana if you like, but don't mix it with opium."

17

Olomouc 1990, 1991

For where would we be
if love were not stronger than poetry
and poetry stronger than love?
  Miroslav Holub *United Flight 1011*

I TAKE THE BUDAPEST-BERLIN express through flat, featureless landscape to
Bratislava. In the station a young woman is selling Slovakia decals—a handsome outline of mountains—to stick on your windshield. A dream—a flag,
postage stamps, embassies in Bangkok and Buenos Aires, our own security
police.

I have a room in a modern hotel on the hill. Soft rock hums on every
floor—where am I? Downstairs there is a kitschy eatery with 'folk' motifs
from an L.L. Bean catalogue—Eastern European Peasant Section. After the
total frustration of Hungarian, however, I enjoy forty minutes' self-delusion
that I understand Slovak with the menu and the shop windows.

Bruce Barton and I stopped for lunch in Bratislava (it was easier to cross
borders in Nazi than in Communist Europe) on our drive, late August 1939,
from Budapest to Vienna. We saw the ruins of the synagogue, vandalized and
burnt by Catholic Fascist Slovaks, not by Germans, reality of the New
Europe. I remember a lingerie shop where the bras on display had little
round holes cut in the cups to make the wearers more interesting.

Bratislava (Pressburg to Austrians, Pozsony to Hungarians) was once the
capital of Hungary at a time when parliamentary debates were held in Latin,
a common language for educated representatives of the various nationalities.
Now a four-lane highway extending from the bridge across the Danube has
plowed through one part of the old city, by coincidence wiping out the remnants of the Jewish quarter and what was left of that same synagogue, but
there are still aristocratic and bourgeois streets to enjoy despite the years of
anti-Slovak teaching I have received from Jiři. I listen to a courtyard concert
of eighteenth-century music and stop in a vinarna—light Slovak wine has no
equal ("Yes, they do have nice wine and pretty girls and nice folk music,
but . . .")—to write letters. Beyond the city are horse chestnut–lined suburbs

of Habsburg prosperity, fantasy creations of gables and balconies and semi-peasant pitched roofs. Their owners can hardly be blamed if history walked over them.

The formal purpose of this visit, however, was to call upon the library of Komensky University. My visit to Poland and Czechoslovakia the past November had persuaded me of the need to make some tangible commitment, however limited, to strengthen the process of democratic change since 1989. Maja Woźniakowska had suggested the group of little private schools in Kraków, and now it might be more useful to choose an institution in Slovakia, which receives little Western attention and where there is such resentment against the pushy, grabby Czechs. To provide funds for foreign book purchases for this Slovak National University was a worthwhile goal. If an angry minority has its legitimate demands respected, it begins to act responsibly—from a life spent as a teacher, one of my fundamental beliefs.

At 12:45 Friday the director has quit for the week ("typical"). His secretaries, one kilometer from Austria across the Danube, speak 1% German as I try to explain my interest. The cramped, undistinguished quarters are not encouraging. Would not extra funds simply disappear? Subscriptions to *The National Geographic*, a word processor—anything else?

Jiři meets my train* in Brno. From his letters, I have some idea of how much of November's hopes have leached away. It is not simply higher prices and the threats of Slovak separatism, fueled by the ambitions of Vladimir Mečiar, the boss who would like to see his wife as Minister of Culture and his mistress's brother as ambassador to Germany. And it is not simply that more was expected from Vaclav Havel than any leader could supply. Does he possess the strength of character to make hard decisions forcefully? There is a new selfishness, anxiety, irritability of colleagues and neighbors. Do Czechs behave reasonably only when they have a common enemy? The Communists have been beaten, but they have a patience and discipline that the democrats lack. When things start to go bad will they, under new names, work their way back into power?

I am invited to speak to the faculty of Jiři's school on Rooseveltová Ulica. What did I try to accomplish at Commonwealth? What is there that I know that might be of any value to Czech teachers at this time? If one can speak freely, what does one have to say? That is the question I have brought back home from every visit to this part of the world.

* Nadraží = railroad station. Na zdraví = to your health (as in Polish, na zdrowie). Americans find it hard to tell the words apart. Therefore, in friendly social gatherings, Czechs are puzzled when their new American acquaintance raises his glass and says, "Railroad station."

Meanwhile, the students have mutinied: they will never study Russian again. The economical decision is to recycle all Russian teachers over the summer.

"Goot mornink, leetle cheeldrum. I learn you Aenglish yazik goot, no?"

New joke: angry father inspects son's report card. "But when I went to the WC, Masaryk was the murderer of the working class, and when I came back he was the little father of our country."

Jiři sets up a lunch for me to meet the new rector of Palacky University, named after the great nineteenth century scholar, Frantisek Palacky, whose history of the Czech lands had a tremendous influence in developing national consciousness. Josef Jařab had studied at Harvard ten years previously. He had written a book on black American authors of the twentieth century. He was an engaging, alert, unpretentious man and we immediately hit it off. Czech universities, like the country itself, have been cut off from the international world of the late twentieth century. Their students, even their professors have weak skills in any language except Russian, which everyone is trying to forget as fast as possible. Even if my library project were a success, he told me, there would be few scholars equipped to read foreign books.

There was little real knowledge of the techniques of modern administration, especially in advanced computer use, Dr. Jařab continued. There was poor resourcefulness in serving students with special needs. He gave the example of a woman he admired, a serious student who had broken her spine in a sports accident. Nowhere in the land did there exist an institution that allowed her easy access to the tools of learning.

All right, maybe it was worth while for me to change the direction and the scale of my thinking. Dr. Jařab was exactly the sort of man I had hoped to find. (He was proud that he had not taken refuge abroad after the Warsaw Pact invasion of 1968: "No one was going to drive me out of my own country.")

Everyone wants to do something exciting in Prague, but at a provincial university like Palacky, which had enjoyed a certain reputation for liberalism because it was 100 miles away from Party headquarters, an intelligent and sustained program might have a more significant impact. Where to begin? What contacts did I have? Where could limited resources go farthest? If I put up hard currency for round-trip transportation from Prague and $1000 apiece for a year's personal costs, could I ask American colleges for soft-currency full tuition and then negotiate board and fees? Any professional would recognize as well as I did the value of having one or two students on campus who spoke from the reality of this newly-opened world. It would be no one-way-only enterprise.

It was also true, though it took me time to realize this, that even Dr. Jařab, newly elected by the professors and students, could do surprisingly little to bring about change at Palacky. The Communist Labor Code made dismissals illegal, and because there were limited funds for expanding the faculty, new teachers could not be hired. What went on in the classrooms was pretty much as before, and the students felt cheated. Merrill's tiny scholarship project had to carry a heavy symbolic weight.

For Jitka, the handicapped woman, I thought of a small college in southeastern North Carolina, St. Andrew's Presbyterian, where by sheer chance I had lectured the preceding February. It was a generous, academically responsible school where literally every class and dormitory room was wheelchair accessible. Perhaps they would invite her.

I started with Moravian College in Bethlehem, Pennsylvania, whose president, Roger Martin, I knew well, which had grown out of a seminary begun two-and-a-half centuries ago by German and Czech-speaking members of the Moravian Brotherhood. Today there are more black Moravians in Jamaica and the Bluefields coast of Nicaragua than white Moravians in America and East Germany, but the college maintained a strong sense of its cultural roots and respect for its patron, Jan Komensky (Comenius), the great seventeenth century educator. Dr. Martin agreed to accept two students.

The president of Wheelock, a women's college in Boston that specialized in early childhood education, committed himself to two more. Over the summer of 1990 I mailed out 2500 fund-raising letters: to family, friends, former students, any person I could locate with a connection to either country, which raised about $10,000 for each of the projects in Kraków and Olomouc.

Don't trust anything. As Milada and Lucie were about to leave for the Prague airport, the State Department panicked at the threat of students squeaking their status into that of immigrants and cancelled their visas to Wheelock. For Moravian, David had already built a firm background in computer science. One State Department agency supported the new policy of encouraging capitalism in former Communist countries by backing such students; another agency followed the old rule of deliberately excluding all Iron Curtain computer specialists. It took hard work from the college's Congressman to unravel this K.u.K. bramble patch so that David might show up only two weeks late.

For the second year we knew the rules better. At the Palacky end Dr. Jařab was served by a first-rate administrator, a young Italian-American, a Florentine educated at Swarthmore, who enjoyed taking responsibility until each problem was solved and who treated her overwrought clients with practical kindness. Nevertheless, since these are hard times for American colleges, the costs ran far higher than I had estimated.

Bohumil and Eva entered Moravian, where they profited from the respect that David and Pavlina had won. What surprises Europeans at a good American college is that genuine friendliness, the privilege of calling a professor by his first name, the readiness to reach out and make sure that a student understands, will be combined with a hard-boiled demand for results. Milada and Lucie did make it this time to Wheelock. Šarka went to Quaker Earlham where she enjoyed the mix of small-town Indiana and Chicago, a center of hospitable Czech families, and found her day at the Art Institute the richest esthetic experience of her life.

Lida and Miriam arrived in Atlanta to enroll at Spelman. For two white Europeans to study at an all-black college had its risks, but the president, Johnetta Cole, believed this was an important step for Spelman to take. For Lida the year was demanding but rewarded an innate sense of adventure. She formed a friendship closer than with anyone she had known before with a woman in her dorm who came from a small town in South Carolina, older than the other students because each year at college had to be paid for by a year of work. Miriam was disillusioned by the weak background and discipline of both students and teachers (that can be true—I've taught at Spelman) and the lack of any interest in the culture she brought with her. After a few months she left and transferred to Georgia State. When the fall-out from May's riots in Los Angeles brought dangerous violence to southwestern Atlanta, Lida was moved by the concern of her black friends for her safety. Miriam saw it as proof of the foolishness of the original expectations.

Jitka arrived at St. Andrew's, Lida and Miriam helping her with the transfer at Atlanta's impossible airport. Yes, every room was readily accessible, there was a large swimming pool 200 meters from her bedroom, nobody saw anything strange about a woman moving around in a wheelchair. A German class had rather ordinary students, but the courses in religion and philosophy exposed her to a depth and freedom of enquiry that she had never hitherto experienced. The pathology of poverty and illiteracy of triracial Scotland County was worse than anything one would find in Czechoslovakia.

Why so many women? Czech women are more aggressive? Or men, more involved in science and technology, are locked into Russian, more worried about careers? Or, on the other hand, the project had too little adventure, no cowboys, no far frontier.

1992–1993 Rostislav and Ondřej attended Moravian. The year made Rostislav think he'd enter politics and work for reunification with Slovakia. The College of the Atlantic, a small school in Bar Harbor, Maine, which specializes in the science and economics of environment, a critical field in Czechoslovakia, accepted Dagmar and sent a student in the other direction. The university does offer courses in English on Czech history and culture. If this works out—and why shouldn't fluent Czech be a useful sign of initiative when American career preparation is so standardized?—the whole program can expand. Katerina followed the encouragement of Lida (now studying at the University of Arizona) to enroll at Spelman. The college has a long tradition of international study, not only at European universities, but expanding to São Paulo, Singapore, Dakar, Tokyo, and Harare in Zimbabwe, but Curtrice from Chicago, whose father is black and whose mother is second-generation Czech, will be the first student at a Slavic university. She is worried about racism. Jiři sees no problem in Olomouc but would not advise a black woman to go about alone now in Prague.

For over thirty years I have helped students from Morehouse and Spelman study in Europe; a year in Paris, Madrid, Edinburgh, Vienna was once the opportunity for human freedom impossible for a black in America. The rules change.

⁂

Dr. Jařab had invited me to receive an honorary doctorate from Palacky's school of pedagogy. I thought it proper to reply in Czech, and for that 12-minute speech had been practicing the last couple of months. Jitka Zehnalova at St. Andrews had written the Czech equivalent within my triple-spaced version. The language is harder to pronounce than Russian or Polish. Worse than the expected disdain for vowels is the idiosyncratic syllable stress which effectively prevents most Czechs abroad from ever hearing their names pronounced correctly. Navratilová, the tennis player, introduces the first syllable with a bang, then scurries over the next three to land with both feet on the final a. For linguists who respect precision, an adjective with three genders and six cases, singular and plural, demands the memorization of thirty-six endings. If you wish to go someplace, is it by bicycle or airplane, every morning or once a month, for pleasure with your girlfriend (pritelkine) or on a business trip? Did you finish the trip or turn around because you mislaid your keys? Charming for poets, but a grade-B American will collect a herd of fifty nouns, two dozen adjectives, ten trusty verbs in their simplest forms, yes and no, please and thank you, and more or less limp from here to there.

Palacky headquarters occupies a palace of the archbishop (who wants it back); I join a procession in colored robes and funny hats to the platform.

Costumed academic processions leave me with mixed feelings. In Boston I have taught too many professors' children, resentful because Dad's old Ph.D., or new book, or tenure anxiety is more important than their problems, and they will pay him back by getting a D in chemistry. Or because the ornate robes of German (Croat, Argentine) professors, representing the scholarly dignities of the past, never hindered them from accepting the liquidation of their Jewish (or any other) colleagues whom authority had proscribed.

Fortunately Jiři's teenagers are in the audience, amused by kindly Pan Merrill's fight with their language.

The two students who had been at Moravian are present as proof of what this program can offer. David teaches a course, in English, in advanced computer procedure to faculty members. Pavlina is my interpreter for an hour's conversation with 40 or 50 family members of students abroad. One must be realistic and not expect, like Mauskewitz from Grodno, that in Amerika there are no cats and the streets are paved with cheese.

It is easier to travel from Kraków or Olomouc to New York than it is to make the three-hour drive to the other city. Like Swedes and Norwegians who scorn each other's stereotypes (Norwegian joke: "Are you a Swede?" "No, I'm a Dane, but I've just got out of the hospital."), Czechs and Poles will not waste time learning each other's language or anything about the other's history and culture, and if mischance puts them across the border, converse in "Me Tarzan, you Jane" or in German or English. The penalty for their obtuseness is the number of weak (more numerous and even weaker after the Slovak foolishness) nations who will be fitted neatly into Grossdeutschland's market basket.

Accordingly, my crusade has been to exploit whatever credit I have accumulated over the years to push for a conscious exchange program such as would be taken for granted in Western Europe and at responsible American colleges. Why not a habit of switching students and staff (not one or two but one or two dozen) between Jagiellonian and Palacky? OK—why not with Komensky University in Bratislava, 80 miles (800) in the opposite direction? ("Slovaks aren't interested.") Build up the numbers until the visitors, like Blacks at American schools, begin to change the atmosphere of the host institution. Why doesn't Jacek Woźniakowski's *Tygodnik Powszechny* establish a policy of including one article on a Czech subject in each printing ("We had a whole issue last year.") or a series of Czech guest editors? People start to yawn.

"Pan Merrill, we have just what you've been speaking about! Come see our Polish exhibit, opening today!"

In the gallery upstairs sprawls a display of self-consciously tragic gigantism: sweeps of black interrupted by random splotches in red and orange. Esthetic pornography. "You dumb Czechs (Americans, etc.) don't understand—can never understand—the suffering that we Poles have endured, the spiritual depths . . ."

There are, of course, New Yorkers who would buy this stuff (Lord knows, the Polish economy needs hard currency), center it in their penthouse parlors for monologues on the Slavic soul, and after a while wonder why their wives are drinking more and their daughters have gotten themselves pregnant.

"Pan Merrill, you like?"

"Well . . ."

Dr. Merrill takes off his robe, puts his diploma under his arm, and returns to Žilinska Ulica. Jiři believes that fluency in English is the absolute first step in his country's re-entry into the world and has organized a volunteer course in a village school outside the city. The principal had taught at the embassy school in Havana ten years ago, and we communicate in a mossy Spanish. The classroom holds about thirty eleven year olds. Czech and Polish children (OK—all children) are beautiful. Then life wears them down.

How to begin?

"How many of you have dogs?"

Most hands go up.

"American dogs say bow wow. What do Czech dogs say?"

"Vaff Vaff."

"Would an American dog need an interpreter (Jiři gives the word) to speak with a Czech dog?"

A joke. Laughter. They shake their heads.

"Cats?"

No problem. Miaou. Pigs? These are country children. "American pigs say oink oink."

Czech pigs employ a more naturalistic language. Pigs are very intelligent. If you gave them a bath first they'd make good pets. Could you teach them to write? No, they couldn't hold a pencil with their feet. (New verbs and nouns). What about reading?

"Pigs not read!" (A policeman's son, a teacher's.)

"Why not?" (The American spirit) "Hold the pig on your lap, start with a simple book, with pictures. You'll see."

❧

Jiři is worried about his job. He hasn't gotten along with the principal, a Communist. Now the boss has changed his spots, presents himself as a patriot and Jiři as the old-fashioned leftist. Maybe he'll quit teaching, become a businessman like everyone else. With the new panic about environmental destruction from both coal mining and nuclear wastes, Czechoslovakia is moving into an energy crisis. How about solar heating? What do I think of that?

"The sun doesn't shine between November 1 and April 30. It's forbidden. Zakazano."

Perhaps I could be a silent partner. And Vera has a good head for finances. There is no infrastructure, no climate for business here. Despite its pre-war know-how, it is a nation of government employees, and entrepreneurs are grab-it-and-run. Jiři shifts back to talking about the Slovaks. Mečiar and some of his gangsters are beginning to claim that Moravia was originally part of the medieval kingdom of Slovakia.

"Don't let it bother you. You'll have to speak Slovak in the living room, but I'm sure they'll let you use Czech in the kitchen and bedroom, at least at first."

He doesn't think that's funny at all.

18

Prague 1939, 1949

People who walk across dark bridges
past saints
with dim, small lights.
Clouds which move across gray skies
past churches
with towers darkened in the dusk.
One who leans against the granite railing
gazing into the evening waters,
his hands resting on old stones.
    Franz Kafka

Prague!
Who has seen her but once
will at least hear her name
always ring in his heart.
. . . and in my ear, suddenly,
sounded a gloomy booming.
that was the roar of bygone centuries.
    Jaroslav Seifert *Verses From an Old Tapestry*

AFTER ALL THE ANTICIPATION and anxiety, Bruce Barton and I crossed the border from Ostmark (Austria's Nazi name) into the Protectorate of Bohemia and Moravia with surprising ease. Brno, where we stopped for lunch at a businessman's hotel, was an almost German city. It was harvest time, however, and though most of the traffic was of army trucks, peasants in gay blue, red, white costumes were marching with wreathes of wheat bedecked with cornflowers and poppies, even dancing in circles. When we stopped to watch, Bruce got out to write 'Viva Beneš!' on the dirty side of our Renault. We nodded graciously as the peasants waved.

Then, rounding a corner, we almost crashed into two SS trucks piled against each other. Wounded soldiers, some of them blood spattered and groaning, lay stretched out on the road. Our car with its shocking slogan jolted to a stop just in front of an angry sergeant.

"Raus mit, Frankreich!" he snarled.

Cringing, terrified, I crept out. My defense, total idiocy, fitted national culture. An entire book, *Good Soldier Švejk*, had been written by Hasek about a seller of stolen mongrels with fake pedigrees who had paralyzed the Austrian war effort by his feeble-minded obedience to all commands. Instead of the dignified challenge to German authority that, I reproached myself afterwards, I should have shown, I relied upon exactly the correct response.

"Gosh, gee whiz, sir, I sure don't know how that got there! Boy, wow, you're sure right! Danke schön! That's a bad deal! Ja, ja, ein zwei drei!" until the German became disgusted and waved us on. Safely out of sight, we rubbed off our defiance.

"The most beautiful city in Europe!" as I have been repeating for half a century, has a banal approach of interchangeably characterless buildings, its streets dominated by street cars—today transformed into charming subways, so that dissidents who flee to New York and ride on *that* system beg to be allowed back home. Our wallets close to empty, we stopped at a nondescript building with *Pension* over its doorway. A view, not of the castle, the river, a spired church, but of a courtyard with a toy dirigible, a birdcage, a pot of geraniums in its windows, an adolescent voice singing *The Donkey Serenade* as its owner pounded on a piano. All right, just as good. Next morning the musician added *Who's Afraid of the Big Bad Wolf*, which sounds better in Czech, and there were carpets beaten and clothes hung out to dry.

We started out. An elderly man, hearing our English, volunteered as guide. There weren't many tourists now, he wouldn't charge us much—though one must always be careful. Gestapo agents masqueraded as foreigners. Truth was spread by hidden radio stations. Arms were being hidden away for the great post-war pogrom of Germans and collaborators. As tourists once returned from Paris with stories of Grand Guignol skits,* later on they retail stories of the new Europe. Prague and Warsaw are the production centers.

German gendarmes who accompanied the occupation in March 1939 are surprised that the tales of chaos and Communism are false and are embarrassed to be treated with such hatred. The guide shows us the statue of the Golem, the monster brought to life by Rabbi Loew as a protector of the Jewish community. Will it free its people from the Germans? We saw the old synagogue, the central space for worshippers, slits in the wall for women to observe the service without distracting the men, and the slum of tombstones in the graveyard.

---

* A couple are arguing about finances. The stage darkens. The wife returns with a prosperous bourgeois. Money is exchanged. Flirtatiously re-adjusting his clothes and hers, she leads him to the now-curtained bed, pulls aside the drapes, revealing the white-faced corpse of her husband. "Don't let it bother you," she apologizes. "I'm just trying to raise burial costs."

We walk across the noble Charles Bridge, are shown the statue of St. John Nepomuk hurled into the Vltava (1393) by Wenceslas IV for refusing to reveal the queen's confession—patron saint of those who suffer in silence. Next up the winding streets to the Hradčany Castle and the Cathedral of St. Vitus with its shimmering stained glass windows.

Somewhere around the castle hill two black-clad SS men pass in opposite directions, but instead of barking 'Heil Hitler,' they hiss, "Sss-sss," "Sss-sss" like snakes. I never forgot that. I was a witness to genuine SS men and their calculated efforts to terrify a subject populace which would stretch all across Europe. I have told that story again and again, and recalled it unpleasantly once in 1987 when I spent a week in Jerusalem. A patrol of three Israeli soldiers carrying machine guns passed me in the Arab quarter of the Old City. "We are the masters—don't you forget it."

Why is everyone so intensely concerned over the newspapers? Stalin has signed a pact of non-intervention with Hitler. Now the Germans will be totally free to invade Poland. The Russians have betrayed us just as the French and English betrayed us.

∽

The wartime story of Prague and Czechoslovakia was entirely different from that of Warsaw and Poland. Shortly after the invasion of Poland, a rather amateurish resistance movement called the Sokols, former lieutenants of the former Czech army, sprang up and was quickly put down. A fighter squadron served with the RAF, persecuted later as pariahs by the Communists up to the arrival of Havel. Jews were rounded up and sent to Terezin, on their way to Auschwitz. Tens of thousands of forced laborers were shipped to Germany. An army corps did fight alongside the Russians. The Slovak uprising was savagely repressed, and the whole nation suffered the iron rake of war as the Red Army fought its way westward from Ruthenia to Prague. On the Italian front a few Czechs and Poles (the latter were immediately enlisted into the two infantry divisions under General Anders) would be captured as kitchen helpers in the infantry companies. After the armistice I met some soldiers in Czech uniforms, who belonged to a division responsible for maintaining rail communications in the Po Valley, gloomy fellows dreading what repatriation might entail.

On the whole, however, the country, the capital were strangely quiet. Be cautious, maintain calm were the instructions from President Beneš in London. Then, stung by the accusations of Czech passivity, he ordered the resistance to kill Reinhard Heydrich, SS boss of the Protectorate, a spectacular action that would raise national pride and encourage resistance. Heydrich was killed on June 4, 1942, and the large mining village of Lidice was razed, every male in it shot, by German security forces five days later.

"1939–1941 marked not only the temporary collapse of the Left in Europe; it marked for the second time the nearly universal failure (the first was in 1914) of the Marxian theory of politics. No matter how cruel, no matter how vulgar, Hitler had a more profound understanding of human nature than had Marx, . . . and Socialism has proven to be the principal political configuration of the century."[*]

And in the 1990s, if you focus your eyes with care, that may still be true. Besides obedience and hatred, National Socialism asks for so very little. You are always taken care of. In a society based on infinite gradations of hierarchy there are always people on the levels below you. There is no holy writ to be appealed to which might confuse the simple or the unnecessarily clever. Its picture of the world has no loose ends. Truth is whatever the Leader says, today. Adolf Hitler was never totally defeated.

Liberalism, expressed in the intrigues and deals of parliamentarians, the venality and self-importance of journalists, offered no reassuring promise for the future of Eastern Europe. It was certainly not healthily represented in Czechoslovakia by the octogenarian ex-professor, Thomas Masaryk, who had resigned the presidency in 1935, nor by the faithful bureaucrat, Edouard Beneš, who followed him. The leadership of the socialist parties was no less elderly and shopworn: deputies who had given too many speeches, brutal union bosses, intellectuals who had long since lost any connection between words and reality.

Though Fascism shared with National Socialism a contempt for parliamentary democracy, laissez-faire capitalism, and Marxism, the conservatives in Spain, Italy, Austria, Hungary, even some in France and Germany formed the first group to offer any resistance to Hitler's wave of the future. The two most effective leaders against Hitler were the patriotic traditionalists, Churchill and DeGaulle. National Socialism, however, especially in Central Europe (Austria, Hungary, Romania, Slovakia), made its main inroads among the industrial working class even more than among the middle classes. The Nazis hated the same people—Jews, politicians, the wealthy, the chattering classes—and were young and tough. Most peoples and all classes of Eastern Europe feared Russian domination more than German, with the exception, Lukacs adds, of perhaps the Czechs—out of an archaic affection

* The most interesting material I have read on the conflicting reactions, both Right and Left, to Hitler and Stalin in the years 1938–1941 comes in the chapter "Movements of Politics" of John Lukacs' *The Last European War.*

for that old foe of the Habsburgs? He also suggests that there was, except for Jews, more individual freedom in National Socialist Germany than in Communist Russia, and I wouldn't disagree.

∞

Prague was never bombed by the Allies. It was known as Hitler's air-raid shelter, and many convalescent hospitals for Wehrmacht wounded were sheltered there. The only real violence was a few days of therapeutic street fighting at the very end when any Czech with a gun joined the Russians to shoot at any soldier wearing a German uniform (by then mainly Ukrainians from the mass of Red Army prisoners raised for the Nazis by General Vlasov) to cleanse themselves of the years of fear and humiliation. One of my colleagues at the Bundesrealschule where I taught, 1951, in Vienna, a Sudetenlander, described a German civilian seized at that time, tied to a lamppost, doused with gasoline and set on fire.

The Nazis had run the city with a surprisingly small number of soldiers and police. Their weapons, like the Communists', were rows of filing cabinets with the names of informers and the names, often the same, of those informed on. If you wanted to know anything, names were available with which to start the search and then to be precisely taken care of. Any immature rashness was immediately paid for by the patriot's family and everyone connected with him. I remember one news item from war's end: the birthrate had suddenly increased. Here was a sign of silent defiance to Hitler's promise to cleanse Europe of Czechs and Poles as he was already doing with Jews and Gypsies and brittle intellectuals.

The war ended. An aged, tired Edouard Beneš returned to the Hradčany. Again president, his first act was to expel every German from the republic. Sympathizers, collaborators, loyal anti-Nazis—no difference. All of them had to go, right away. Perhaps for a man who almost all his life had served as Masaryk's private secretary, who had experienced bone deep the impotence of being one of Britain's stable of refugee heads of state, here was the chance to show himself as strong, ruthless, a molder of European history, not simply its victim. He might impress the Red Army generals, the Communist unions, Stalin. His allies, who had, after all, wiped out Dresden and Hiroshima, scarcely noticed.

To give dignity to his ambiguous status, Beneš proposed his country as the bridge between East and West, one that might allow the capitalist democracies and the people's republics to understand each other.

That hope spoke to me. I was finishing my first year of teaching in St. Louis, at the school based on book VII of Plato's *Republic*, the education of the guardians, offered to me on Monte Rotondo above San Pietro, the promise of a possible future. We had opened with eleven boys from Pawhuska and Tulsa, Houston and Manila. I taught Ibsen and Shakespeare, American history, Spanish grammar, where a sudden realization that the city council facing Dr. Stockman in *Enemy of the People* was just like the one in Pawhuska probably provoked the first analytical thought in Melvin's life. I worked hard in my narrow classroom over the garage and took part in the self-important faculty meetings where we expelled boys lacking the brains or character to deserve Thomas Jefferson School. If America is to lead a new free world then it must develop a new ruling class, and we set these young men to learning Greek and memorizing Shakespeare. The seniors read *The Republic* for Plato's lessons upon discipline and conformity, and his arguments for total control of every part of life and the priority of the Ideal over any false reality given by one's senses. It took me some years before I realized how close these were to Stalinism.

Nevertheless, this job had little to do with the broken Europe I had seen in Italy and the determination then that it was my duty to share the task of rebuilding. (In the fall of 1948, however, Thomas Jefferson was the first school in the entire United States to enroll a Japanese student. Jun Sakurai had been sent us by my Mississippi employer, Sam Franklin, who after serving as a Navy chaplain in the Pacific, returned to Tokyo as a teacher and pastor. I was proud of my school's participation in this first step towards reconciliation.)

I went to the Czech consulate in New York City. The cultural attaché, a sensitive young man (as doomed, I thought later, as the Jewish family I had called upon in Berlin—or had he been clever enough to keep shifting and to keep supplying new lists of friends' names?) was sympathetic to my proposal of teaching for a year in Prague, my response to Beneš' hope.

"The Iron Curtain, you must realize, exists only in the minds of American journalists."

Why not?

In July of 1949, with my wife and six-year-old Catherine back at our drab hotel on Vaclavske Namesti, I went around to the Ministry of Education trying to locate the official mentioned by the helpful attache. A year and a half had passed since our meeting. Gottwald had seized control, his picture hung on every wall. Beneš had died. Was this an idea or simply the pretense of an idea?

For an hour one sunny morning Mary and I sat in a little hillside garden by the castle while Catherine involved herself in a complicated game. A carillon of bells from a church tower and the view of the spires and towers of the city below us were magical and made everything seem possible again.

Briefly. We had arrived here from Milan, which had suffered its own war, but where style, craftsmanship, imagination, color, precision were being put to use for building a new society. Plumpig* was the word for this gray city. In a store where we bought beautiful printed linen, a sad man offered me an encapsulated history of Communism. Right after liberation, all enterprises with more than 500 employees were nationalized, properly, for any corporation that large had inevitably collaborated with the Germans. Then, shortly, any firm with more than fifty: department stores, medium-sized factories, big hotels, the insurance company where Franz Kafka had been an unhappy claims adjuster—the foundation blocks of capitalism. Then more than five employees. The system is ended. The state knows best, as Josef II insisted. The reassuring façades remain, but it is at a ministry in Prague, which in turn receives its orders from the appropriate desk at the Soviet embassy, that the decisions are made. But the machine cannot stop. No grocery store, no shoe repair shop, no beer parlor is small enough to escape. No citizen can be trusted alone. Why? What is the ultimate goal?

I was out of my depth.

I would, however, perform an intellectual's next best act: write a novel. The last night, leaving wife and sick child, I ran through the streets, past the Hus monument in the Old Town square, past the Golem, down to the river, with the outline of the Charles Bridge to my left, the profile of the castle roofs facing me, trying to take in and hold every detail of the city—streetcar noises, restaurant smells, voices.

At the airport for the plane to London, the policeman pawing through our clothes and souvenirs took out each book and riffled through it.

"Some people are so cheap they will give their letters to be mailed abroad because they won't buy postage stamps."

That remark became my textbook example of Communist argument.

So, I carried my Olivetti to the classroom on top of the garage and started *Catch a Falling Star*. Roger, who had lost a leg in Italy, takes Lucia and their three children (the oldest by her first husband, shot down over Germany) to Prague at the end of summer 1948 to fulfill a teaching contract. The government has changed, his official has disappeared, he is really not welcome, by anybody, though he doesn't—nor did I then—realize the fact. A cramped apartment is found and Pan Direktor Dr. Elersiek grudgingly allots him a couple of classes. Roger works hard, learns Czech, makes a few friends, wins respect from his sullen pupils. Lucia becomes a Prague housewife and with

---

* German: clumsy, crude, ungainly.

her ration books learns to wait in line. There are not many rewards, but when he stands on the magical bridge, swans on one side, gulls on the other, as he looks downriver to the castle, to the spires and towers, he sees *his* Europe, which he paid for with his blood.

During the winter of 1944–1945 when I had been stationed near Florence, the question of survival became real for me—food, clothing, warmth, the moral survival of the girls who rented themselves out to American soldiers for two cans of beans and a bar of soap, the survival of people who read books and painted pictures, of those who had lost their families at Auschwitz.

Roger and his family make it through the winter, but spring brings an even grimmer climate. A vulgar American named Joe Chorley appears. Roger is the only American firmly enough placed within Czech society to know trustworthy individuals to be approached as possible CIA contacts. Furiously Roger dismisses him, but had that man loitering at the other end of the park a hearing device strong enough ... Secret police* are given magical powers. He is arrested, interrogated, strapped into what looks like a dentist's chair while a needle is inserted under his finger nails, but continues to say No. Reluctantly the elegantly groomed embassy official secures his release by trading off a Czech agent held in Munich. Lucia learns the grotesque sentence—"Devte mi nohu meho manžela" ("Give me the leg of my husband")—to retrieve his artificial limb from the police.

The book closes as they pull out of the same railway station where they had arrived. Lucia is in tears. Roger has been defeated. The ideal of love and freedom is as fleeting as a falling star, but something of Will, of spirit—perhaps—endures.

The book absorbed a solid amount of writing and rewriting, even if from my resourcelessness it never reached a publisher and disappeared without a trace on the upper shelf of a closet. A few friends read it. One German who had been a socialist refugee in Prague during the 1930s said it captured the feel of the city—praise I appreciated. Teaching in Austria a couple of years later was a more realistic way of putting that fantasy into practice.

It needed some years, however, for me to become embarrassed by, even ashamed of the story. First at the naïveté—simple people have dignity, not the naive—of hero and author who believed that such an enterprise could have taken place. Then as I became more aware of the realities of Czech Communism, horrified at the lethal destruction that Roger, a plague carrier,

* Statni tajna Bezpecnost

would have brought with him. Every colleague who had spoken to him, his favorite student, Miloš, who had visited their home, Milada, the ground-floor tenant's daughter who had been their baby sitter, would have been hunted down.

Despite his crude, old-fashioned factory-worker's 'trust-me' face, Klement Gottwald carried out his Party purges with Shakespearean cruelty that rivaled Stalin's. The faithful brutality of a hard-liner like Rudolf Slansky, who had been vice-premier and secretary of the Party, did not protect him from being arrested, tried, and eventually hanged as a Trotskyite, Titoist, Zionist bourgeois nationalist. In his *Czechoslovakia Since World War II*,* Tad Szulc offers an obsessive description of the hermetically isolated security teams given the task of liquidating each other. Team B is assigned the preparation of the machinery that will trap Team A, now enjoying its sunshine of power. Unknown to them, however, perhaps on the floor above in the internal security building on Bartalomejska Ulica, is Team C gathering the evidence that will bring B to socialist justice six months later. And Gottwald has already started quiet conversations with one or two trusted colleagues who will form the nucleus of Team D.

The silent preparation, the friendly assurances, the sudden pounce and rapid liquidation of those not in the long-range game plan are not totally unlike the choreography of an American corporate takeover. The accused had the obligation, which their whole political career had trained them not to question, of participating in the theatre, dramatically blaming themselves with just the correct vocabulary, and, after a hard day in court, asking their handlers if they had behaved properly, even if none of this slowed down their executions.

Both Hemingway and Orwell describe the cold-blooded activities of the Communist operatives—Spanish and Russian—in Madrid who were much more concerned with eliminating socialists and anarchists than in maintaining a united front against Franco's Fascists. What those writers could not foretell, however, was that almost all of the Russians were themselves arrested and quickly put to death when they returned home. Stalin and postwar leaders in East Germany, Czechoslovakia, Hungary, Romania did not trust Party members who had served in Spain, even in the strictest police roles. They had become too internationally oriented, intrigued even by new definitions of class struggle. Tito had been an officer of the Croat battalion in an international brigade, no recommendation.

* Viking Press, N.Y., 1971.

Wander through the charming streets of Prague, listen to Mozart practice in one of the Rococo houses of Mala Strana, catch the tap-tap of Kafka's word processor from the Street of the Alchemists, drop in on Dvořak's favorite bierstube or Smetana's vinarna, spend an evening at a recital of Brahms quartets or a performance of Chekhov, enjoy the exhibit of children's watercolors, the art nouveau ornamentations of the *Europa's* café or the classic Calvin Coolidge of the *Alcron*—what a civilized city! Nothing of this ornament, *nothing* had the slightest impact on the precision and cruelty of Communist control.

Should one even rethink some traditional conclusions about Joe McCarthy? He frightened politicians and movie producers, paralyzed the State Department, deluded the ignorant, seduced the venal, and exposed the spinelessness of American leadership when faced by a ruthless tough who knew what he wanted. Any figure who had even questioned the totalitarian conformism of the American Way of Life was in almost as much danger as if he had lived in Prague. Not true: you might lose your job, but you probably didn't go to jail, and few were hanged. Class antagonisms were shrewdly exploited, and products of state teachers' colleges were turned against their betters from Harvard. Leftists despised dumb Catholics and bumpkin bigots as McCarthy sympathizers did the gullible enthusiasts. It was not our country's finest hour.

But Americans had never run up against a man like Stalin before. Hitler had told lies—"the only claim I make is for the German Sudetenland!"—and confronting his lies had cost a terrible price. Stalin had spoken of peace and the brotherhood of the toiling masses, and with his pipe and friendly moustache had hoodwinked the most pretentious intellectuals, who preferred to believe his words rather than look for the facts.

I despised the Communists I met at college in the 1930s: "Soviet troops were forced to cross the Finnish border to forestall a British invasion." And the Berkeley Maoists of the 1960s who asked no questions about the spontaneous surrender of the total personality of his followers. Radicals exploit whatever battle cries come to hand and become a Chassid, a vegetarian, a pot-smoking guitarist, whatever most dramatically sends their parents up the wall. My memory is good enough to recall my own postures. At eighteen I fell in love with the Spanish republic and bitterly regretted, I told myself, that I had been too young to fight for it. In my sixties I gave an emotional loyalty to the Sandinistas and regretted that I was too old to do more than write checks.

It is better to wrap oneself in unquestioning acceptance? What is, is what should be?

The most brilliant professor I had at Harvard was Paul Sweezey, who taught a course on the economics of socialism. I remember my sense of humility at being privileged to learn from a man like him. This was 1941. Ulbricht, Gottwald, Ceaușescu, the Budapest uprising and the Warsaw Pact invasion, Brezhnev and Kim Il Sung could not be foretold.

And yet no one better informed than we warned us that Stalin's lies, his insistence on total control, the cruelty of his Party purges and the need not only to kill but to humiliate his enemies absolutely, the cruelty of his extermination of the Ukrainian peasantry (bad taste to mention) were not only the basis of his style of leadership but existed as the intensification of Lenin's principles of administration. They were even the inevitable result of Marx's refusal to tolerate the slightest disagreement. Yes, terror might be a historical necessity, the university sympathizers agreed, but did not care to ask what that actually meant, nor to discuss that their own safety depended on their despised French or American passports.

I remember an article on Sartre and Picasso in *Preuves*, the French monthly (bankrolled by the Congress for Cultural Freedom, later revealed as a CIA front), written by Czesław Miłosz in 1957. These two were the cultural stars of France, proof of Communism's distinction in intellect and art. If, Miłosz insisted, any gifted Russian had wished to follow out the threads of Sartre's definition of freedom or base his graphic style on Picasso's, the cost could have been lethal. Sartre explained that he did not wish to distance himself from the French proletariat by disturbing their loyalty to the Party, and he hated America so intensely that any alternative was permissible. It is impossible for any individual to carry on daily life in a bipolar world with an equal hatred for both sides. Nevertheless, one might insist on higher standards for telling the truth.

> *In times that have no present we stick to the future's image of old*
> *   memories.*
>   Ivo Smoldas *Snapshot*

> *Unbreakable Union of Mighty Republics*
> *Has wielded forever the Great Russia*
> *Glory Glory to Great Stalin*
> *Who showed us the path of Freedom*
>   Michalkov, from the Soviet national anthem.
>   "It sounds better in Russian."

19

Prague 1968, 1974, 1978

Prague never lets you go. This little mother has claws.
Franz Kafka

A startling metaphor is worth more
than a ring on one's finger.
Jaroslav Seifert *To Be a Poet*

Why now the visit
middle of the winter, in this city
so long joined to frost.
   Hurried everybody empties his mouth
of sentences and flees the streets
for a warmer place.
A coffee in the café, the wait
for a friend who never arrives . . .
Someone wraps a face in a scarf
the scratching noise of a needle
on a never-ending record.
   Lutz Rathenau *To the Poet Franz Kafka*

I DID NOT RETURN to Prague until February 1968. Gottwald had died of pneumonia caught at Stalin's funeral, 1953. He was followed by Antonin Novotny, a lifelong Communist, once a worker in an armaments factory, a prisoner for four years at Mauthausen, a dedicated Stalinist, unwilling to adjust to the peasant tantrums of Khrushchev, and increasingly isolated and unpopular. Though a brutal and often vulgar man, Khrushchev was a human being and insisted on better behavior and even a minimum of truth telling.

Some years earlier, at a discussion evening of MIT students in Boston, I had met a tired, badly worn visitor from Novotny's Prague. He was the pastor of a church of the Bohemian Brethren, and each Sunday in the large building that had once been filled with well-dressed parishioners greeting their neighbors, exchanging smiles with their sweethearts, showing their piety to their employers, and worrying about the roast duck, he ran a service for a small congregation as worn as he was.

"You know, under the Austrians, under their Catholic domination, we had to learn some skills then, too, of survival."

"But what do you see as your function? What role do you play as a Christian minister in a Communist country?" came the earnest American question.

He replied after a moment's thought: "I suppose we come together to consider important matters in a serious way. What you read every day in the newspapers, what you hear on the radio is neither important nor serious. All we have to rely on now is each other and what we can still take from our Christian inheritance. In a way, though it's hard sometimes to maintain a belief in this, we are better off than in the days when everyone called himself a Christian."

We come together to consider important matters in a serious way. How many American clergy would have envied him. And since the police already knew who the members of the congregation were, what they said and did, and since they asked little from the society around them, they were, in a strange way, rather free.

Student and intellectuals' opposition had weakened Novotny's authority by autumn of 1967, and in early January he was replaced as first secretary of the Communist Party by Alexander Dubček, a Slovak. Dubček favored a reduction in the totalitarian character of the Party without the loss of its predominance, but popular loathing for the whole system was so universal that any hard-liner, certainly in Moscow, might well fear that the movement could not be reined in.

For a visitor just arrived from Boston and Zurich, none of this dynamic was visible. I remember cold wet feet in the slushy streets of February, streetcars, scaffolding over the Tyn Church, smoke-filled restaurants, the exhaustion of having left my school at a difficult time, damp gray overcoats and gray faces, and then the surprise of an unexpected Van Gogh in the National Gallery, a bright, intense garden of line and color that I had seen in a hundred other of his paintings, which brought a wave of joy to my heart and convinced me that I was at home.

A dear friend, a close colleague, was dying of cancer, and I had promised his wife that I would interrupt my sabbatical to conduct the memorial service. That cable reached me two days later, and when I returned to Europe it was to Warsaw.

Socialism with a human face? Communism? We move from Marx to Lenin. Socialism is an interesting topic, and we argue about economic and social priorities. Communism is about power. And Leninism—forget the professors and militants—is lies and fear. There is no toleration, there can never be toleration of any demand from any voice on the outside for sharing this power. And, if one wishes to survive, as a colleague, even as a human being, any discussion of the sharing of power among the insiders must be meticulously worded.

Kronstadt is the name to remember. That was Peter the Great's naval base on the approach to Leningrad.* The sailors there had played a highly publicized role in defending Petrograd from an attack by Caucasian troops under General Kornilov, and are always pictured in Communist iconography of Lenin's seizure of power in 1917.

Nevertheless, in March 1921 the same Kronstadt garrison rose against the Party's dictatorship. The revolt was wiped out by the Red Army and the Tcheka (Communism's first security police). Communist leadership may never be challenged by any individual, any group, Left or Right.

Dubček's economic reforms in 1968 were reasonable: decisions are better made by workers and local management than by central authority. His political decisions—relaxation of control over intellectual, journalistic, artistic life—were humane and overdue. It seemed clear to Czechs and sympathetic foreigners that this reasonableness—there were no demands for independence from Party supremacy or from the Warsaw Pact, as Imre Nagy had foolishly made in 1956—would be seen by Brezhnev's government for what it was.

The Communists held Leninist standards of measurement: what appears reasonable at one moment may become, shortly, intolerable. On the night of August 20, Soviet tanks, with contingents from East Germany, Poland (Gomułka, a liberal in 1956, had become a hardliner), and Hungary rolled across the borders and ended the heresy. Dubček was not executed, as Nagy had been, but stayed in office for a while,† served briefly as ambassador to Turkey, and then was allowed a desk clerk's job in the Slovak Forestry Ministry till the upheavals of 1989. The Americans, as they had about Hungary in 1956, protested cautiously.

The line tightened. It was not simply a matter of accepting the Communist victory as Czechs had accepted the Habsburg victory of the White

---

* St. Petersburg until 1914, then Petrograd because it sounded less German. With the October Revolution, it became Leningrad, to return to St. Petersburg after the collapse of the Communists.

† In Dubček's posthumous autobiography, he gives the scenario of a formidable Soviet ice hockey team beaten by Czechoslovakia in a world title match at Stockholm. Then with KGB connivance, rioters stoned the Aeroflot office in Prague, which provided the pretext for his forced resignation in April 1969.

Mountain in 1620. If one held any position of the slightest status, one had to sign a formal paper approving this action to save Czechoslovakia from a Fascist threat backed by the American and West German secret police. If not, the doctor became a window washer, the actor a trash collector.

A student named Jan Palach refused to accept the habit of compromise and in January of 1969 doused himself with gasoline and set himself on fire in Wenceslas Square. He was buried in Prague's Olšany Cemetery, but so many mourners came to his grave to light candles and lay wreaths with the motto 'We remember' that the Husak regime had his remains removed to a country graveyard and a new headstone and a new body, of an unknown woman, placed in the empty space.*

> *A human torch*
> *races through Prague.*
>   *Today's heretics are spared*
>   *the long journey to Constance.†*
> *Prague, city of the schism,*
> *has become the city of the Council of Conscience*
>   *the dead philosophy student*
>   *testifies louder*
> *than debates in the Party Secretariat or in Parliament*
> *where words are swept on the rubbish heap of history.*
>   Ondra Lysokorsky *Ballad of Jan Palach, Student and Heretic*

The Brezhnev Doctrine gave the invasion its rationalization: it was the obligation of every socialist nation to go to the aid of any fraternal power whose integrity was threatened by counter revolution.

An American cursed with a historical memory sighs. Guatemala, 1954: Eisenhower had the C.I.A support the military-landowner putsch that toppled the elected Arbenz government, which had threatened the properties of the United Fruit Company. Over the next thirty years this military dictatorship murdered more than 100,000 Indios. Cuba, 1961: Kennedy allowed the CIA to back, up to a point, the Bay of Pigs invasion and dealt with Mafia allies to try to poison Castro's cigars. Administration after administration copied the Arab boycott of Israel in its international blockade of Cuba and with a Stalinist para-

---

* Timothy Garton Ash, "Prague—a poem, not disappearing," an essay in Vaclav Havel, *Living in Truth*, Faber and Faber, London and Boston, 1989.

† The Swiss-German city where in 1415, despite an imperial safe conduct, Jan Hus, the Czech reformer who led the way to Martin Luther, was burnt as a heretic.

noia tried to prevent any citizen contact. Chile, 1971-1973: Nixon and Kissinger ordered the CIA to destabilize the Allende government, provoking the turmoil that led the way for General Pinochet's seizure of power.* El Salvador, the mid-1970s until 1991: Americans financed and armed the military-landowner side in a civil war as lethal as the Soviet takeover of Afghanistan, with the same bombs, mines, napalm. Nicaragua, mid-1980s: "Managua is a two-day drive from the Texas border" was Reagan's justification for support of Contra attacks upon the Sandinistas. The Ortega government had flaws that American liberals preferred not to know, but it was by destroying schools and clinics that the Contras prevented Soviet-Cuban domination of the hemisphere.

The State Department denounced such comparisons as Moral Equivalency (Goebbels and Stalin preferred False Objectivity), and it would cost your job if you indulged in it. Essentially Brezhnev and Reagan were saying the same thing: This is Our Turf. No change in management will be tolerated. Don't confuse policy with facts.

In the Western Hemisphere today, the most murderous revolutionary movement is Peru's *Sendero Luminoso*. The person to be killed is not the society princess but the woman who runs a soup kitchen, not the foolish tourist but the French volunteer in village development, not the police chief but the hard-working mayor of a barriada. Orthodox Stalinism insists that the first enemy to be wiped out is the one similar enough to confuse the masses and dilute their loyalty. Because it has been United States' policy to destroy any form of democratic socialism (a concept feared equally in Washington and yesterday's Moscow), only uncompromising savagery can survive.

∞

I returned to Czechoslovakia for a few days in 1974, mainly to make a pilgrimage to Telč, a beautiful town in southern Moravia whose vast arcaded market square is a gem of popular architecture. I had rented a car in Munich that allowed me to cross the border between Passau and Strakonice. It is only by road that one grasps the monstrosity of Communist management: the 20-foot-high double wall† of electrified barbed wire that stretches on both sides as far as the eye can see, a guard tower every 200 meters, in front a ribbon perhaps 20 to 30 feet wide for mines. Whether one tries to understand what

---

* Henry Kissinger, September 15, 1970: "I don't see why we have to let a country go Marxist just because its people are irresponsible." Walter Isaacson, *Kissinger*, Simon and Schuster, N.Y., 1992.

† The 1992 Republican party platform advocated the construction of a steel fence along the Mexican border from San Diego to Brownsville. In 1996 Pat Buchanan proposed the same idea, though when attacked for its cost hinted that maybe he had been fooling.

this barrier across the entire length of the Austrian-West German borders cost to erect and maintain or the theory behind this colossal effort to keep one's citizens from running away, the impact is staggering.

I hiked up and down Vaclavske Namesti, past the hotels and bookstores, past the unchanging excavations for the subway and the scaffolding over the Tyn Church, across the Charles Bridge, winding up Nerudova Ulica to the Hradčany. Or one can turn left down Loretanska Ulica to the Černin Palac, with its monstrous columns and its window moldings like tombstones, one of the most brutal impulses of megalomaniacal *Staatsmacht* (the word needs no translation) that the Habsburgs or any other dynasty ever indulged. It contains the Ministry of Foreign Affairs from one of whose windows Masaryk's son Jan jumped or was thrown to his death, March 10, 1948.

> *The play is over,*
> *the workday begins.*
> *A gray wall obscures the sun from us.*
> *But once the day will arrive*
> *When we'll walk out of the ghetto,*
> *And life will smile at us.*
> Anonymous *A Song for the Feast of Purim, Terezin 1943*

Back across the Vltava one walks along Pariźska Ulica through the Josefov, the old ghetto quarter, named after its eighteenth century protector, the only area of central Prague to be massively progressed, its sordidly picturesque alleys replaced around 1907 by Art Nouveau battlements, gables, Ionic columns, and balconies as of Loire Valley chateaux, where wealthy Jewish families could enjoy their oriental carpets in perfect security. The nearness of Wealth to Death invites in the fifteenth century. Unbidden, he enters, his bones clacking, and after pausing to light up a Havana cigar, he addresses the frightened, overweight family,

"May I invite you — "

"But we're all packed, we're on our way to Karlsbad."

"But really, Auschwitz is not far. You won't need all that luggage. My, what a charming hat."

A block away from Paris Street is the Alt-Neu Synagogue, dating from the thirteenth century, where I go to visit the little museum of drawings and poems by Jewish children in Terezin.

Terezin, thirty miles west of Prague, a fortress built by Maria Theresa against the Prussians, was Hell's antechamber, the 'nice' camp to persuade Swedes, for example, that the Germans were not simply monsters. Gullible inspectors would arrive from Stockholm, listen to the children's songs, visit their neat dormitories, pat their heads, hand out bars of chocolate, nod to the friendly guards, and return home. Then the guards confiscated the chocolate (they have children of their own who enjoy little presents), ordered the children to pack up and climb into the trucks that took them to the train that would transport them to Auschwitz. As my granddaughters were reaching the age of these children, I found the museum unbearable. It was too easy to imagine their faces after the visitors and the guards said good-bye, and step by step they came to realize where they would be going. Did any child start to scream? Were they always well behaved?

And as everywhere, the memorials set up by the Communists mentioned the nationalities of those who died there, but not that there were Jews.

Who made the decision about Auschwitz? OK, who gave the orders to use napalm on Vietnamese villages? Didn't anyone say he was sorry?

Once in Peru I met a German woman from a suburb of Frankfurt. She used to cycle to school while American planes roared up and down those roads shooting at anything that moved, including eleven-year-old girls cycling to school.

"Nie wieder Krieg," writes a visitor in the museum's comment book. Easy to say.

> But if I recall how helplessly I watched
> as they dragged off the Jews,
> even the crying children,
> I still shudder with horror
> and a chill runs down my spine.
>   We were living in hell
>   yet no one dared to strike the weapon
>   from the murderers' hands
>   Jaroslav Seifert *Lost Paradise*
>
> And death looks on with a casual eye
> And picks at the dirt under his fingernail
>   Anne Sexton *After Auschwitz*

∽

Back again with Mary in 1978 on our way between village churches in East Anglia and a conference in Istanbul. Instead of the row of shabby hotels along Vaclavske Namesti, we had chosen the *Alcron* on a side street leading towards Nove Mesto (the New Town). It was a textbook example of Early Coolidge, a self-conscious modernism of elevator design and cut-glass light fixtures, curving tubular railings alongside the stairs leading to the front lobby, evoking nostalgic memories of office buildings and department stores on Michigan Avenue, gay parties setting off in their Pierce Arrows—something more?—yes, a luxury liner crossing the North Atlantic. Ginger Rogers descends the grand stairway to the first-class dining salon attired in flowing chiffon, Fred Astaire in white tie and easy dignity a few steps behind.

The Czechs, who even in K.u.K. days could enjoy only a tenuous connection with Triest (whose officials spoke German, merchants Italian, and marketwomen Slovene) for a ride down the Adriatic, had clearly chosen this hint of the *Ile-de-France* and *Aquitania*.

The claim to cosmopolitanism of any Eastern European restaurant is the menu in four languages (sometimes five, to reach the hypothetical soprano from Paris), even if fewer than half the items are available. In theory, however. . . . For the Soviet delegations, though they despised the Czechs as colonials, a visit to Prague and to the *Alcron* with its clean tablecloths and waiters' fingernails and its light fixtures that worked was exposure to Culture.

Even before 1939 the brightly lit *Alcron* lobby was not a place for Jews or intellectuals, who preferred the coffee-fragranced Art Nouveau public rooms of the *Europa*. On a later visit I remember a laughing dozen of young people, the men in tuxedos, the women in bright ball dresses, running along an alley leading off the *Alcron's* entrance, late for some wonderful party being given by F. Scott Fitzgerald. As an old-line semi-Marxist I wanted to stop one of these *jeunesse dorée* and ask his class background. Would only the children of the highest Communist officials have the money and confidence to wear such garments?

The lobby of the *Alcron*, where I order slivovitz instead of a martini, speaks for two American presidents, not only Calvin Coolidge, but Woodrow Wilson. By 1915 Thomas Masaryk had set himself the task of selling England, France, and Russia on the concept of an independent Czechoslovakia as a republic out of the ruins of the Austro-Hungarian empire. Since there had never been such a nation, this was more difficult to imagine than an independent Poland. By 1918 Masaryk had become increasingly involved with America in order to gain financial support from the Czechs of Chicago and the Slovaks of Pittsburgh and political support from President Wilson. The latter's *14 Points* pledged to a Europe of democratic national entities clearly agreed with Masaryk's own dreams. In fact, when the post-war dust settled, Masaryk's Czechoslovakia was and remained just about the only democracy that fitted Wilson's expectations. The two tall, slender, dignified professors even looked surprisingly like each other.

"We need a president and we get a university professor," became a comment. The Poles and Hungarians had a land-owning nobility. The Czechs had to make do with professors. One could do worse, but President Masaryk had a lot of problems on his desk that had to be solved at the same time—immediately.*

To work out Prague's relations with its national minorities, he had to face the paradox that each one of the *14 Points'* successor states—Poland, Romania, Yugoslavia, as well as Czechoslovakia—found itself a miniature Austro-Hungary, treating its own minorities often worse than the former empires had treated theirs. The Poles in Tešin, the Hungarians in southern Slovakia, which for a while meant heavy fighting with Bela Kun's Communists, the Germans along the Sudeten borders and in every city, the Ukrainians in distant Ruthenia, accidentally tacked on, and the Slovaks, just emerging from centuries of Hungarian oppression—they came to have some trust in Masaryk personally, not much in his government.

To rebuild a war-worn industrial structure and create a financial and commercial system worthy of a European capital, helped by French and American loans, far ahead now of Vienna, bled dry by 1918, the Hauptstadt only of a tiny republic . . . we are back in the lobby of the *Alcron*.

To construct a viable political system. Czechs defined politics as opposing the Austrians, disrupting the parliament in Vienna with fiery speeches and banging their desktops. Now they had their own parliament but not new ways of working in it. During the years of Nazi and Communist oppression it was easy to romanticize the civilized quality of Masaryk and Beneš's republic, but there were up to 16 egocentric political parties, in the first 12 years ten different governments, an unpleasant smell of corruption, and outside in the streets clashes between police and students and strikers, a never resolved relation with the Communist labor unions. Masaryk found himself bypassing parliament as the Habsburgs had and running the country with the bureaucracy, trying to create a genuine democracy by authoritarian methods.

---

* Much of this between-the-two-wars material comes from Z. Zeman, *The Masaryks, The Making of Czechoslovakia*, Weidenfeld & Nicholson, London, 1976, as well as Rothschild, *Op. cit.*

His first priority was to make Prague a Czech city. That meant renaming the streets and changing the signs, requiring that government and law, business and education be managed in the new language. When the Quebéc government forbade shop signs in English and insisted that business meetings be held in French, firms shifted their headquarters from Montreal to Toronto. The Algerians took on the harder job to de-Gallicise Algiers and Oran. Arabic must become the language of the elite, not just of servants and politicians. Forget Europe. Talk to the people on your street. Hindu women switched from frocks to saris, from Rosalyn as their daughter's name to Radika, from mutton chops to curry, and poured their husband's Scotch down the sink. This started in Prague.

Trees make Arabs nervous, and a patriotic gesture within newly independent Morocco and Libya after World War II was the cutting down of the forests planted by their former French and Italian masters.

Masaryk also felt compelled to confront the reality that for 300 years the Habsburgs had ruled his country not only by their police sergeants and schoolteachers, but by an authoritarian Catholicism. Its priests had counseled obedience to rulers anointed by God, at times had also been willing to reveal to the police the secret that some unwary girl might have told in confessional about her headstrong brother. To create a new nation, in Masaryk's thinking, it was necessary to rebuild the democratic Protestant traditions dating back to the 15th-century Hussites: intellectual freedom as well as the right to search for truth against any authority (and like most Central European populist crusades, with bloody attacks on the Jews.) The Czechs, not always strengthened by the out-of-step Catholic Slovaks, would always comprise a small nation, but they had the good fortune, nevertheless, to be free of a hereditary aristocracy and a military tradition, and through education and the habit of hard work would make a place for themselves among the nations.*

In Masaryk one can see traits carried over from the old headmaster, Josef II, who knew what was best for his peoples whether they agreed or not, and these tenets would be seen again in Konrad Adenauer, who rebuilt a devastated West Germany by the force of his moral authority.

As the Coolidge years ended so did the inflow of foreign capital. The collapse in 1930 of the Vienna Creditanstalt broke the backs of Central Europe's banks. Each nation, punished now for the loss of the K.u.K. free-trade imperium, protected itself by erecting ever higher tariffs. In a nation of

---

* Much of this material comes from a paper by Candida Mannozzi, *Masaryk and Havel: The Czechoslovak President as an Authoritarian Figure*, written for Johns Hopkins University's School of Advanced International Studies Bologna Center, 1992, pp. 5–13.

eleven million, Czechoslovakia had one million unemployed. As economic conditions got worse, the political bonds came unglued. The coffee houses of Prague—Czech, German, Jewish—became hermetic. No one ventured across the boundaries. The Slovak nationalists withdrew support. The Sudeten Germans, blaming their unemployment on the Czechs, shifted their allegiance to Konrad Henlein's Nazis. An aged Masaryk resigned in 1935, leaving the sinking ship to his permanent #2, Edouard Beneš.

Suppose the Czech army had fought instead of surrendering in October 1938? Stalin had made fulsome pledges of support, knowing that Polish refusal to allow Russian troops to cross their territory and French weaseling out of their share of the mutual aid treaty protected him from turning words into action. Hitler had promised to bomb Prague into rubble, but would things have been any worse than they became?

The heaviest wheel rolls across our foreheads
to bury itself deep somewhere inside our memories.
Mif *Terezin 1944*

20

Prague 1983, 1985

Give us news
of all the screams which we do not hear
all the murders to which we're accustomed.
Remain strong in your weakness
permit the word its enormous power: to be honest
in its impotence, glorify nothing
of its impotence. Remain in your room
join us in future battles: Give us courage
with your fear
      Lutz Rathenau *To the Poet Franz Kafka*

Hey, you on the corner,
we already know the story
of the loneliness of modern man
So don't stand there all night
on that windy corner!
      Peter Handke *An End to Idling*

I ARRIVED IN PRAGUE again on July 1, 1983, a hundred years to the day of Franz Kafka's birth. That seemed special. Would there be parades of introspective, alienated young men, some wearing fanciful cockroach costumes, followed by files of patient but quietly demanding women? Would President Husak, whose imprisonment by Gottwald for heresy in the 1950s during the Slansky purges might have given him a tolerance for non-conformists but didn't, proclaim some 24-hour celebration of ambiguity in honor of Czechoslovakia's most famous writer? No dice. I made some remark about this to the taxi driver taking me from the airport, but he preferred to discuss a murder committed the day before by a Vietnamese.

By 1991 the sale of Kafka T-shirts to tourists would become a way to earn hard currency. In 1983 he didn't exist. The Communists could not deal with any artist, such as Dostoyevski, on an alien wavelength. Is indecisive, ineffectual Kafka, fletcherizing each bite of food into mush, repelled by the stained and crumpled linen of his parents' bed, fearful that his fiancée's vagina had teeth, the totem of our unhappy century?

In his exhaustive, often repetitious biography, Frederick Karl* continually makes the point that it was Kafka's inability to respond in any reasonable way to the humiliating ambiguities of life in his parents' apartment and in his daily toil at the Workers' Accident Insurance Institute that enabled him to write so perceptively of the alienation of our time. Any exasperated therapist whose "Pull up your socks, dammit!" had brought about a more wholesome lifestyle would have crippled an artist as sensitive as Kafka. The Castle, after all, does not reply when we try to ascertain its will. We seldom understand the indictment under which we are brought to court. The constraints of daily life turn us, more often than we care to admit, into cockroaches. Kafka's fear, resentment, contempt, and loathing directed towards his father plus variants of these feelings directed towards his long-suffering fiancées supplied the energy released in his writing, which allowed him to keep on writing despite his slow destruction by tuberculosis.

Those who accepted surface appearances without too much questioning, who followed the rules of building a career and building a family within an accepted social framework, found themselves after Franz Ferdinand's murder in Sarajevo immersed in a war whose horror and duration they had never imagined. Kafka's countrymen were slaughtered in Galicia around Lemberg and Przemysl fighting the Russians, in typhus-plagued villages in Serbia, in the Alps and along the Isonzo River, slaughtered to protect an empire they despised, while that empire gradually disintegrated beneath their feet.

Any serious study of who Kafka was would also lead to a complexity that no Marxist (and few Americans) would care to examine. He was a German-speaking Jew of a city being fought over by Czechs and Germans. Despite his vulgar Prager accent he wrote in a pure German worthy of Goethe, his ideal, but that refinement did not protect him from the contempt that Austro-Germans had for all Jews. The Jewish loyalty to the Habsburg Empire was considered betrayal by the Czechs who, when beaten back by the police, took out their frustration by sacking Jewish stores—as rioting American blacks sack Chinese and Korean stores. Kafka himself, belonging to an attenuated, Westernized Jewish culture, gave his own loyalty to an Eastern shtetl world that his father had been anxious to leave and that he knew only theoretically. How are these complications explained by any all-or-nothing ideology? Better to pretend he never existed.

As a Jew Kafka's freedom of political choice was, of course, limited, but it is inaccurate to see such marginal personalities purely as victims of the twentieth century. Any number of unloved neurotics, failed pedants, passed-over

* *Franz Kafka, Representative Man*, Ticknor and Fields, N.Y., 1991.

bureaucrats and would-be artists found meaning, direction, comradeship, and wholesome activity wearing a brown shirt and black boots or else conducting a meticulous examination on whether the accused's recent statements followed the correct interpretation of Lenin's total program.

> *The only qualification that people need in order to perceive more*
> *clearly the dangers of 'big-lie' politics is to be powerless.*
> Milan Simecka

Some months before that hundredth birthday of Franz Kafka, I had spent a week in Nicaragua. I had been so disgusted by Reagan's disregard of any fairness and accountability in facing America's needs that I wanted to make a pilgrimage to this country whose government he was so bent on breaking. Would the professed Christian Socialism (a term which in Central Europe means simply *no Jews*) of the Sandinistas be a workable alternative not only to self-indulgent, imperial capitalism but also to Warsaw and Prague's rancid Communism? Managua, largely destroyed in the 1973 earthquake, is a mix of Los Angeles and Warsaw in its formlessness, and the endless blocks of California bungalows had disguised a dictatorship by the Somoza family, friends of Washington ("He may be a son-of-a-bitch, but he's *our* son-of-a-bitch," Roosevelt said after awarding a medal to Anastasio Somoza in 1942), far more murderous than the Communist one in Prague's charming streets.

What can one see? The steel and concrete cathedral remains a ruin, weeds growing out of its aisles. More uniforms, more guns of its militia, many of them women, protecting the people, as in Prague, against the United States. It is a poor country, as everywhere else in Latin America, from both Marxist mismanagement and the anaconda of ever-tightening United States' strangulation. The streets of the two market zones are as exhaustingly bustling as any in Istanbul, but the equivalent of a mosque is the reading room of the Bulgarian People's Republic. Bulgaria became, oddly, a big brother to revolutionary Nicaragua, particularly with regard to large-scale, mechanized agriculture, and its silent library has shelves filled with volumes in Spanish on the heroic struggle against fascism, but the rooms are empty and one can sit quietly.

I carry letters of recommendation. One is to a student center, but I cannot understand the dialect of anyone under thirty. Another is to the deputy minister of culture, a Jesuit priest whose office is the remodeled bathroom in Señora Somoza's former bungalow. He pulls up his pant leg to show a pistol strapped to his ankle. "To remind me of the realities of our situation," he jokes. A third is to the sister-in-law of a former student of mine. Kathleen came as volunteer at a Catholic day-care center but proved so skilled with language that she was transferred to the historical section documenting the revolution. She speaks frankly about Sandinista errors and the dangerous pressures from the hardliners, but who expects a revolution to be easy, or safe?

"You don't quit. You work very hard. Nicaraguans are intelligent people—they learn who they can trust and who they can't."

The most impressive person I meet is a woman in her thirties, daughter of a German woman and of a West Point graduate killed as a lieutenant colonel in Vietnam. Sarah is in charge of the United States desk at the Ministry of Foreign Affairs, is clearly exhausted (her week's job includes standing night guard, Sunday drill with grenades and machine guns, as well as six ten-hour days of office work), speaks very rapidly with a sardonic humor at the irony of herself, of all people, occupying so high a position, and at the ridiculousness of Nicaragua thinking it can stand up to America.

"I wish we ran things better. I have my worries about the Communists, too, but they came to our aid when we were flat on our faces and you guys didn't. Basically we're trying to do simple things, like cutting down on infant diarrhea, the real killer in every Third World country, and by showing the campesinos that they can deal with this, reasonably, themselves, by digging wells and latrines and washing their hands, not waiting for miracles from a doctor with a black box. The losses were terrible during our fight against Somoza. There isn't a family which didn't lose a son or a daughter during those years (I think of Warsaw—later, one of our own inner cities), and I don't think anyone's standard of living has improved all that much since then. Last week, though, I met an old campesina out in a village. She was still very poor, that was clear, but I was struck by her pride. 'I feel I'm a citizen of a free country. I've learned to read, I can vote. People respect me. The revolution gave me that.'

That's what makes my job worth it."

The secret police is dangerous, hard to control, but maybe still necessary—there's a lot of sabotage. The Communists like to make threatening gestures, which encourages the Reagan administration to respond with even tougher policies: it's the symbiosis you read about in high school biology. Maybe both sides' hardliners get together secretly and plan out what they'll do next so as to protect their jobs.

Sarah is proud of the Sandinista love of poetry. "Even at the cash register there are these little books for sale, bought by and written by, often, quite simple people. 'A revolutionary is a poet, a poet is a revolutionary' is an official slogan. The intensity of poetry is the only way to match the intensity of our times. It frees people from passivity and despair, it keeps the mind alive searching for an exciting word, a new metaphor. It proves we haven't been dehumanized by the forces against us."

I am reminded again of Warsaw, what Czesław Miłosz said about the verses written during the uprising and the cold years under the Communists. And of young blacks I've known, former students often, whose artless verses were a gesture of defiance, a proof that their authors had not given up.

I am glad to leave the tensions of Managua at the end of my week, but sad. It is a fragile revolution, to be taken over by the police and apparatchiks, with the poets and volunteers put in their place. Or to collapse into misery and chaos from the limitations of its amateur leaders, and be ground to pieces by the vindictive rage of the Americans, my people.

⌒∞⌒

In a tiny Prague apartment there lived, as one might expect, a Commonwealth School graduate and his Czech wife. They had two tiny rooms: one as living, dining and parents' bedroom and the other a cell where their two boys bickered with each other all day. Tony played a jazz guitar and worked for the embassy as impresario for visiting music and dance groups. He lived there because he respected the city's culture, believed that his own role was more significant in Prague than it would be as just another academic at a California university, wanted his sons to grow up with two nationalities. He disliked the ghetto isolation of the international school (the older boy's teacher knew fewer than two dozen Czech words) while fearing the authoritarianism of the public school, which the boys had also attended. Czech teachers did not welcome any interference from parents, which, therefore, forced the boys to learn how to deal with adults entirely on their own. Hardest for them were visits to their grandmother in deepest Bohemia. "Eat! Eat!" the old lady shouted at the two thin little Americans sullenly chewing their way through the dumplings and noodles she forced on them. She had lived in the republic during the depression years: a child who did not eat whatever was put on his plate might not survive. Nevertheless, Tony appreciated the way a child in this culture might remain a child. It was not forced into a premature adolescence of sex and money.

He and Helen took me with them to a gig at a Plzen jazz club. Plzen, the famous beer town, was the one Czech city liberated by Eisenhower's troops, though that fact was not officially admitted by the government until 1990. It was also the home of the great Škoda plant, bombed in late spring of 1945 quite obviously to keep it from falling into the hands of the Russians, though not, it appears, earlier when it was arming the Wehrmacht.

United States' popularity was well served by this generous musician. For young working people in their country's dingiest city, here was a genuine American artist, not only a guitarist of Big Town quality, but with his jokes and slang completely at home in their language. (Tony spoke Czech so well that when he reserved a restaurant table he used English so his vestigial accent would not place him as a Slovak and therefore next to the kitchen door.)

On the drive back we stopped at a new 'Chinese' restaurant. Dr. Husak understood his subjects' longing for cosmopolitan adventures and had a standard eatery on the Prague-Plzen road repainted vermillion and gold, with local herons on the walls converted into oriental cranes, scroll work tacked in the corners, Czech food chopped into tiny pieces and given Chinese-type names, served by the same glum staff wearing embroidered skull caps, and lo—Šanghai!

1983 was the year when perhaps 200,000* Vietnamese 'guest workers' arrived in Czechoslovakia 'to be trained in the techniques of twentieth century industrialism,' in reality, like Turks in Germany, Algerians in France, Hispanics in the United States, to perform the shit jobs their hosts would no longer accept. They lived in barracks outside the major cities, actually received about 20% of their (small) wages; the remaining 80% were deposited in korun accounts for purchase of trucks, motorcycles, machine guns by the Vietnamese government, the equivalent in local currency then released to the workers' families at home. A neat theory, but the half-dozen industrial apprentices I passed filling a hole in a Prague street under the eye of a bored Czech foreman could have been Republican caricatures of workers from the New Deal's WPA.

I shared a compartment with two Vietnamese on the train to Olomouc. Neither side had ever encountered a member of the other nationality, but we carried out minimum courtesies with our respective Czech dictionaries. At a station one of them jumped off to return with half-a-dozen bottles of beer that he deferentially offered the other passengers. I found that sad—though I had a bar of Swiss chocolate to trade—for I could guess what their monthly wage might be, and here they were trying to be nice to these whites who treated them like scum.

It was always exciting to arrive in Prague or Warsaw, run along the familiar streets, catch the sounds and smells, try out, one more time, my language skills, which never improved no matter how loyally I pretended to study. After a couple of weeks the charm and sharpness faded, the language became

---

* This figure has come down to 60,000 in the mid-1990s but even the Czech embassy in Washington cannot agree on a correct number.

frustration rather than accomplishment, I saw the shabbiness and felt the restrictions that formed the background. It was always a relief to find myself in a seat on the plane.

The Frankfurt airport is, of course, the cathedral of twentieth-century consumer culture. Anything you might possibly want—watches, alcohol, Hermes scarves, cameras, cute toys—can be yours. Pairs of strolling police, he with a submachine gun, she with a pistol, add spice. Purgatory for a Czech not bad enough for Hell would be to run for eternity past these gorgeous vitrines with fistfuls of non-convertible korun.

On this arrival in Freiheitsland, however, the first boutique on the right advertised "24-hour adult movies!" Suddenly I understood. The billions we poured into NATO, the beautiful intercontinental rockets and fighter planes and masculine tanks were to protect our constitutional right to watch, despite all the Communist threats, pornographic movies. You learn so much from traveling abroad.

My visit in 1985 started in Zurich. The city held strong memories for me out of my arrival from Munich in the last days before the invasion of Poland. The brown shirts and black boots, swastikas and 'Heil Hitlers' of this 'tomorrow the World' war that was going to crash upon Europe had been left behind as Bruce and I crossed the Swiss border that night. The next morning brought not only sunshine but the sight of citizen soldiers, still in civilian clothes, rifles across their backs, cycling to their mobilization stations. It was a middle-class performance, nothing grand, but clearly well planned, a sign of trust (each citizen kept his own rifle in his closet), of shared responsibility, so that a potential aggressor would think twice before he crossed the borders. It was the proof that a civilized society could still exist.

Zurich was proud of its role as a guardian of German culture during the Nazi years, as a shelter for (some of) the refugees—its border wasn't easy to penetrate. The Swiss were proud of their well-organized pig and potato economy (the beautiful herds of brown cows were a luxury in wartime) that kept the country fed. Coal was imported from the Germans in exchange for Oerlikon anti-aircraft guns. The country also remained independent because so many important Germans and Italians had stashed their money in Swiss banks.

Beyond all this historical prose, however, is the reality that Europe has few cities more beautiful than the old quarters of Zurich. Why didn't I stay there instead of compulsively heading to Warsaw? I always booked at the *Storch*, comfortable but unpretentious, taking a small room looking out at a church tower and a winding street or, for some francs more, at the ducks and swans on the fast-flowing, green Limmat. Across the river is the noble Herrenmunster with its windows of reds and blues, Bible stories in high relief on its doors (Joseph turns away in shame from Mrs. Potiphar's importunity). A few blocks further is the sweet little square, bordered with geranium boxes and antique shops, where a sweet little house carries the plaque informing that here lived Lenin in 1916. Was that good taste simply wasted on him? Couldn't the bourgeois manners that surrounded him, cleanliness and courtesy, respect for the police, have modified some of his actions in subsequent years?

After rethinking these reflections I walk past the Spanish restaurant, more and more expensive, where I always have dinner, on to the Kunst Haus. This is a favorite museum, refreshingly non-French, where there is an exhibit of Chagall with fewer floating brides and instead the flames and tragedy of his Jewish towns. I always visit Hodler's room, the students putting on their greatcoats and picking up their rifles before the battle of Leipzig, the breathless early mornings over Lake Geneva, the portraits, deeper and deeper, of his mistress as she lay dying of cancer.

The young women who direct traffic were trained as temple dancers in Bangkok for their formal gracefulness. I stop at an elegant delicatessen to buy a bouquet of gifts for Warsaw: tins of olive oil, aromatic packets of coffee, a tiny bottle of cognac, a pineapple, candied apricots, Emmenthaler and Gruyère.

Since my plane leaves in early afternoon I have the morning for a walk along Bahnhofstrasse, safe self-indulgence since the prices are too high even for Texans. In the bank windows are blow-ups of thousand mark, thousand franc notes, more perfect than any work on the walls of the Kunst Haus, then sable coats and Persian rugs, until in one window the most beautiful pair of pyjamas I have ever seen, of the finest cotton, pale green, mauve, yellow stripes, woven by princesses.

Suddenly, I have enough—to hell with it! As in Copenhagen when I'd run away from Warsaw, as in Vienna later on, I am seized with surfeit. What sort of person will spend his days going in and out of the establishments on Bahnhofstrasse, laying down the thousand franc notes that will let him carry home that pair of pyjamas. The city made a difference back in 1939, in 1942. What difference does it make now? What of any value does the Herrenmunster's preacher have to say on Sundays?

The elegant banks will accept all money—from dictators who robbed it from peasants, from cocaine entrepreneurs, from Arabs who bathe in oil—and will issue them secret numbers and ask no questions.

The plane leaves for Prague and a couple of days later when I take the next one to Warsaw, I realize that I have left all those delightful gifts in the luggage compartment of the taxi.

∽

At the airport the inspector does not open my bags—doesn't he care? One explanation is that the customs police are angry because they did not receive the same raise as other staffs. This leniency is a sort of strike.

"Pornography? Toronto?"

("Mister, I don't even have a pornograph.")

The taboo against pornography may be the last remaining gesture of Czech Marxism. In Poland during the mid-1980s there was a lively public debate regarding individual freedom versus social discipline, though the poet Wisława Szymborska thought the debate a fabrication to distract attention from genuine taboos. An American equivalent was the great post office plebiscite on choosing the young Elvis or the old Elvis for his 1993 commemorative.

Toronto has become the capital of the Czech intellectual diaspora. Kundera and Skvorecki are its best known residents, though Havel's work has been published there too. The English translations are the channel for Czech writing around the world. Originals are smuggled back in quite easily.

I was here, as in Poland, to purchase miniature etchings for the show of Polish-Czech graphics at a gallery in Boston. Americans need to learn greater respect for the craftsmanship and imagination of these nations' heritage, amplify the income of individuals, make some contribution to their economy. I take an aged, circular metal staircase up to the cramped office of a state arts agency, inspect the precise little etchings of architectural and fanciful objects. A thin, bent woman enters with an exquisite dry point engraving of a flower at $6 for the rich American. "No price less than $10!" I insist generously and am later ashamed of my pettiness.

∽

Vaclav Havel was born in 1936 to well-to-do parents. What must it have been like for a sensitive child to live, from his earliest consciousness, with a father and mother who were always afraid: of the Germans, of the Red Army's coming, of the Communists, of the anecdotes and adjectives passed on by their neighbors and "friends," and without the security—tomorrow will be like today—upon which bourgeois life is based? Since his class background did not justify higher education at state expense (his proletarian wife, Olga, traveled much further along the academic road), what were the books and experiences by which Havel educated himself?

One liberating influence mentioned by Milan Kundera in *Living in Truth*, a collection of essays by and about Havel, is the theatre of the absurd and its star, the Romanian-Parisian writer Eugene Ionesco. "We were suffocating under art conceived as educational, moral or political. Ionesco's plays fascinated us by their radically anti-ideological nature. They returned autonomy to art and beckoned it to take again the path of freedom and creativity. . . . But if Ionesco's absurdity finds its inspiration in the depths of the irrational, Havel is fascinated by the absurdity of the rational. And if Ionesco's theatre is a critique of language, the totalitarian regime has made such a parody of language that Havel's critique of language became at once a demystification of social relations."*

Here one thinks of George Orwell and the Polish poets from Adam Ważyk to Szymborska and Barańczak in their obsessive dissection of language as both the bulwark of and the first step to destruction of totalitarianism. The first production that Havel put on during the 1960s at his theatre in Prague, *Na Zabradli*, was Ionesco's *The Bald Prima Donna* and *The Lesson*, which my wife and I had seen in Paris in 1956.†

Havel's sensitivity to language made him realize, again in Kundera's words, that the difference between what one declares and what one does is not a *fault* that can be corrected by appropriate therapy, but rather it is the *foundation* of Russian totalitarianism, which is built on that contradiction and could not exist without it. The same sensitivity to honest and dishonest language was not only the basic theme of his plays but also provoked his confrontation with the Communist regime of Dr. Husak and eventually led to Havel's becoming president of Czechoslovakia.

In July of 1975 a European Security Conference was held in Helsinki attended by political leaders from thirty-five nations, including the Soviet Union and Czechoslovakia. One of its agreements was an understanding on closer contacts between peoples of different nations together with a reaffirmation of respect for human rights. In 1977 Havel became one of the principal movers behind, creators of, and spokesmen for Charter 77, which stated simply that if the Czech government had signed that Helsinki accord, then it should live up to its words. This logical conclusion was attacked as "commissioned by the centers of anti-Communism and Zionism and delivered to certain agents of the West by a small group of people from the ruined reactionary bourgeoisie . . . and bankrupt organizers of the counter-revolution

---

* Faber and Faber, London, 1987, p. 260.

† "Perhaps it is part of the plebian tradition of Czech culture, but here we tend to be more acutely aware of the fact that anyone who takes himself too seriously soon becomes ridiculous, while anyone who always manages to laugh at himself cannot be truly ridiculous," Havel, Anatomy of Reticence in *Living in Truth*, p. 182.

of 1968." For his obsession with language Havel was arrested and in autumn 1979 sentenced to four and a half years in prison.

Like the South Africans who kept Nelson Mandela in jail, the Czechs with Vaclav Havel on their hands must have felt they had a tiger by the tail. It would not do to appear too accommodating, and yet the face-saving compromises that any reasonable man would accept—"Just sign this very small piece of paper and we'd be more than happy to let you make that interesting trip to New York where you've been invited to speak"—were stubbornly turned down by both men. And gradually the authorities, to their dismay, realize that these two trouble-makers behind bars or under house arrest have turned from being prisoners to becoming the heads of governments in exile.

Like Mozart with his last three unperformed symphonies, Beethoven too deaf to hear what he has written, the playwright cannot witness his own creations, but his plays are put on in half a dozen different languages, including Polish until the proclamation of martial law. He keeps on writing at his farmhouse in northern Bohemia, even if constantly watched by the police, who might suddenly break in and confiscate a year's work. (He has crept out into the woods at night and buried parts of his typescript in the hole of a tree.) The fear of a house search concentrates the mind wonderfully. Far more effective than any publisher's deadline.*

"What has happened to the idea that a man should live in full enjoyment of social and legal justice, have a creative share in economic and political power, be raised on high in his human dignity and become truly himself? Instead of free economic decision-sharing, free participation in political life and free intellectual advancement, all he is actually offered is a chance freely to choose which washing machine or refrigerator he wants to buy."†

One envies a country whose leader can express himself with such moral sensitivity and precision. But watch out. A man who can employ language of that richness may be willing to let words take the place of useful action.

* Timothy Garton Ash, *Living in Truth*, p. 218.
† Havel, Letter to Dr. Gustav Husak, in Timothy Garton Ash, *Living in Truth*, 1975 p. 13.

21

Prague 1989, 1990, 1991

Pravda a laska musi zvitezit nad lzi a nenavisti.
Truth and love must prevail over evil and hate.
  Vaclav Havel 1989

Civilization and Profits go hand in hand.
  Calvin Coolidge 1920

Os ricos são brancos
Os pobres são prietos

The rich are white
The poor are black
  Brazilian proverb

I HAD TAKEN THE TRAIN from Dresden through the black mountains and past the ugly towns of the Sudetenland where all the trouble had started. Although the worst soft-coal gouges are not visible from the train, the landscape is so devastated that when East German television wanted to film a new version of *All Quiet on the Western Front*, they could simply dig trenches and string barbed wire on their side of the border, put their actors into 1917 helmets: instant no man's land. Statistics say that men from these areas have a life-span ten years' shorter than elsewhere, plus the highest rate of divorce and alcoholism. Under the Communists it was taboo to discuss environmental pollution, a disease only of capitalist countries. Simple folk must be nostalgic for those days.

A pair of East German and Czech border police move along the aisle to check our passports, young, correct, interchangeable in their fake-fur hats. I miss the pariah quality of DDR police in 1960. I have a long conversation, trying to upgrade my Austrian German of almost 40 years past, with a hydroelectric engineer who travels often between East Germany and Russia. He criticizes the government freely, so proud of its world sports record, but if one of these stars ceases to win, he is thrown away like garbage.

The first K.u.K. building of yellow ochre, with white moldings curled around its windows and doors, gave me a sense of joy: I was within the Empire once again, rolling along the Elbe and then the Moldau. My hotel this time was the *Pařiž*, built in 1907, the same year as the *Francuski* in Kraków, the *Bristol* in Warsaw, the *George* in Lemberg, when to be a part of a Paris of the East was the hope of any cultured entrepreneur, at the height of Prague art nouveau: fanciful floral designs in glass over the doors, Mucha's vague women with flowing hair upon the walls, the birdcage elevator creeping up and down. I am ridiculously happy. Emancipated from the *Alcron* and Calvin Coolidge, only a few hundred meters from the Stare Mesto. The scaffolding—after 40 years!—is off the Tyn church, and a great tricolor is draped around the base of the Hus monument.

When Jiři visited Boston on the 4th of July, 1987, he had been struck not merely by the skyscrapers, the old Chinese woman bent over a trash can to hunt for scraps of food, the alarm of a young black teacher when he asked to take a snapshot of her bi-racial children playing together, but by the easy-going flag-carrying of the multi-ethnic crowd picnicking along the Charles. "The Communists have stolen all our patriotic symbols—our flag, our anthem, *The Bartered Bride*. When a national holiday comes, we stay home and work in the garden."

There is a tension in the crowded streets. This is a time when something, at last, will be happening. Havel na Hrad—to the Hradčany Castle, the president's palace on the hill—is plastered on wall after wall. Stop Dogmatizmu. I shall carry that to my Harvard reunion. I should be halting passersby and asking them to tell me the story of their lives. How prepared are they for this? Instead I am, as usual, on the Charles Bridge, carried away by a lonely impulse of delight. The end of a November afternoon has brought a pale orange sky at the western end, with a black outline of wooded hills on the left, the castle and St. Vitus' roofs and towers on the right. The orange glistens on the river, swans swimming on the right, gulls hovering and sweeping in the air on the left. One can only utter some wordless thanks for this gift, as when a deer runs across the road in front of you or the newest grandchild staggers up to your chair and says, "Play with me." The breath of sadness in Mozart: how often will this come again?

Jiři and his family arrive the next evening: Jirka now taller than me, Jana strikingly pretty. They are filled with excitement about the demonstrations, sparked by the university students, even in provincial Olomouc. On the streets there they had helped to make things happen instead of silently accepting what was forced upon them, throwing away the old and dirty, putting on clean new clothes.

From the *Paříž* we walk to Na Příkope, avenue of the decisive student demonstration a fortnight ago. In Olomouc the authorities had not fought back: they had simply disappeared. Here the police had gone out of control and attacked the students. A revolutionary dialogue, such as had occurred in Vienna after Metternich's removal in 1848, came about between the demonstrators in Prague and East Berlin, widened a few days later to Bucharest and Sofia, sped up by television, but again with the surprise that the unimaginable had been natural. Along the edge of the sidewalk are bunches of red carnations, flickering candles for the students beaten and killed by the police, like the little Warsaw shrines back in 1957. In a couple of places, television screens show over and over the chaotic images, the cries and shouts of that night.

And this time the leadership and direction are purely Czech. Gorbachev had visited Prague in July 1987, welcomed enthusiastically everywhere because the people believed that he had come to free them from Husak. Their nationhood had been given them by the victorious Allies in 1918. Another generous foreigner might do the same now. The 300 years of Austrian domination, the years of Nazi and Communist domination had eroded any conviction that they could determine their own fate by themselves.*

Any adult also remembered the humiliation of having given in, without a shot fired, to the German seizure of the Sudetenland in 1938, having acquiesced to the Communist seizure of power in 1948 and again to the Warsaw Pact invasion in 1968. There was nothing in a half-century's history to give any Czech a sense of pride. Americans who endured the scars our nation suffered out of Vietnam should feel sympathy.

The first snowflakes of winter come against our faces. Jiři the teacher is explaining the events to his children, and I think I catch the words that this combat, this suffering and victory, was won by students just a few years older than they. They were the ones who stood up to the police and after that no one could go backwards. I think we are all close to tears. Chceme Pravdu—we want truth! After all the times that I have seen Prague silent, humiliated—and now they have won. *We* have won. One utters a silent prayer.

I take a taxi to the airport, past new apartment houses and tourist hotels with their swimming pools and fax machines. The farther away from the center the fewer flags and posters. "Havel is paid by the Americans," the driver remarks.

---

* Mannozzi, *Op. cit.*, p. 22.

❦

Tva vlada, lide, se k tobe navratila!

People, your government has returned to you!
Vaclav Havel 1990 New Year's Address, quoting from Thomas
Masaryk's Inaugural, 1918.

*The struggle against power is the struggle of memory against
forgetting.*
Milan Kundera *The Book of Laughter and Forgetting*

May 1990

Prague has suddenly become the tourist capital of the world. Czech chic.
Hotel keepers double their prices and still can laugh at those searching for a
room. Apply long in advance and they haven't made up their schedules.
Apply later and everything's full.

Jiří finds me a room in elderly Pani Zufničkova's apartment on Na Valech,
an uninteresting avenue behind the Hradčany. "How much would you care
to pay?" For $25 a night I receive also a breakfast of coffee, bread and cheese.
Brittle is the word for the furnishings as for the thin, silent widow. We bow
and exchange morning formalities. Her occupation is to sit at a small table
with a small photograph of her husband facing her while she paints a platoon
of lead soldiers in K.u.K. uniforms.

I walk down the hill towards the cathedral and through the formal gardens, graced with magnificent horse chestnut trees and lilacs in bloom, foun-
tains and geometric plantings, the sentries in generic Central European, no
longer Soviet, uniforms. A gaggle of teenagers slouches by wearing Snoopy
and Hawaii Surf Girls T-shirts made in Singapore. We have won the battle
for the future. *You, Jean-Paul Sartre, have lost.*

At the foot of Vaclavski Namesti is a new statue of the old professor,
Thomas Masaryk. He exists, not merely on street signs in Zagreb and Mexico City. Along Na Příkope are kiosks with large photographs of smiling
American soldiers in Plzen, May 1945: another taboo down. Further along
is a display of plywood busts of all the Communist bosses from Stalin and
Gottwald to Mao and Kim Il Sung. Brezhnev has a special model because the
top half of his head is missing—never really used. I pass a group of Japanese
entering the *Paríz* to take "my" room and wish them well.

Though I resent these tourists shuffling down the Champs Elysées on their way to the Piazza San Marco, the streets are crowded in holiday fashion, and I like to think of their marks, yen, dollars, francs rebuilding the Czech economy. A tall young man accosts me in a friendly, bullying way. "Change dollars?" "I already have"—in the taxi from the station. He is Yugoslav. "I give you thirty for a dollar"—three times, not twice the official rate. Greed! I hand him $50 for a wad of hundreds and start to check. "No, very dangerous. Police," he warns me and disappears. I slip into a doorway to add up my booty, and there beneath the fatherly 100 korun note is a fistful of tens. I am punished, as I should be. Would that all the sharp-toothed foxes on Wall Street. . . .

The useful fact from this mini-morality drama, however, is that when naive Americans talk about creating democratic capitalism, it will be entrepreneurs like this money changer, plus the Party bosses who took their łapówka (Polish—sweep of the paw) or mordida (Mexican—bite) off each hard-currency transaction who will have the wherewithal to exploit the new rules. If you add in the humble who know that the only thing to be trusted in life is an envelope of $5 bills under the mattress, and the sophisticated who open a bank account in Zurich, Vaclav Klaus, Havel's Minister of Finance, may see less of this flotsam and jetsam than you imagine.

My modest hope is that this localized prosperity may allow a coating of civility to the knives these amateur politicians are using on each other. Havel is a decent and sensible man, still surprised at himself, of all people, walking from prison to the Castle, standing up even against Plato's *Republic*, ("The rulers are the only ones who should have the privilege of lying") in rejecting the sacred privilege of the state to violate the rules enforced upon the individual. First of all it should tell the truth. *Pravda vitezi*—Truth will prevail, Masaryk's choice for the new republic's motto against Lenin's "Truth is a bourgeois prejudice." ("No one will ask the victor if he told the truth."— Adolf Hitler, *Mein Kampf*.) How grateful Americans would be if their presidents spoke fewer lies

If a policy is morally responsible, then it should be followed even when the cost is high. Therefore, since the spread of armaments throughout the world is a source of misery, Czechoslovakia should refuse to have any further involvement with weapons export. Such was the conclusion of Jiři Dienstbier, who had become Havel's Minister of Foreign Affairs straight from his previous job as boiler tender at a factory. Since the Communists had tried to build up Slovakia's industrial capital by placing the new arms factories there, it is Slovaks who pay the price for Dienstbier's moral sense. The

Americans are quite willing to take advantage of this new vacuum in the international market, joined in their open-ended garage sale of military junk by former republics of the Soviet Union. (By 1993 Dienstbier's prohibition had been repealed as quixotic.)

Havel felt obliged to apologize for the harshness of President Beneš's mass expulsion of all Germans in 1946. That example made him cautious about a wholesale purge (*Epurazione*, in post-Fascist Italy) of Communist collaborators. That, along with the fact that the network of informers in Czechoslovakia was as pervasive as in East Germany, meant fewer bodies hanging from lampposts, but more of the same foxy faces sitting behind the same desks with minimal cosmetic changes. Havel was backing good people like Josef Jařab at Palacky. When would individuals of this caliber become a critical mass to demonstrate the quality of the nation's new leadership?

Havel was also running up against the same problem that Masaryk faced after 1918. Czechs show civic courage in opposition: against the Austrians, against the Communists. When they are asked to work *for* a political movement, they, like the Poles, lack traditions of cooperation and compromise.

⌀

"He is still very popular."

The surface is tarnished and people take democracy for granted.

"You can say what you want, but what difference does it make?"

The disease of the West, already. Democratic politics is Vaclav Klaus trying to hammer through a deflationary policy that will enforce competitive standards of industrial production even at the expense of serious unemployment. Perhaps he will try to parlay success there into a home in the Hradčany. It is Vladimir Mečiar attacking this irresponsible capitalism for its impact on his workers, so typical of historic Czech contempt for Slovak interests, culture, dignity. Now is the time to discuss, at last, the reality of Slovak independence. Mečiar, proud of having started life as a prize fighter but angry when the media dwells on the fact, has the apparatchik's impatience with opposition. The Slovak press will not be allowed to tell lies or foreigners to make provocative statements that will simply encourage spontaneous anger. Slovakia must become a unified nation. (The Jews are dead—that makes things easier.) It is divisive to allow Hungarians to have their own secondary schools. *They* didn't let *Us* have *Our* schools!

"He is a decent, sensible man."

That we know. That every street in a democratic country should have a pub and a couple of bakeries and sweet shops is his model, without wastelands like Warsaw or the South Bronx.

"It is not true that people of high principle are ill-suited for politics. The high principles have only to be accompanied by patience, consideration, a sense of measure and understanding for others. It is not true that only cold-hearted, cynical, arrogant, haughty or brawling persons can succeed in politics. In the end, politeness and good manners weigh more."*

We need, everywhere, to hear such words. But when in those years in prison Havel had all that leisure for reading, why didn't someone give him a good biography of Franklin Roosevelt? FDR had high goals in fighting poverty, inequality, injustice—words that became taboo in the 1980s—but he had a hard-boiled understanding of practical methods, and he was willing to work hard. Fundamentally Czechs and Slovaks are willing to accept compromises in order to hold their country together. They recognize the threat from Grossdeutschland and the dangerous rubble heap of what used to be the USSR. They would accept a higher level of cooperation with the Poles and Hungarians if geniune leadership expressed its importance. Havel could go over the heads of Klaus and Mečiar if he paid the price, as Roosevelt or Truman would, of barnstorming every town from Plzen to Košice, and insisting face to face that union includes justice and mutual respect.

In the October 19, 1992 *New Yorker*, Lawrence Weschler, whose book on Solidarity and martial law in Poland I found so insightful, wrote a long, troubling article on post-revolutionary Czechoslovakia. Unlike Poland and Hungary, the attainment of freedom came to Czechoslovakia so rapidly that no one was prepared. Unlike Poland, where Solidarity had been a mass movement, the Czech anti-Communist, post-1968 opposition never possessed more than a few thousand members. Jan Palach had burnt himself to death in January 1969 as a symbol of revolt, but revolt itself had been limited to a few Prague rock groups like the *Plastic People of the Universe*, songs with ambiguous lyrics, books published in Toronto, and Havel sitting in jail.

If the seizure of freedom in Czechoslovakia as well as in East Germany had come so rapidly, with so little resistance, why not earlier? Were the security police—*Statni tajna Bezpecnost*[†]—so dangerous, or was that alleged danger an excuse? Was it shameful to admit how easily one was frightened?

---

* Address at New York University, October 27, 1991.

[†] In 1993 Jiři received an official statement that he had never had any contact with them.

What is the American equivalent of the taboos that contaminate post-Communist society, like this gonorrhea of informing? Perhaps it is our health-care system, which has been not only paralyzed within the gridlock of competing interests but so shrouded by ideas that cannot be examined and words that must not be spoken that it might as well have been designed by Stalinists.

The sister of the elderly Italian barber who cuts my hair had a stroke, was taken to the local hospital where she was put in intensive care. After twelve days, without recovering consciousness, she died. The next day her daughter was presented with a bill of $140,000. Different varieties of insurance paid for most of that, but the story's point is the ghastly disregard of economic, medical and moral values that permits such a typical American travesty.

Each system has its built-in benefits. That electrified barbed-wire fence around the Czech borders meant a lot of good jobs. Low-skill employees found honest work listening to phone calls and reading other people's mail. American computer clerks, insurance executives, lab technicians, and brain surgeons are not going to sit back and let their jobs be taken away.

1991

This time I stay at an old-fashioned little hotel behind the Tyn Church, only a block from the main square that I walk round and round, trying to hold fast every beloved façade and tower. The Hus monument is hung with banners demanding solidarity with the Chinese dissidents, and there are Christmas booths selling puppets and decorations.

I pay a pilgrim's visit to the *Bertramka*, where Mozart stayed, and attend an elegant presentation of *Cosí Fan Tutte* by an Italian company. That level of culture, of course, will be kept alive for and by tourists. How about the theatres and jazz clubs for which Prague, like Warsaw, was famous as a way to remind its people that leaden-footed authority didn't always have the last answer—and which are going out of business in the brave new world of bottom-line economics?

I make a trip to Wilsonovo Nadrazí to check my 7 A.M. ticket to Vienna. This leads me past the oriental Spanish synagogue on Jerusalem Street and its two bulb-topped minaret towers from Granada and Fez. Closed, in decay— Prague has only one synagogue worth dressing up for tourists. At lunchtime I enter a pretentiously façaded restaurant untouched by Euroniceness. After making sure I've waited long enough, a sullen waitress plunks down a plate holding a slab of fat through which crawls a pink worm of "meat." Next to it, face down, a fistful of greasy sauerkraut. The poor girl, who reminds aged German and Jewish returnees nostalgically of the slatterns with whom they had had their first adolescent adventures, will be scolded for forgetting to put her thumbprint on my spoon. It is sad to think of this picturesque slovenliness menaced inexorably by McDonald's and Burger King.

"Haffa nize deh."

On the way to the Karluv Most and its Christmas time souvenirs is a store that sells Kafka T-shirts. Welcome home! One makes a gift list of literary and Jewish friends, for there are also shirts with Rabbi Loew and the Golem.

That night, passing the, *Europa Hotel* on my way to the opera, I see my first hard-core prostitute: tight tight mini skirt, spike heels, low cut blouse, meticulously applied eye shadow, vermillion lipstick.

When I lecture at obscure colleges on political theory, I begin with Lenin as the supreme figure of our century. It is he who establishes the totalitarian state as the vehicle and ultimately the goal for 100% rationalization of human life, far beyond Josef II's vision and Plato's. Hitler and Stalin were his pupils. The alternative to Lenin is Franklin Roosevelt, pragmatic, human, realistic about his methods and allies, and with a realizable vision of a just society.

Not true. It is Calvin Coolidge and his ideals of profit that bestride the narrow world like a colossus. If rich people become richer that's the way it should be. If poor people become poorer they are easy to ignore. In our time the banner has been carried aloft by Ronald Reagan and his girlfriend, Margaret Thatcher, the Lenin and the Stalin of the capitalist counterattack, but some day the world will recognize the lobby of the *Alcron* as the cradle of our century.

President Bush proclaims, "The Cold War is over and we won it!" Mikhail Sergeyevich Gorbachev is already a figure of history. Vaclav Havel is the decent and sensible president of a small land—we don't need a vast amount of real estate—some one quite different from the stable of leaders we know, but his country is slipping through his hands.

> *but:*
> *will freedom know how to sing*
> *the way slaves used to sing of freedom*
> Branko Miljkovic *EverybodyWill Write Poetry*

22

Vienna 1937, 1939, 1951

1939

The namelessly dead
the meticulously murdered
on ghetto sidewalks
were covered with newspapers
until they were carted off

Newspapers since then
with increasing circulation
have diligently served
to cover up the truth
that's lying spread-eagled on its back.

As long as it's not breathing
and doesn't raise its head
otherwise the swarming letters
the blowflies, the fleshflies of words
would rise up buzzing from the startled sheets
in search of other prey
      Jerzy Ficowski *From the History of Journalism*

IT WAS 1939 AND MID-AUGUST when Bruce and I reached Vienna after our three-week circle to the southeast: Budapest, Bucharest, Sofia, Belgrade. "The wheat is harvested—now there will be war." Would Bulgaria and Hungary team up on Romania? How would Yugoslavia go, or would Croats and Serbs just fight each other? Was a volunteer regiment of Hungarians secretly training to fight alongside the Poles? With the young Americans one could try out one's rumors as well as one's English.

We had collected a fair basket of impressions since leaving Poland. The French-speaking Czech cook of a small Hungarian inn in what had once been Slovakia helped us fill out our papers. He had formerly been manager of two large hotels in Prague and Bratislava and said goodbye with "We'll meet again in the trenches fighting against Germany." Black buffaloes, fields of sunflowers in Transylvania, and our first onion-towered Orthodox churches. Signs in Romanian restaurants: "Do not discuss politics." A barefoot peasant girl in Bucharest with a basket of vegetables on her head walking past a ritzy hotel, dames in their underwear who leaned out a window and whistled at us. Soldiers in Sofia with caps on the side of their heads, shoulder boards, belted tunics, black boots, straight from St. Petersburg. Officers wearing sabers and curled moustaches on their way to call upon Madame Karenina.

Lost at night on a dirt road in a Serbian village, we made contact with an immigrant America. "Twelve years in Pittsburgh"—about the only words that remained. "My uncle lives in Toledo, you know him?" From a woman: "You stay in our house if you want." Their breaths were heavy with garlic. What would the outhouse be like? We begged off, a shame. Later on I was sorry.

There was no hiding place. In perfect English a cultured Romanian told us, "The war against the Jews is the war for Christianity." Every human being on the continent was waiting for Adolf Hitler to make up his mind. Nevertheless, even protected Americans felt a sense of dread to see the swastika again at the Austrian border, to hear Heil Hitler, see His face on the wall, and receive the contempt for these dumb Americans in their dirty French car.

Vienna was our first conquered city. The desk clerk at the *Bristol* (next day we switched to a cheaper place) smiled and said, "We are Ostmark now." A neat "Juden unerwunscht" stood at his elbow.

It was a strange visit. I wanted to show Bruce the charming parts of Vienna that I remembered from a Grand Tour two years before with my cousin and his tutor. ("All men wear uniform little moustaches" is a diary comment from 1937.)

That tour, stopping only in hotels like the *Bristol* had included a pilgrimage to the Karl Marx Hof apartment complex in the western suburbs, which the heroic socialists had tried to defend in 1934—rifles versus cannon—against the brutal army of Engelbert Dollfuss, almost the first political awakening for a romantic 13 year old. Dollfuss was an earnest man so short that he prompted all sorts of jokes: "That's not a turtle, that's the chancellor wearing a steel helmet." In winter he went ice skating on the frozen surface of his chamberpot. He was murdered by Austrian Nazis in July of 1934, but Mussolini's mobilization prevented Hitler from seizing control. Don't rush things. Dollfuss was followed by Kurt von Schuschnigg, who ran an old-man's dictatorship until broken by Hitler at the Anschluss in 1938. I met Schuschnigg after my return from Austria in 1952, at a swimming pool in St. Louis, where he taught. His only question was of the current price of shoes in Vienna.

Bruce and I visited the noble cathedral of St. Stephen and the elegant summer palace (Austrian yellow walls with green shutters) and formal gardens of Schönbrunn, ate chocolate éclairs at *Dehmel's* and stood before the Johann Strauss monument, the ingratiating artist playing his violin within a sort of stone doughnut, where sentimental girls had placed sad little bouquets after the Nazi takeover. But these courteous people feeding pigeons were our enemies now. The boys our age, fewer wearing uniforms than in Germany, would become soldiers fighting us. We took an afternoon drive up the Danube through beautiful towns like Durnstein and Krems, stopping at a garden restaurant filled with laughing people drinking new wine, till the huge sign—JUDEN VERBOT—as if it were the establishment's name, made us get back in the car.

We found ourselves talking about Fritz, our friend at Deerfield, and his parents who taught at Smith College. They had invited us one Sunday to their house in Northampton for lunch, which included a whipped cream and chocolate cake roll made by their Swiss cook, and talked of the cities in which they had traveled, studied, made music, and which now, save for Zurich, were finished. What would the Jacobis say of this, or that, was always with us.

Despite the frictions of a long journey with only each other to rely on, Bruce and I were still getting along surprisingly well. His French was better than mine; I knew fifty words of German. He was more aware of the human side of the drama we passed, but sometimes failed to remember that, having spent a year at Harvard, I knew much more about history and culture.

The formal reason for our stay, of course, was to pick up at Gestapo headquarters the three day permit for Prague that we had requested in Berlin. We made our way to the *Hotel Metropol*, found the proper office, were handed the visa. The process was easy, no one frightened us. On our way out we passed an old couple dressed in black, each with a yellow armband and Star of David, clutching each other as they tried to climb the stairs. The fragility of the two old people, their nearness to death, like the Teich family in their empty Berlin apartment, the frantic antheap in Warsaw—what to say?

A rainy Saturday afternoon, bored and restless, the permit for Prague not valid until the next day, we were drifting through the Stadtpark. Two rows of green benches, empty, stretched to infinity, one yellow bench with four people on it. They could have sat on a green bench. No one was there to stop them. They did not have yellow arm bands or hooked noses, but they had been told it was forbidden. (I thought of the rules when I worked in Mississippi a couple of years later.) Three men, a woman were sitting on the yellow bench waiting—literally—until someone decided to put them to death.

∞

I chanced upon Austrians a couple of times when I was a soldier in Italy. The 36th (Texas National Guard) Division was trying to force its way through the mountains between Naples and Rome, stumbling around the town of San Pietro. We were faced by German mountain troops, one of whose divisions was the 44th, largely composed of Austrians. A prisoner was brought back to 141st regimental headquarters, and a half circle of maybe forty or fifty Americans had gathered around him, staring silently at the zoo animal, clad in a blue-green uniform with a peaked wool cap, exactly what Austrians had worn back in 1917.

When the German forces in Italy surrendered in May 1945, the task of Headquarters G-2 was to keep track of the passage of German regiments into prison camps. A staff officer came to our headquarters outside Verona, a beautiful aristocrat speaking better English than the Americans he dealt with, who let himself be known as an Austrian, complaining how he had been forced to serve under the Germans.

> *He was evil and ruined everything;*
> *they were good;*
> *whenever he dishonored and dulled the sword,*
> *they presented it newly sharpened*
> *and handed it to him again and again.*
> Michael Guttenbrunner *Hitler and the Generals*

∞

1951

In 1951, after five years of teaching, I had applied for a position in France under the Fulbright Program. That seemed a way to recharge the batteries and test what I knew with a different audience. We were sent to Austria, funded, in local currency, for the purchase of surplus American army equipment, and my modest salary in Vienna and Graz represented a second-hand jeep and perhaps 300 blankets.

With three children (eight, four, and two, the youngest still in diapers), Mary and I drove east from Cherbourg, not always easy, though if you travel with little girls, of course, every cathedral becomes a glorious stage for hopscotch: "Not down the main aisle, dear."

We arrived in Vienna. The Fulbright authorities on Rooseveltplatz, formerly Goeringplatz, formerly Dollfussplatz, helped place us in an apartment in Hietzing, beyond Schöbrunn, an old-fashioned suburb lined with horse-chestnut trees. September's sound was the crack of shiny brown nuts hitting the sidewalk, each child had its own collection. With the apartment came Frau Anna, an elderly cleaning woman. The landlady cautioned us not to pay her wages that would upset the neighborhood pattern, though we could make her a nice gift when we left. Mary learned enough housewife German to buy provisions. An aged gentleman she nodded to at the corner store addressed her with "I used to be a general in the Imperial Army, and now I must do the shopping." Each time they met he said the same thing.

The 8-year-old we enrolled in the local school. For a few days she was picked up as mascot, a sort of teddy bear, by the third grade's social set—she had interesting toys, her mother offered cookies. Then they became bored— "Du redest so blöd" ("You talk so dumb.")—and dropped her. The building caretaker had a lonely eleven-year-old niece who used to drop in at teatime and pedal around the apartment on Bruce's tricycle. After a while Irmgard became Catherine's closest friend and almost a member of the family.

I took the Stadtbahn each morning to my Gymnasium (academic secondary school) near the Ring. My teaching at Thomas Jefferson did not prepare me for this job. It was strictly Us versus Them, no American self-delusion about working together. The teacher was Boss, sometimes quite rational, the next moment yelling at his pupils like a Marine sergeant. I sat in the back row, filled with guilt for being shouted at, but the boys did not mind. They cheated compulsively. Any boy called on would stand at his seat while all his classmates whispered the answers. A good teacher, however—I remember a couple of brilliant classes on *Faust*—had no trouble.

My position was marginal. The teacher would look at his watch and state that Herr Professor Merrill will tell us about Indians. All the boys had read Karl May and his uplifting tales of Winnetou and Old Shatterhand, just as Polish boys had read Sienkiewicz's blood-drenched *Trilogy*, and in carefully enunciated phrases I told them about the Navajo. Later on I added classes on the life of a student at Kirkwood High and 'A walk around New York City,' starting at German Yorkville in the East 80s, down past the Irish bars and

Italian restaurants to the streets of Polish Jews and Chinatown and then up the West Side, ending at the *Éclair* on West 72nd where we sat down for coffee and pastry.

All my colleagues were Wehrmacht alumni, most of them on the Russian front—yes, I too had been an infantryman. They went on and on about the hardships of winter, their fear of capture. We said nothing about politics. The Nazis were Germans—Piefke. I was polite and listened, like a woman in the hostess's kitchen. In German I could not get angry or tell jokes.

Boys with Slavic names, the art teacher said, draw pictures in red and blue. Boys with German names use green, brown and yellow. Why weren't we Americans smart enough in 1945 to realize who were our real enemies? If they'd had our planes and tanks behind them, the Wehrmacht veterans would have been willing to fight under American generals, and together the two of us could have rolled back the Russians. One man had served as tutor for quite a few Jewish boys. "You gain a totally different picture of Jews when you see them with their families." In my year of teaching in Austria, including six months in Graz after leaving Vienna, I met *one* man who mentioned the death camps. He told me that a guard who could not stand it any more had been transferred to his anti-aircraft battery in the Ukraine. From him my friend had learned about Auschwitz.

Everyone except Jews, Communists, some intellectuals, and reactionary Catholics had been in favor of Anschluss. Nationalists were glad to be part of greater Germany, socialists hated Schuschnigg's dictatorship. Protestants became citizens of the nation of Martin Luther. In the Austrian republic there were no jobs. After Anschluss, there seemed no limit to how far a young man of energy and ability could climb.

Little bits of history slipped out. In 1952 the winter Olympics were held in Norway—"But Austrians can't get visas!" Hours later I remembered the ugly reason. After 1918 many Norwegians took malnourished Viennese children into their homes to feed them back to proper strength. When the Germans invaded Norway in 1940, many of those soldiers were Viennese who still remembered the language a bit. In 1952 they were still not welcome.

I taught at four different Gymnasien that fall, one of them for girls on the Maria Hilfe Strasse, where the nicer Jewish shops used to be. The star of the English department was a dramatic, red-haired Jewish woman, who had preserved herself from Auschwitz and Majdanek by taking refuge in England, and then, not totally rationally, had returned to Vienna, where some of her acquaintances resented the way she had escaped their sufferings.

Those different work places forced me to know different slices of the Innere Bezirk (central city). Though Vienna as a whole was divided into four sections (Hietzing was British) within the Russian zone (which we could cross by one highway only), the central area was policed by the famous jeeps carrying their British, American, French, and Russian MPs, useful for arresting drunken soldiers, but primarily ceremonial as the last symbol of Allied collaboration.

1951 saw the start-up of the Marshall Plan, surprisingly far-sighted and in Austria well-administered and generously acknowledged. What were the Austrian resources, like mountains and Mozart, the American officials asked, and then how could these be best utilized by remodeled hotels and theaters, new roads and hydroelectric plants, with investment even within the Russian zone. One had reason to be proud of one's country.

Twice a week Mary took German lessons with a Sudeten refugee, Frau Gavora, who had married a Slovak during the war—"a Catholic monsignor and a Lutheran bishop were guests at our wedding and peasant girls danced the csardas in their petticoats"—he was now in a Communist jail in Bratislava, on the other side of the moon.

From these lessons, my colleagues, shopping, even our children, we learned Viennese language and life, in patches, like tiles in a mosaic. Because most people, except for timber exporters, opera singers, contractors, and wholesale meat dealers, were poor, and for formal occasions still wore clothes they had purchased before the war, the currency was different varieties of ceremony. For academics a doctorate was fairly easy to obtain and not of much value, but every holder, even if he sold neckties, received the correct title. "G'nadige Frau" ("gracious lady") was old-fashioned Austrian; Germans, and by the 1990s Austrians, were amused by this musty habit I still employed. A purist kissed the hand, or made at least a downward swoop, as gentlefolk do in Kraków, and if you had made the acquaintance of your colleague's wife it was hoflich (courtly) to use at parting, "schön Handküss zu Haus," a vicarious (beautiful) kissing of her hand to be passed on when the other man reached home.

Other terms, usually pejorative, were fun to employ. Ein blödsinniger Kerl (a profoundly stupid lout), in fact ein echte schlampig* hochnäsiger Schlurf (a genuine, slovenly, stuck-up hippy such as hung around the entrance to my school twenty years later) spoke Quatsch (nonsense) and would end his days as ein hoffnungsloser Knecht (a hopeless failure). The special accents in which these terms could be used, nasal and whining if you

---

* It was impossible for any self-respecting German to talk about Austrians without using Schlamperei—all-purpose slovenliness.

were middle class, grob (coarse) if you were proletarian, would either be delightful or obnoxious according to how much wine and coffee you had recently drunk.

With November Vienna became colder, rainier, poorer, even less of a tourist spot, but more firmly mine as Staatsangestelter (state employee) in my brown raincoat and Alpine green hat, moving in the dispirited trudge of Nachkriegszeit* (post-war times). I knew that I belonged. I had a useful role to play teaching these adolescent boys and girls, sharing with them my conviction that the task was important, and more than that, they were important.

The base point of my city was the Stefansdom, its roof still under repair from shelling the last month of the war. (For the Eastern cities—Budapest, Poznań, Breslau, Vienna, Berlin—the Germans had fought doggedly.) The silence and dark with the flickering candle flames reflecting off the altars' gold shielded each visitor from the misery of the streets. In good times a cathedral is a postcard stop, a paragraph for a sophomore course in art history. In hard times it becomes a sanctuary. I thought about my winter visits to the Duomo in Florence when I came down from army headquarters on the road to Bologna, and of what I found again and again in the somber church of St. Mary in Kraków.

Does God exist? How do you know? What difference does it make?

A second stop, beyond the Ring, was the Baroque dome and the two great columns of the Karlskirche, to honor the victories of Charles VI's† armies under Prinz Eugen of Savoy against the Turks, a statement of Habsburg right and duty to protect Christandom. The Karlskirche, unlike the Stefansdom, was a daylight, good-times church, no place for a humble heart, appropriately enough bordered by a monument to the heroes of the Red Army, with its own victory column and grave stones, Russian guardsman and nervous Austrian policeman. A bit beyond stretched the formal gardens and graveled walks of the elegant Belvedere Palais, a gift to Prinz Eugen, where the sun shone more often than in the city. It sheltered now a museum of Austrian art, with Gustav Klimt's chestnut trees and florid ladies and Egon Schiele's agonized nudes.

---

* My Uncle Harden, who had started life as an opera singer but lost his voice in the trenches of France, studied piano in his nachkriegs Wien. His memory was of the hungry girls who formed a circle around any obvious foreigner and would not let him escape till he promised to go home with one of them and give her enough money to buy food.

† Charles was the father of Maria Theresa, who set her stamp on Austria's eighteenth century as Victoria did on England's nineteenth, and grandfather of rational Josef II and foolish Marie Antoinette.

Third was the great block of the Hofburg, the center of Habsburg Staats-macht, rivaled only by the Černin palace south of the Hradčany, with no apology for power—represented here by the equestrian statue in Roman garb of Josef II. On the edge of the Josefplatz was the restaurant *Zur Stadt Brunn*, in memory of the generations when Brno was an Austrian city and Czech simply the language of the dishwashers. For 15 schillings (60 cents) I would have a modest lunch of goulasch, a saltzstangerl (a hard roll with large salt grains on its crust), a glass of wine, and a kompot of apricots or gooseberries.

In my daily travel back and forth from my Stadtbahn station, I could readily enter the Russian sector in the working-class part of the city. Legal, yes, but some violation of propriety. This was the second year of the Korean War, with always a shade of fear that that might turn into World War III, Austria, and our family, the first Soviet targets. Matthew Ridgeway, the American general in command, was accused of having launched germ warfare, and any large stretch of wall that could be reached by the Communists sported a huge scrawl of Ridgeway=Pestkrieg. Russian soldiers and their families were forbidden to have any contacts with civilians, American families were afraid to. Austrian employees at the PX were forbidden to speak German: the foreign words upset army wives. Eight-year-old Catherine and I worked out a sentimental story of sharing a building with the family of a Russian officer, another version of the novel I wrote about Prague. While he is away his wife falls sick, and it is up to us to look after the children. The parents return and gradually the two families become friends. This was during the last terror-wrapped years of Stalin, and Americans could not realize that even one social call by a Russian officer to an American home would have cost him his job, his freedom, and perhaps his life.

I spent an afternoon in the Russian reading room. Black was white. The Marshall Plan was imperial exploitation, the Americans had invaded North Korea, the Russians had brought democracy and prosperity to Eastern Europe. I was in *1984*. Was there a single fact that I could hold as true? Then in one illustrated magazine I found an article on brilliant examples of Russian modernism in the architecture of Moscow today. Why did the building that received the highest praise seem familiar? The Wrigley Building in Chicago—1912. They could not imagine something more creative than that. There was my fact.

For Mary and myself the richest gift of that autumn was opera. On almost the last major raid upon Vienna before the Red Army closed in, American bombers had destroyed the great mit Pracht (magnificence) und Prunk (ostentation) Opernhaus of 1869, so we attended the smaller Theater an der Wien, built by Schikaneder, Mozart's impresario. Twice a week we took the Stadtbahn from Hietzing for our 28 schilling (a bit more than $1) seats.

We heard everything: *Marriage of Figaro* and *Don Giovanni, Boris Godunov* with George London, which brought out the Russian officers and their wives, *Aida* which brought out the Americans. An over-ripe Ljuba Welitsch in *Salome* and Franz Lehar's *Giuditta* which suited every critic's dismissal of Viennese decadence—"Meine Lippen sie küssen so heiss!" What we had seen formed the week's conversation.

Magic Flute, Rosenkavalier and *Fidelio* were the three favorites. The fairy tale costumes and characters of *Zauberflöte* included moments of pure beauty like the duet between Papageno the bird man and Princess Pamina (Erich Kunz and Irmgard Seefried, who stole our hearts) on the love between man and woman. When we have had our fill of self-centered intellectuals, whether Harvard Business School professors or Politburo planners, we are less impressed by the noble rationalism of Sarastro's priests. Perhaps the typically female fury of the Queen of the Night may be, in the long run, less costly. Monostatos the Moor is both evil and cowardly because he is black, but his cry—Cannot a black man love?—is less laughable than it seemed in Mozart's day. How well will Princess Pamina get along with the constipated purity of Prince Tamino? The fun-loving Papageno and Papagena's sexiness, planned to produce a lot of little kids just like Mom and Dad, is refreshing. The tale is told that *Zauberflöte* was being given the night that Mozart lay dying. He held a watch in his hand so that he knew what aria, what chorus was then being sung, and he beat time with his finger and whispered the words of the songs.

Rosenkavalier was Mary's choice. Time threatens the Marschallin and her love for the young Count Octavian (a contralto in trousers)—all the clocks in her house have been stopped. Another threat is the loutish Baron Ochs von Lerchenau, who wants Octavian to carry the silver rose of courtship to Sophie, daughter of rich Herr Faninal, who in turn would like a titled son-in-law. Sophie and Octavian, of course, fall in love instead, the baron is humiliated, and the Marschallin graciously releases Octavian to his new love. The story and the music were too rich for my taste. One is all too aware of the daughters of foolish fathers who did *not* escape a Baron Ochs in the Vienna of Maria Theresa that Hugo von Hofmansthal and Richard Strauss brought to life, but the final trio of the three women is the most beautiful work of all late Viennese music.

For me the greatest experience was *Fidelio*. Its message of loyalty and courage, of defiance to evil made it unwelcome to the Nazis. In the anonymous dark the audience applauded in the wrong places, as they did in Warsaw for Mickiewicz's words against corrupt old men who take bribes and grovel before the Russians. *Fidelio* was the consecration piece for each rebuilt opera house in post-war Germany and Austria, and its audience could put behind them for a moment the misery of war and post-war, and forget their own moral shabbiness.

Fidelio demands a suspension of disbelief. Leonora, disguised as a boy, becomes Rocco the gaoler's assistant in hopes of learning whether her husband Florestan is the secret prisoner of evil Don Pizarro—and in so doing attracts the love of Marcellina, Rocco's daughter. Any woman, of course, who can sing the music that Beethoven hands Leonora is not going to slip into a boy's disguise. Will Florestan be able afterwards to put aside masculine ego at owing life and freedom to his wife? Critics fault the terrible vocal strain Beethoven puts upon both Florestan and Leonora, the symphonic burden of the orchestra. It doesn't matter. The off-stage horn call as the messenger arrives from the king is the call of hope, the promise of justice. The overture, which doesn't fit the mechanics of the opera, is, nevertheless, the noblest piece of music ever written.

Catherine, Amy, and Bruce did not complain when their parents left for the opera in the evening because they knew that Elli would come. Elli, a law student at the university, recommended to us by the Fulbright office, was our door opener to Vienna. She lived in her mother's cluttered Ring apartment with her older sister, a somber medical student. They came from a cultured, well-to-do Catholic background. Although Herr Back was 'racially' Jewish, he had relied, as the Nazi threat deepened, not only upon his Catholic baptism but upon his record as a cavalry officer in the first World War to protect him, and had not tried to take his family to safety abroad. He was mistaken. Then, to give his wife and daughters a little better chance to survive, he killed himself. The first years of the war the family lived in the somewhat greater safety of Hungary, but as the battle lines moved westward they came back to Vienna. Elli's sister Hannah had obsessively tried to understand the demonic quality of the Nazis by buying every book she could about Hitler and his partners. Now, with the Red Army in the eastern suburbs, they must burn all of these in their great tiled stove. The first Russian soldier who stumbled down the stairs to the basement where they were hiding was a boy, like so many of the front-line troops, often with bandages over recent wounds, and asked only for a drink of water.

Hannah was the one who foraged for food during the ensuing days. What could they get for linen, china, silver, as the housewives of Warsaw had done? Where, after peace came, could one pick up a piece of charity from Sweden or America? It was the agony of those days that had scarred her spirit.

For Elli the indestructible richness of Vienna was her nourishment. Who were the leading singers and conductors (Karajan, taboo in America for belonging to the Soviet Friendship Society), what were the best theaters and restaurants (which she could not afford to enter), the authors and architects, the lights and shadows of the famous mayor, Karl Lueger? Every opera we saw, almost every new street we walked down must be presented for her opinion.

In my wandering along the narrow streets behind the Stefansdom I came upon a bookstore with a large display of art books, from the libraries of Ringstrasse apartments, I suppose, or of vanished Jews. A volume on Austrian architecture caught my eye. In the dark behind the counter sat a young woman who turned on the light for me. She was in her late twenties, with dark hair, an oval, sallow face; and her courteous manner, gentle voice and reserved smile struck my heart. We talked about the book I had purchased, other books. I mentioned my teaching position at the Gymnasium, which even introduced the subject that I had been a soldier in Italy.

I came back to the store and bought other books and a mysterious ink and wash drawing by Kubin. Reserved about her own life, she was curious in asking about mine. Yes, she had lived in Vienna all during the war. It was hard, those first years afterwards even more so. People did not have the money to buy luxuries like books, but perhaps things now were becoming a bit better.

When I left the store—I never saw another customer—she turned the light off. Her eyes, her smile were as fragile as a fire of paper in an iron stove, but she had survived.

What was she like? How had the Nazi years, the bite of the war, the coming of the Russians touched her? Suppose I had been a soldier then—how would we have met, what would we have offered each other? A story started to grow in my mind that I could not escape.

It is early 1946. Sergeant Giles Bauer works at a headquarters unit around Rooseveltplatz but has volunteered to serve at a warehouse for Volksdeutsch Sudetenlanders expelled from Czechoslovakia. He has a fiancée, Barbara, back in Isona, Oklahoma, but—he speaks German—he has been asked to stay on. With his friend, Sgt. Thaelmann, a cynical Jewish combat interrogator from Leipzig who despises all Austrians but from amusement or boredom shares Giles' work—they coach soccer for the boys—he remains at the warehouse.

Giles goes to the same bookstore, buys the same book, meets the same young woman seated in the cold as I did. The darkness is swept away by the same courteous, reserved smile. He works up courage to invite her to a

Mozart concert at the Musikverein, and shares the worn red carpets, the flaking white and gold paint, the glistening brown, silver and gold instruments. He is introduced to her aunt at their cluttered Ringstrasse apartment, offers them a cheese sent by Barbara from Isona. Irmgard Oertl becomes nervous at being courted by an American soldier with such gifts. The stereotype of what she is expected to offer in response is too evident. It is too hard to be simply Irmgard and Giles.

She had a fiancé, Witold Kratochwil (a Viennese name), a lieutenant of artillery whose battery had been overrun in a Russian attack. Is he still alive? He was on the losing as well as on the wrong side. Both of them knew that from early on.

"I live in nothingness and call it my life."

Giles has come to love a little girl at the warehouse with a blue hair ribbon. He will organize a Faschings (carnival) party for the children. He locates a beautiful red rocking horse (Irmgard is not amused by his boast that he used to be a cavalryman), hires a thin old Schrammel (a 12-string guitar with a double neck) player to sing for the children, and scrounges food and gifts for a party. The party ends. Dark cold hopelessness rushes back to take over the warehouse, and that night a woman smothers her child, wraps herself in a blanket, and slits her wrists.

Giles will start a school—the Tannenbaum Schule, the fir tree, ever green. No one believes in this dream, but people more or less help him out of curiosity as to how it will fail. Failure we understand. Success is threatening—a conclusion shared by any number of hippies and blacks I taught during the Vietnam years. The school does survive, however, and the Army comes to patronize it as an example of American big heartedness.

Irmgard eventually accepts him as her lover, and after she becomes pregnant they are married. Giles returns to Isona and eventually she follows. The story becomes more difficult now. Returning to his hometown is not easy. He finds a low-paying job at the high school, but there seems no opening for his energy and idealism. I had taught enough boys from towns like Isona to know how mediocre were the standards. Irmgard is disappointed by his inferior position—aren't all Americans rich?—but starts her own successful business painting furniture in Austrian peasant style. They have two more children. She becomes able to endure Oklahoma summers. She overlooks the emptiness of Isona because she really does not look for anything beyond her family, her home, the work she has found for herself. Though the book ends, the story continues. She is amused as well as irritated that Catholics in such a Protestant town are looked upon as a secret society, but she makes friends with an Italian war bride who drives her to the church of a Mexican congregation in Ponca City. Like Natasha at the end of *War and Peace* she puts on weight. She is unimpressed by Giles' loathing of Senator McCarthy. Anyone sympathetic to the Communists and the Russians is simply a fool.

Without my being able to do anything about it, Irmgard became the dominant figure. Giles faded. When the Fulbright office sent me to teach in Graz, with Hungary (and the Russian zone) a few miles to the east, Tito's Slovenia and Croatia a few miles to the south, I wrote and rewrote *A Prize of Value*. I felt close to Irmgard and respected the life she had made for herself. Shouldn't Giles stop complaining and make use of his GI Bill for an advanced degree and go into college teaching? Get out of Isona!

When spring came and the chestnuts leafed out and blossomed, then the lilacs, I would buy a cup of coffee and a tiny cognac that allowed me two hours of writing at a café table. This is why Americans went to Europe. Graz had a mountain with a castle and a river in the middle of the city—the Mur, flowing from the Alps into the Drava and eventually the Danube. In the Hauptplatz the market ladies sold wurst, plums from Serbia, paprika-salat from Hungary, oranges from Israel. Graz was a beautiful city to live in as a state employee, a part of society, not as a tourist. Our family comprised 20% of the total American population of a city of 200,000. 1913 had been its peak year—the year my Realschule had been founded and its laboratory gear purchased, the style of the hats worn by widows of K.u.K. officials. Graz was the cheapest city of the republic. It was the southeasternmost German-speaking city of the empire, and therefore strongly Pan-German before 1914, strongly pro-Nazi before 1938.

A beautiful city, a novel that was a pleasure to write, but it turned out to be the story of failure.

23

Vienna and Graz 1952, 1991

Grub first, then ethics.
    Bertolt Brecht

THOUGH WE RETURNED TO VIENNA for short visits several times after that stay in 1951, it was Graz, in Steiermark, where we spent a longer time, that became *our* city, not shared with a million other visitors.

My boss, Herr Direktor Hofrat Dr. Nager was an imposing man with bald head and rich white beard. Russian soldiers, thinking he was an Orthodox priest, used to salute him. His three loves were his school, the Socialist party, and the English language. He had not been trusted by the Nazis, who forbade him to teach English but allowed him to stay on in Latin and Greek. Most of the people inside that self-important building—a monument to the creative discipline of Austro-German culture in 1913—were afraid of him, but he was generous to me.

Our apartment in a new jerry-built structure beyond Conrad von Hötzendorfstrasse overlooked the pink-walled city prison. For our landlord, an elderly priest, that three-room apartment represented his life's savings. One time he showed up very disturbed that if war came the Russians would not let us return to America, and he would not be able to get his apartment back. Austrian law was heavily stacked in favor of tenants. I assured him that the Russians would immediately ship all Americans to Siberia—he was safe. Later on Father Friedl returned to apologize for such suspiciousness. It was not his real nature.

Because the local public school lay on the other side of a dangerous streetcar switching center, we enrolled Catherine in a Catholic school. When the children were told to say Lenten prayers for the sins they had committed during Faschingszeit (Carnival), that brought an interesting conversation on Sin. She enjoyed the folk songs they learned, came to speak good German, and was a bit condescending that Amy at nursery school used Steyrisch. During the winter, when cellar-smelling cabbage, potatoes and apples plus sauerkraut, cheese, sausage were about the only items for sale at the corner grocery (Eckegeschäft), the milk turned blue so that wealthy foreign skiers in the Tyrol (Americans and at that time also Egyptians and Argentines) could put whipped cream on their coffee. There was a lot of snow that year, and Bruce enjoyed being pulled along the streets in his sled while Mother did her shopping.

Although Graz had a diversified industrial base—the Puch motorcycle works the best known—with iron and steel, instrument manufacture and railways, the closing off after 1918 of its natural markets in Yugoslavia, the loss of Trieste to the Italians, locked the city inside the cramped economy of the Austrian republic. The endless depression of the 1930s made a bad situation worse, and the noisy promises of the Nazis seemed the only way out. At Anschluss the Grazer Rathaus was the first in Austria to fly the swastika. Yugoslavia was even poorer and cheaper than Austria, however, and a monthly Sunday for any organization (opera subscribers, Friends of Nature, veterans of the 141st Regiment) was to rent a bus, drive across the border to Maribor and consume colossal quantities of food, wine, slivovitz until they rolled unconscious back home.*

Although a tiny alley named Judengasse wound through the old town (30 miles away in the mountains was Judenburg—imagine being a Wehrmacht soldier from that town), Graz had a minuscule Jewish population and escaped the ugly mob scenes of Vienna in March 1938. The invasion of Yugoslavia three years later was the city's most appropriate involvement in the war, though their soldiers paid for it during the terrible Russian winters. Our baby sitter, who was writing her doctoral thesis on F. Scott Fitzgerald, was the daughter of a well-to-do Volksdeutsch peasant in Slovenia. The Germans had controlled the days, the partisans, the nights. (Vietnam?) When the Wehrmacht withdrew, her father was arrested by the Communists and was never seen again, and Ingrid and her mother were eventually pushed across the border into Austria carrying only the clothes they wore.

As the Red Army fought its way ever nearer, Graz's hardline Gauleiter proclaimed that the city would fight block by block, house by house to defend the homeland (die Heimat, a feminine noun, by 1945 had replaced der Vaterland), and then jumped in his Mercedes and drove off at top speed to surrender to the Americans in the Tyrol. The city fell silent. Street cars stopped running. Austrian flags began to appear. The first Russian soldier entered Graz on a galloping horse. Then came the tanks with infantry riding on their tops, followed by horse-drawn wagons carrying supplies and more infantry.

---

* In spring of 1993 members of the Graz Wagner Society paid a visit not to Maribor but to strife-ridden, near bankrupt New York City in order to attend the Metropolitan's Ring cycle. Of course the music is just as good in the opera house of any German-speaking city, but these affluent conservatives were tired of Wotan as industrialist, Siegfried in blue jeans, and wanted Wagner's traditional fur wraps.

The Austrians were terrified, but the conquerors—perhaps because they hadn't had to fight for the city—did not behave as badly as in Budapest and Vienna. The items most wanted were watches (sometimes a soldier would wear four or five on his wrists), faucets, and door handles.

After the armistice (Waffenstillstand) southeastern Austria became the British zone, which made Americans more popular, although most of the British soldiers were stationed around Klagenfurt, 100 miles west. The Austrians, unlike the French and Italians, having seen the Russians at first hand, had little interest in Communism, and the country was run with mechanical fairness by the Socialist and the Catholic People's parties. The president was Socialist, the prime minister Volkspartei. At our school there was the same balance, down to the janitor and assistant janitor, reversed at the conservative Gymnasium across the river.

Austria, accordingly, celebrated both Socialist and Catholic holidays. For May Day the police took elaborate precautions to make sure that the Socialist and Communist parades did not collide, and on the Ascension Day (Christihimmelfahrt) long weekend, Mary and I flew southeast to Sarajevo. It was a beautiful, civilized city. The muezzin's cry from the minaret outside our hotel window awakened us, and we could see men washing themselves in the little mosque's fountain before going in for prayers. From tiny outdoor restaurants came the smell of roast lamb šiš kebob and raznici (tiny pork chops). An aged man seated at his doorstep was playing a one-string guzla. Jews, who still spoke, or counted, in Ladino, the language they had brought from Spain by way of Morocco and Turkey, had disappeared, but it seemed a city that accepted its mixed population in a reasonable way. It is sad to have seen Sarajevo turned into one more rubble heap, to hear about 'ethnic cleansing' again, and to see the comfortable nations unable, unwilling to halt the destruction.

⁊⊘⁊

In the summer of 1956 we rented a villa on the Attersee, a lake near Salzburg, among the chestnut and fruit trees that Gustav Klimt loved to paint, next to Steinbach where Mahler wrote his third symphony, spiritual and profound, each ensuing movement even more spiritual and profound. Our landlady put shoe polish on the roses to keep deer from eating them. 1956, of course, was the year of the Hungarian uprising against the Communists and then against Red Army tanks. From the brave words of Eisenhower and John Foster Dulles, the Hungarians expected American help that never came, but as the fugitives stumbled across the Austrian border, they were welcomed generously with such an outpouring of food and clothing that a fear grew of guns being hidden within some package of winter underwear that would set off the wrath of the Russians.

Mary and I returned briefly to Vienna and Graz in 1960, and I came again with Amy and Bruce in 1964 on our way to and from Warsaw and Olomouc. All the foreign soldiers had gone. Vienna had become again an expensive cosmopolitan capital. From our windows at the Hotel *Ambassador* on the Kärntnerstrasse, in rooms lined with crimson damask, we witnessed a thin parade of blue-shirted Communist Youth with self-consciously serious faces on their way, probably, to pay homage at the memorial to the heroes of the Red Army. By now the march-past was silly.

Again Mary and I were in both cities, March 1968, on our way to Yugoslavia and a mini-sabbatical in my brother's house in Athens. We were traveling with David and Paul, at fourteen and thirteen, old enough to be interested in what they saw, young enough still to enjoy traveling with their parents.

In Vienna came the news that LBJ would not run for re-election and would try to make peace in Vietnam. In Graz were headlines that Martin Luther King had been murdered. The murderer had not been found, mobs of angry blacks were looting the stores and burning cities. We bought every paper we could, though the stories were the same—*America in flames!*—puzzling out the words of newspaper German we had forgotten. To the Austrians, though, it was an exciting event, like some crazy riot after a super rock-and-roll concert, and there was a note of malicious superiority, too. Those Americans, always so damn sure of themselves, were tearing themselves apart. To our hotel concierge, who seemed a thoughtful man, I tried to tell a bit about King's life (we had served together on the board of Morehouse College in Atlanta). "What a tragedy, Herr Professor!" but his conclusion was that one couldn't expect anything different from black people, who were, let's face it, pretty primitive. Essentially, of course, he didn't care. King and the burning cities meant little to him, he had problems of his own. And there was no reason for kidding myself. In Graz or any other city in Austria or anywhere else I was a tourist, and the only country where I had anything of value to say and do was at home.*

---

* In 1982 I happened to meet the assassin, James Earl Ray. A friend who had turned his life into a crusade against the death penalty had two clients on death row of Tennessee State Penitentiary outside Nashville. Coming thru its L-shaped outer lobby, we passed a glum, shapeless man shuffling down one 40-foot arm of the L, then turning around to shuffle down the other-25. He had to be kept within the death building since a black prisoner in any regular cell block would have killed him within 24 hours. To shuffle silently (no one gave him a word) back and forth, for as long as he lived—there could be no more awful picture of Hell.

At home there was Vietnam. It began as a war belonging to the government and the news magazines. And young men who saw themselves faced by barracks life, ambushes and raids in swamps, and perhaps death, when no one else seemed touched at all. But after a while we were all touched—even Commonwealth School. Our boys were coming close to the army, as they realized. We were an independent institution and should make up our minds where we stood.

Those who did take a stand in the early years of the war seemed painfully innocent—scruffy kids with long hair. As one of William Lloyd Garrison's abolitionists said in the 1840s: "We are not to blame that wiser, better men did not espouse the cause of our oppressed colored countrymen. We Abolitionists are what we are—obscure men and silly women and we shall manage this matter as might be expected from such persons as we are."

Our oldest daughter, Catherine, living in San Francisco then, was caught up in radical politics. What shocked her in her first serious demonstration were the *sounds* of violence: the smack of a policeman's hand on the side of a face, a man's cries when he was hurt, the crash of a body hitting the metal floor of a truck after a demonstrator had been struck, his arms pinioned, his eyes sprayed with mace, then thrown into a police van like a sack of coal. Later she and some friends lay down side by side in the road outside the Oakland army base to block a troop convoy bound for the docks. The trucks were stopped, for five minutes, by these obscure and silly people, who were sent to jail, where Catherine planned to give lessons in modern dance and conversational French. The reality of the Santa Rita Rehabilitation Center was not what she had imagined. The Politicals wanted the curtains open so they could see the hills, and the Criminals, for whom the center was a sort of home, kept the curtains shut so that the place would seem more cozy. Catherine's two weeks at Santa Rita ended her involvement with politics.

The demonstrations, everywhere, as time went on, grew uglier and seemed more futile. If in my classroom I tried to stress the resiliency and good will of so much of American history and the need for responsible citizenship, I was confronted with Richard, a troubled sixteen-year-old who happened to be on the Cambridge Common when a demonstration against the war had turned into a riot. With his hair down to his shoulders he was the enemy and a policeman hit him in the face. How to talk to Richard about citizenship?

The police had become Pigs, victims of their own fear and hate, but more dangerous yet were the self-appointed Robespierres with their peculiar mix of virtue and terror, their own search and destroy missions, their total disregard of the right-wing counter-attacks those actions would provoke.

∞

Well, the overnight visit by Mary and me in 1978 was by error: we had missed the direct plane from Warsaw to Istanbul and taken the one instead to Vienna. Already the prices, the shop windows, the elegant visitors from Milan and Paris were moving the city out of the range of memories we retained, and the opera tickets were too costly to consider. It was 1991 before I came back.

By then a curious change had come over international opinion concerning Austria. In the 1950s I had loved Austria because it seemed to contain all that was best of German culture without German Staatsmacht and the guilt of the Nazis. By the 1980s the argument ran that the Germans had, to some extent, in uneven and painful ways, often by the actions of obscure men and silly women whom they despised, come to terms with their responsibility for the Nazis and the war. The Austrians, on the other hand, had wrapped themselves in the cocoon of fellow victim: "We were Hitler's first conquest." That was a foolproof gimmick for evading responsibility for the screaming mobs that welcomed Anschluss and enjoyed themselves to the hilt watching Jews scrub the sidewalks of Vienna. The uncovering of the hidden war-time role of Kurt Waldheim, secretary general of the United Nations and then president of the republic, whose Wehrmacht unit had used savage methods against Yugoslav partisans, epitomized this evasion. Austrians were angry, not at his actions, but at the criticism of them by foreigners—New York Jews. The sad, elegant officer who had come to 5th Army Headquarters at Verona acted differently, I am sure, when he dealt with Poles and Serbs.

What to forget? What to remember? When the German woman I had met on a train in Peru talked with me about the history of great nations, she told how she tried to give her children an understanding of the reality of Germany's past, which was at times pretty awful. But there were events in German history and German qualities worthy of respect and trust. You could not raise children bound, crippled by guilt. She had been an eleven-year-old girl cycling to school when fighter planes roared overhead firing at anything that moved. One forgives the American pilots. One forgives the young artillery officer on the Russian front whom she eventually married. That long conversation with Frau Solf helped free me from my own bonds of anti-Germanism.

Come let us reason together, sayeth the Lord,
though your sins be as scarlet
they may become white as snow.

But before that the sinner, as Isaiah reminds him, must come to an awareness—"Lord, what have I done?"—of the reality of his own actions. Had the
Austrians done this?

It wasn't until Gorbachev's last year in power that the Russians admitted
what everyone knew, that it was Stalin's security police, not the Germans,
who had murdered the Polish officers in the forest of Katyn. It wasn't until
1992 that the Japanese, whose culture does not welcome the open discussion
of ugly truths, admitted the enslavement and torture of tens of thousands of
Korean and Chinese women forced to serve in the army brothels. It was
almost 1994 before the United States government admitted that both soldiers
and civilians, including pregnant women and retarded boys, had been scien-
tifically exposed without their knowledge to cancer-causing levels of radia-
tion: the Western mind's fascination with experimental procedure.

Who is keeping score? On the technicians (one can hardly call them soldiers) in American planes who massacred the columns, mainly unarmed by
then, of fleeing Iraqi soldiers? On our careful government which made certain that no dead enemy face appeared on television. What was the reward for
the unsung genius who suggested that if bomb casings were made of plastic
instead of steel, they would be just as lethal but would not show up on the x-
ray machines given Hanoi by the Swedes and Russians? What American president—forget the Russians and Japanese—ever apologized to Americans as
well as to Vietnamese for the futility as well as the cruelty of that war?

Why blame Kurt Waldheim and the other young gentlemen of the Wehrmacht for what they may have done in Yugoslavia which does not compare
with what the Croats, Serbs, Bosnians have done to each other?

⟨∞⟩

In 1991 I wanted to spend two days in Vienna after my standard zigzag—Warsaw,
Kraków, Olomouc, Prague—in order to visit those streets, churches, muse-
ums, wine cellars I used to know and to distance myself from a weary load
of reflections.

The previous two weeks had left me surprisingly troubled. Two years
before, the Poles and Czechs knew who were their enemies, what the rules
were and how to get around them, and had the conviction that they were on
the winning side. We shall overcome. Now, who was the enemy? The guys
who said they were in charge and didn't know how to manage anything? Ex-

Communists, Germans, Slovaks, the fellow next door? There were no rules, or they changed every day. OK, some people had opened little boutiques and restaurants and computer service stations and charged high prices for what they offered, but it wasn't *us*. One could write or say anything one wanted. Nobody cared.

What were the good things that Freedom had brought from the West along with T-shirts and the *New York Times*? Striptease competitions in the establishment on Spitalna Ulica. Violence in the streets of Warsaw and Prague, from fewer policemen and fewer jobs, from skinheads and old-fashioned hoodlums finding a mission in beating up orientals and gypsies since there were no longer enough Jews to go around. Get-rich-quick sharpies and con-artists.

Just as the ideals of Socialism had been hijacked by the Communists, the ideals of Democracy were being hijacked by these vulgarians and the grab-it-and-run profiteers. Socialism had many ideals, starting with the fact that every child should have a pair of shoes. People are not products to be thrown away when used up or out of fashion. To coin a phrase, to each according to his needs, from each according to his abilities.

The Communists used the choreography of Socialism and jammed it into a model of deceit, conformity, police control plus luxury for the elderly bosses at a Vanderbilt-Rockefeller level, hatreds and loyalties turned off and on like faucets, in a system painted over with bright colors, appealing only to the gullible and stupid, mocked at and exploited by the sharpies.

One cannot escape Calvin Coolidge. "The business of America is business." "Civilization is based on profits." Magnificent in the narrowness of his interests, the modesty of his values, the limits of his imagination. Hammered silver cocktail shakers, Pierce Arrow touring cars, flat-chested girls in short skirts doing the Charleston—the world beats a pilgrimage to the lobby of the *Alcron*.

The 6 A.M. train from Prague rolled across a drab November plain. The dining car did not accept Czech currency—the value system had not changed. We crossed the border at Gmund, not Austria's most interesting town, though the standard of living rose, in cars, shop windows, clothes.

I checked into *Der Rohmisches Kaiser*, off the Kärntnerstrasse, between the Opera and the Cathedral. People had warned me that Vienna was changed. Disneyland. As Ronald Reagan and Walt Disney had labored together to create a Platonic abstraction of an America that never was, so here was a model of purchasable happiness beyond any reality. For $160 I could buy a nice shirt. I could go on voyages to tropical beaches, eat pheasant with endive salad, drink Gumpoldskirchner and Rémy Martin, wear tweed jackets soft as maidens' kisses. Poor old John Paul, tired of denouncing Nicaraguan revolutionaries and uppity nuns, pregnant girls and population planners, waves his arms at the West's consumption obsession. He's wasting his time. Poles and Czechs would sell their souls to live in Vienna.

I hurry past street musicians towards the Stefansdom. The neighborhood has been upmarketed into Milan, the little street where Irmgard had her bookstore progressed away. Here it is, at night, with a few surfaces brightened from the street lights, the same black shadows, a hint of purple and dark red from candles behind the stained glass windows, but I cannot call it back. Two scrawny mothers and their babies—Romanians? Croats?—have been hired by the Tourist Bureau to crumple at the entrance and stick their hands out. St. Santaclaus.

At my age, this will probably be my last call upon Vienna. What could I find of my city? At the Creditanstalt, where a traveler's check is cashed for not many Schilling, the clerk speaks with the nasal whine of no other town. Then to the Karlskirche built to celebrate our capture of Belgrade in 1721. People were not as grateful as they should have been that Austria freed them from the Turks. Charles had no son. Frederick of Prussia had agreed to respect Maria Theresa's right to be empress, but broke his word, and Prinz Eugen of Savoy was no longer alive to teach him manners. I can forget the shop windows on the Kärntnerstrasse while walking along the gravel paths before the Belvedere Palais and visiting again the self-indulgent ladies of Gustav Klimt.

I lunch at a modest Turkish restaurant to show solidarity with these by now unwelcome guests (remember the Jews from Galicia, the villagers from Moravia?), whose remittances keep their families afloat here and there in Anatolia. As I measure one more city with my feet, past the square of the Hofburg and its statue of Josef II, a headmaster who'd also had to deal with rough times, energy leaches away, but I reach the Hollywood grandeur of the Kunsthistorisches Museum and slowly climb the marble staircase to the Brueghel room.

This is the room I have been heading for, and the painting. *Guernica* is our century's work of art, Picasso's screaming horses and women in the ruins of the Basque town that Hitler's bombers have just destroyed, but Brueghel's Flemish village and its Spanish soldiers have always been around. King Herod has heard that somewhere a child has been born hailed as king of the Jews and he is taking no chances. Neither are his employees: boys and girls, babies and third graders—in a workmanlike, unemotional way they are being sliced and stabbed and speared even though the hysterical mothers and desperately reasonable fathers are making a nuisance of themselves. In the lower left-hand corner an elegant officer with scarlet cape on top of a spirited, well-fed horse is being harassed by two women begging him to stop the slaughter.

Massacre of the Innocents.

"Lady, I'm only obeying orders. There's nothing I can do. Don't blame me!"

"Look at this! Do something!"—there is nothing else to say. For over fifty years I've been walking through these cities, at the edge of history, looking around me, talking to myself, reading history and poetry, answering the letters written by Flemish villagers who happen to be black mothers in Roxbury and Jamaica Plain. What words can you use?

> *Those who are not angry at things they should be angry at*
>   *are deemed fools.*
>   Aristotle *Nicomachaean Ethics IV*

PART IV

LATER

FEBRUARY 1993

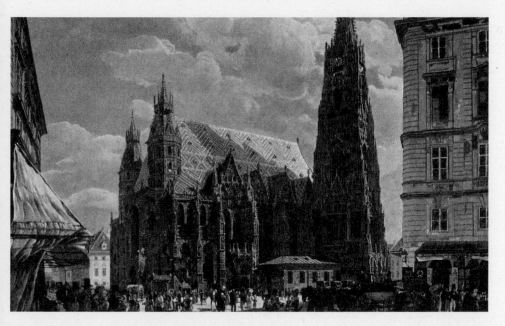

Vienna—Stefansdom. Rudolf von Alt, 1832.

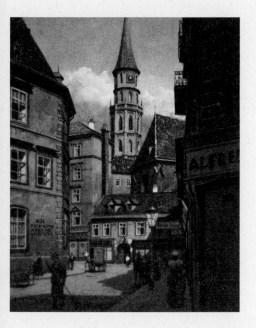

*Vienna—the Michaeler church after
a water color by Richard Pokorny.*

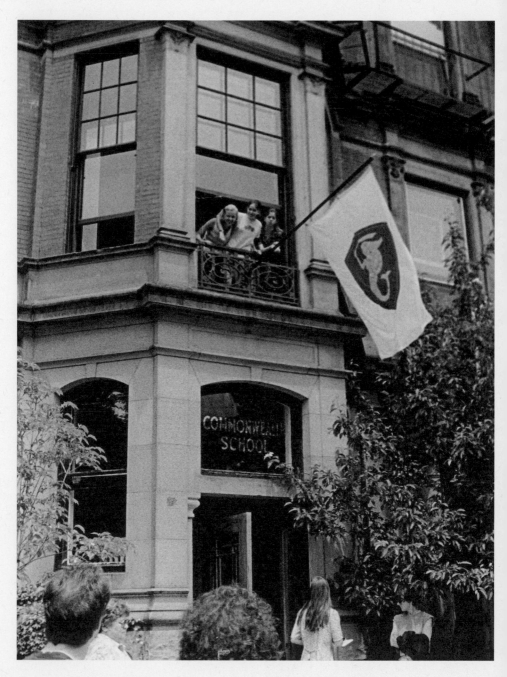

Commonwealth School with its Warsaw mermaid banner, commencement, June 2, 1995. Walter Crump.

24

LVOV 1993

To go to Lvov. Which station
for Lvov, if not in a dream, at dawn, when dew
gleams on a suitcase, when express
trains and bullet trains are being born. To leave
in haste for Lvov, night or day, in September
or in March. But only if Lvov exists.
   Adam Zagajewski *To Go to Lvov*

Jedna atomowa,
Druga atomowa
  i dojdziemy do Lwówa

One atom bomb
A second atom bomb
  And we're on our way to Lwów.
   Polish pop tune 1960s

THE TRIP BEGAN IN WARSAW, so I must be dressed by 6 to leave the *Bristol* in time to catch the plane, a pleasure of sorts driving along the empty, dawn-gray avenues. We were an hour late waiting for connecting passengers from Singapore and Bangkok (important heroin executives?), which allowed time for a fierce snow squall to blow up. With zero visibility, an American pilot would have simply gone back to bed, but the glorious 'what the hell!' tradition of Polish enterprise carried us above the storm clouds, and by the time we crossed the border the ground had become visible.

Lvov (Russian spelling and easiest to pronounce) was the formal goal of this trip. As a historian fascinated by Habsburg and Polish civilization, I wanted to see what might remain of those two cultures in their easternmost city, that barrier against the barbarians coming off the plains of Asia. My visits to Poland had usually begun or ended in a German-speaking city like Frankfort, Zurich, Vienna, leaving the traveler with condescending comparisons as to bathrooms and currency. A trip, however brief, to the Ukraine might offer an opportunity to measure Poland, in contrast, as a reasonably well-managed entity. Finally, I have had my fill of the homogenized credit-card cities of Western Europe, adding on now Prague with its McDonald's, Warsaw with the stupefying luxury of its *Bristol*. Perhaps Lwów, untouched by Beautiful People, might still retain its own personality.

The first generalization from the aging prop planes of Air Ukraine, the shabby airport, uniforms, was that I was back in Poland of 30 years ago. The second was that the Soviet Union had disappeared without a trace. Blue and yellow are the flag's colors, a yellow trident on a blue background the insignia—*one* red button with hammer and sickle was all I saw. The jerry-built suburban apartment buildings, as everywhere, are standard, but the city itself, where the battle lines always moved east and west too fast, where there wasn't enough money for Progress, has Polish church towers and the façades of Renaissance palaces built by the Italians who designed Lublin and Zamość, the statue, of course, of Mickiewicz, but then the state and business structures, the opera house, the balconied hotel come straight, if not from Vienna, from Brunn and Graz.

The *Grand Hotel* is high-season Franz Josef. Wait a moment and there will appear K.u.K. officers in black boots and tight white jackets, with waxed moustaches, swords, and corseted wives wearing complex hats. Another moment and the officers wear khaki and diamond-shaped caps, and in this weather capes that reach to their ankles. What sort of hats for their wives? Moustaches? The Polish army was influenced by the French, and moustaches have become smaller. From my bedroom window I wait for the afternoon march-past of the Deutschmeister regimental band or perhaps a cavalry picket carrying little white and red flags on their lances.

Lwów (the Polish spelling) was conquered from Kraków by Casimir the Great in the 14th century, achieved a virtual monopoly of all Eastern trade, and became the most important city of Poland. It suffered two sieges by Chmielnicki's cossacks in 1648 and 1655, was plundered by the Swedes in 1704. It received a Roman Catholic cathedral in 1412, an Armenian in 1626, a Greek Catholic, (the subject people's religion) not until 1903, as well as a synagogue in 1582. Lwów's importance as a trading center meant that early on it became a New York of nationalities: Poles and Ukrainians, Germans and Jews, Armenians and Greeks, Hungarians and Romanians, Gypsies and Tatars, even a few Scottish Catholic exiles who found employment as samurai in the magnates' private armies. Lithuanian Wilno was the only rival. Eastern Galicia and Lwów were taken by the Austrians in the first partition—1772—of Poland, and eventually Lemberg (its German name) attracted nine railroads and became the major industrial, as well as commercial, city of the western Ukraine.

Lemberg/Lwów offers an example of acceptance and conflict far more complex than Olomouc's bipolar confrontation between Germans and Czechs. Its German-speaking presence was pretty well limited to military and railroad administration, business was Jewish, culture Polish, toilet-cleaning Ukrainian. As tsarist rule radiating out from Warsaw became steadily more oppressive after the failure of the 1863 uprising, especially in the relentless Russification of the entire education system, Lwów's university, under more tolerant Austrian control, became the intellectual center of Poland. Only Jagiellonian in Kraków had more prestige. At the same time Austrian tolerance towards the nascent nationalism of the Ukrainians made Lemberg a city of refuge for patriots fleeing the Russians. Once across the border, however, these refugees found that the Poles, like Kossuth's Hungarians with the Slovaks, denied to the Ukrainians the freedoms that the Poles themselves demanded from the Austrians.

The Austrians appreciated Polish anti-Russian, anti-Prussian resentments and employed their cultured aristocrats in high-level diplomatic posts. They were also willing to practice Habsburg skills of giving police subsidies to Ukrainian intellectuals and politicians as a way to keep the Poles in check. As Slovak and Romanian nationalists were secretly encouraged to frustrate the Hungarians.

For a border city like Lemberg, like Posen, the question arises about the extent to which official authority imposes its culture by means of police sergeants, headnurses, headwaiters, teachers, orchestra conductors. And to what extent, in part unknowingly, does it adopt the culture of its subjects, like the English in India and French in Morocco, through food and music, the servants' amusing oaths and ways of handling horses, the master's mistress. Lemberg was the end of the road; the officials posted there were even more anxious to display the civilizing richness of Vienna: a Brahms symphony for Sunday afternoon followed by a Sachertorte with whipped cream at the *Grand Hotel*. During my 24 hours the Parisian-Viennese opera house was giving *Karmen*, promising Tchaikovski's *Evgeny Onegin* and Borodin's *Prince Igor*, and the theater, where Sarah Bernhardt had played, was giving *Makbet* by Shekspir and Ibsen's *Gedda Gabler*. Ukrainian culture was the little stand selling intricately designed wooden eggs and nests of matryosha dolls* outside the hotel.

The new imperial culture—not an improvement—is American. The *Grand Hotel's* bar sells Smirnoff vodka and Miller beer. CNN, which brought our Iraqi victory to the world, plays non-stop, with advertisements

---

* Tourists are bored with these, likewise the new model nests from Gorbachev and his big red birthmark down to a tiny Lenin. How about combining American capital with Ukrainian craftsmanship to put out a whole new line: Bill and Hillary, Bush and Reagan, down to Nixon and Kennedy?

for the *Wall Street Journal* and Marlboro cigarettes. I had brought along a half-dozen packs as tips, but see a man walking by carrying five cartons in his net sack, their price not much higher than in Boston. (The other side of the New Economics is a haircut for eight cents.) Across the dining room, three young American women, one of them black, are talking animatedly. Always the scholar, I ask who they are. Their role is to monitor the sale of government properties to private investors.

"Any entrepreneur with enough hard currency to buy such property has probably gained it illegally," I offer.

"That's not our concern."

"And be a tough customer to deal with."

"We've had experience."

It's nice to have Communism and the KGB behind us, but how does any former Soviet citizen feel to see the revolution he is enduring refereed by young American females? And the Soviet Union, once the terror of the world, reduced to the status of village drunk?

> *Goodbye our Red Flag*
> *You were our brother and our enemy.*
> *You were a soldier's comrade in trenches*
> *you were the hope of all captive Europe.*
> *But like a red curtain you concealed behind you*
> *the Gulag,*
> *stuffed with frozen dead bodies.*
> *Why did you do it,*
> *our Red Flag?*
> Yevgeny Yevtushenko *Goodbye our Red Flag*

Street life on Lwów is indeed Poland of 30 years ago. There are queues outside the Gastronom food stores, a clot around the little stand where a woman sells yogurt, buses crowded to the last cubic centimeter. In 1957 Warsaw passengers used to cling to every outside toe and finger hold, and Miłosz told of hooligans—'kowboys'—amused at making lariats to rope these riders, jerk them off the bus, and laugh at their cries. The *George Hotel*, the finest of this 'Paris of the East,' dating from the time of the *Bristol* in Warsaw, has balconies from which the captain's young wife made coded hand gestures to the hussar lieutenant across the street as to *when* and *where*. Now it is a slum of Intourist offices, money changers, and cheap souvenir shops.

My guide was a Harvard student from Syracuse, New York, of Ukrainian parentage, working for his doctorate on the topic of religious oppression and freedom. For both Poles and Russians, the Ukrainian Catholic Church was a lower-class hybrid, like the Ukrainian sense of nationality, which existed, as the two superior races insisted, only because subsidized by Austrian and German police. Speaking Ukrainian outside your home could hurt your career, like wearing a cross in Communist Olomouc. Although the Poles did not permit an official Ukrainian university, Masaryk encouraged their intellectuals to study in Prague, and the credits they earned at the secret school in Lwów were recognized by Charles University. Once the Russians had assumed formal possession of the Western Ukraine after the post-war arrangements at Yalta, this cathedral was handed over to the Russian Orthodox, not to be returned to the Ukrainians until 1988 by Gorbachev. The present nation is headed by an ex-Communist thug named Leonid Kravchuk, inflation runs about 50 to 200% per month, independence is 'safeguarded' by a nuclear collection left behind by the Red Army; but for a while people can be gratified that at last they have their own state, language and church.

Borys and I walked back and forth across Lviv (its Ukrainian name) lecturing to each other. All this Habsburg pretension was abandoned in September 1914 to the Russians after little real fighting. Here was the location, the foe that Field Marshall Conrad von Hötzendorf and every last bit of imperial Staatsmacht had been preparing for—Hegel: War is the health of the State. Conrad was admired as a strategist "blending the spirit of an artist with the suppleness of an acrobat" by Liddell Hart, the foremost historian of World War I, as well as by Churchill. "He simply lacked a sense of tactical reality and would attempt feats of strategic virtuosity for which his instrument was inherently unfitted. When it bent under the strain, he merely pressed on it the harder . . . until it broke in his hands."[*]

Abstract war, however, turned into real artillery and bloody bodies torn apart. Real and merciless Cossacks. The Russians did not run away when attacked by Austrian infantry; Conrad's vast waves of cavalry were pushed over so broad a front that their battle fitness was lost before they even made contact with the enemy. His soldiers became exhausted in these zigzag marches that wore out their boots and legs, and the officers wore out their authority trying to enforce orders that no longer had contact with reality.

[*] B.H. Liddell-Hart, *A History of the World War*, Faber and Faber, London. 1934, p. 147.

The Austrians retreated* to the fortress complex of Przemysl, leaving Lemberg to the Russians. Conrad had lost 350,000 of his 900,000 men on the Galician front, and when the Austrians came on the offensive again in 1915 it was with a broken army held together by German glue.

After the Russian surrender to the Germans at Brest-Litovsk in March of 1918, Lwów re-entered history as one of the prizes of a three-sided war between the Poles under Piłsudski, the Ukrainian nationalists allied more or less with the White Russian forces, and the Bolsheviks, all three armies plundering the towns and villages and murdering Jews. The city was also a jumping off place for 1920's fantasy effort to seize Kiev. And when the Red Army reseized the offensive in July and August, Lwów became the fortress that blocked Lenin's fantasy of breaking into Galicia and from there setting Czechosolovakia, Hungary, and Romania on fire.† With a certain peace established between Poles and Russians, the city became the center for a Polish colonial empire, harsher to the Ukrainians, Jews and other minorities than Austria had been. Or from another point of view, enjoying a spontaneity in its cosmopolitan culture lacking in official Warsaw.

How much came across to its inhabitants of the terrible sufferings Stalin wrought on the rest of the Ukraine? Those peasants had not accepted the collectivization program launched at the end of the 1920s. They preferred to kill their cattle and horses than deliver them to the collective farms. This meant starvation in the cities, and a challenge to Soviet authority that Stalin could not tolerate. From hunger, from cruelty, the long journeys by freight train to Siberia, and the exhaustion and cold of the camps there, perhaps five to six million Ukrainians perished. How much of this agony reached Lwów? Not much of it reached Harvard, in the interesting course I was taking on Fascism and Communism in 1938.

To keep this blindness up to date: as the next generation of left-wing intellectuals did not wish to know about Mao's Great Leap Forward's famine in the 1950s nor the deaths and humiliations to their class in his Cultural Revolution. And at the present time, the reluctance of Arab intellectuals to condemn Saddam Hussein's savagery to his own people or the reluctance of African American intellectuals to condemn the corruption and megalomania among the current crop of African tyrants—and the atrocity of clitoridectomy.

---

* "The cavalry regiments, like horsemen of the Apocalypse, in molten confusion, made their way on, their presence palpable from afar by the penetrating smell of the festering galls of their horses." Liddell Hart, *Op. cit.*, p. 158, quoting the Austrian Official History.

† Richard Pipes, *Op. cit.*, Alfred A. Knopf, N. Y., 1993. pp. 190–191.

Two weeks after the German invasion of western Poland, September 1939, the Russians occupied the whole eastern borderland, "protecting the Bielorussian and Ukrainian peasantry against the savage oppression of their Polish landlords," and inaugurated a festival of cleansing in this history-saturated city. Officers, gentry, businessmen, priests, cosmopolitans like stamp collectors and Esperanto scholars, hotel concierges, Jews, poets. Primary targets were local leftists, who thought they were safe if they called themselves Communists. "It's just a mistake, we'll be free by tomorrow," they told each other and kept up their spirits by singing the *International* over and over.

> *When death is cheap food is expensive.*
> Jan Kot *Lvov 1940*

In *My Century*, Alexander Wat, once a hard-line Communist who served many months in Russian prisons in Lvov, describes the frantic desperation of those trying to survive. The złoty had been invalidated by the Communists so speculators from Warsaw, mainly Jews, slipped across the border at frightful risk to buy them with gold or hard currency, dirt cheap, and then smuggle them back for resale in German-held Warsaw. When the Russians abandoned the city, without resistance, to the Germans on the invasion of June 22, 1941, they still took the time to slaughter their prisoners with machine guns or by throwing grenades into their cells. It is always worth while to exterminate any possibly dangerous ruling class.

Ukrainians, who could not imagine anything worse than Stalin, and did not mind at all if Jews were taken away, welcomed the Germans as liberators and hung blue and yellow flags outside their houses. In Trieste I knew an Italian, father of an exchange student I taught, who had been an officer in the force sent by Mussolini to fight alongside the Germans on their march to Stalingrad. Somehow the rumor had spread that these soldiers held church services, and a prize souvenir that he handed me was the photograph of a group of peasant women who had walked all night to attend an early morning mass held by Lieutenant Chersi's company.

Hitler did not see a great difference between good Ukrainians and bad Poles and Russians. All of them formed the mass of Slavic helots who would toil some day on the great feudal farms managed by Germans in the Eastern lands. Ukrainian soldiers in Wehrmacht uniforms did fight for Hitler,[*] but he did not trust them or treat them with humanity, and in the same way that each German staring at the ceiling at 3 A.M. had to reach a private conclusion

[*] General G. A. Vlasov's force was made up of Red Army Ukrainians captured by the Germans.

that his side would lose the war, each Ukrainian had to come to his own decision that Stalin was more bearable than Hitler. That was not always easy to prove. A militant decorated for his courage in standing up to the Poles might be the following month imprisoned, or shot, as a bourgeois nationalist.

Well, I had made all the historical reflections that I could. Lviv is a beautiful city, and with Borys' help I might meet interesting people (Jacek had offered a letter to the Catholic bishop), but I had to be in Kraków the following evening on a train from Przemysl, 80 kilometers to the west. Although theoretically a train did go from Lviv to Poland—"watch out for gun fights between Mafia gangs"—it seemed wiser to hire a driver with proper papers and gasoline* and pay his hefty fee in dollars.

We drove west, passing a few blue-painted izbas out of the deep past, and graceless but solid brick houses, all, with few exceptions, sporting a television aerial. We passed motionless lines of trucks and cars, but the driver shouted "Amerikanski passport!" to the uncertain police officers and waved my blue booklet at them until our luck ran out and we must wait ninety minutes to travel the last hundred yards. "Things will go fine in Poland!"—they did, and we were moved through that post in a couple of minutes. ($50 to $200 will facilitate a border crossing, but after pocketing the bribe, the Ukrainian guards phone their Polish colleagues that illegals are on the way.)

⚬◈⚬

My driver was anxious to start his return trip and get back across the border before night came on, and after useless driving back and forth looking for a hotel, I was urged to start out on my own.

Przemysl was a base point for plugging into the Polish railway system, but I was also looking for contact with its star role as headquarters for Field Marshall von Hotzendorf in 1914. Around the city's outskirts there still stood the remains of the fortifications he had been relying upon, but at night, carrying three bags laden with marmalade jars and alligator/pelican T-shirts (I had started off from Florida), I would hardly reach that far. Wasn't there some restaurant, some kawiarnia where he had stopped for a schnitzel and a warming glass of brandy?

The image I was seeing of that Russo-Austrian campaign was of two weary men fighting with sledge hammers. They could do a lot of damage to each

---

* Gasoline is often sold by soldiers who drain it from their trucks and armored vehicles. To turn cash flow into capital accumulation they mix it with water, leaving a driver in the middle of a snow field with a ruined motor. How to tell the difference? "Drink it," a friend advised. "If it goes down OK, it's diluted. If you're sent into convulsions, it's probably adequate." Who can resist a culture like that?

other and to the villages their armies overran, but the process had little in common with all the plans of pre-war days. Still without any story-book fighting,
as was then taking place at Tannenberg in eastern Prussia or along the Marne,
the Austrian army was simply disintegrating. The German army under Hin-
denburg and Ludendorff had smashed the Russians at Tannenberg, avenging
the Prussian defeat in 1410, and despised the Austrians. "We are handcuffed to
a corpse," was Ludendorff's comment. Nevertheless, that beautifully rational
force was frustrated by the French on the Marne, and in 1916 at Verdun and
the Somme the German army and the German nation were put through the
same meat-grinder that had destroyed Britain and France.

My "own real" war was at San Pietro in the late autumn of 1943. The 36th
Division had the job of taking that town which blocked the Allied passage to
Cassino and eventually Rome. The first Italian regiment that fought on the
Allied side was twinned with the 141st, their communications soldiers shared
our gully, trading their wine for our cigarettes, and as second-string platoon
interpreter it was my job to instruct them tactfully, unsuccessfully, in latrine
discipline. Assaults from every angle on that miserable town all failed, including sending the Italians to be slaughtered on a flank attack upon Monte
Lungo to the south, committing a special elite Canadian-American paratroop
regiment in a night attack, supported by just about every piece of 5th Army
artillery until their mountain blazed away like a Chinese New Year—and that
didn't work either. The Germans dug precise fox holes in the rocky ground,
with a slight overhang so that when we used sophisticated and very expensive
proximity fuses that burst a few yards above ground they were quite safe. The
Germans had been fighting for a long time. They knew how.

Abandoning the ruins of San Pietro, they dug in again at the next town, and
my sub-unit of the 141st's reconnaissance platoon made coffee for the colonel
whose battalion constituted the can opener to winkle them out. The show
opened with the standard artillery bombardment, which did little good
against soldiers as professional as the Germans. Then came the frontal attack
against machine gun and mortar fire by the unhappy, slow-moving American
infantry. The coffee makers could overhear the colonel's phone conversations,
which were mainly reports of the death of one officer after another—most of
whom he seemed to know personally. In his own limited way he was as helpless as Field Marshal von Hotzendorf, and after a while he phoned down to
call off the attack and direct the survivors to fall back to the line of departure.

⌒∞⌒

"Prosze pana, gdzie dobry hotel?"
"Nie ma."

There aren't any. Simple, straightforward, profoundly Polish. Hypocrites pointed me down one street and another, which always ended at the barracks-like Głowny Dworzec (Hauptbahnhof), until from lack of alternatives I entered the cavernous house of the dead that called itself *Hotel Dworzec*. This meant a bare, high-ceilinged room, a bulb hanging from a cord, a door without a lock, a hall toilet that didn't flush, drunks that stumbled up the stairs at midnight. No need to become dramatic—no prostitutes fought in the hallway, no dead rat lay under my bed. While eating my supper of an apple, some crackers and chocolate, and the inevitable little bottle of Rémy Martin cadged from the transatlantic plane, I found a bleak humor that I had come to Przemysl willingly, a fugitive only from the *Bristol's* luxury. In this sad border town no happy people ever stayed at the *Dworzec:* fugitives fleeing the tsarist police, Austrians and Poles fleeing Lemberg in 1914, middle class fugitives of every nationality fleeing the chaos of the post-war years, fugitives from Lenin's and Stalin's police, a Communist or Jew fleeing in the other direction from Piłsudski's police—the first stop, the last stop.

A last desperate crowd beat on the doors the first two weeks of September 1939. Twenty-four hours after war began, with the Polish air force wiped out on the ground and German tanks clearly not made of plywood, reality was evident for anyone with eyes to see, and an automobile and gasoline. Generals and cabinet ministers, bankers and opera singers raced for Przemysl and Lwów and the Romanian border. A Czetwertinski, a Zamoyski, a Poniatowski became simply a frightened old man (sons were cavalry officers) trying to comfort his wife, his daughter-in-law, his grandchildren crowded into my bedroom with the broken lock and the hall toilet that didn't flush.

Is there enough gas? Is the spare tire any good? Is the milk spoiling? Misiu's fever is worse. How much will the Jews give for your earrings? (They were my mother's.) If the Romanians do let us into Czernowitz, then what? I'm afraid of Lwów—it's too close to Russia. Nonsense, Stalin won't let himself get involved with Hitler.

⌘

Those who stay at the *Dworzec*, however, are the fortunate. Przemysl's main hotel is the station itself with its weary inhabitants and their children, waiting, wondering what to do next. If they arrive from the Ukraine, Poland is the land of opportunity. When you add 2 + 2 the answer comes reasonably close to 4, even if that isn't very much.

In a first-class compartment purchased from the travel bureau in Boston, I was back in a world where people like me moved comfortably. We rolled across a snow-dusted flatness created for Cossacks and tanks. One dreary town of warehouses and trucks had the familiar name of Przeworsk. Yes, I had, somehow, exchanged a couple of letters with a woman, an accountant by profession, who had wanted to give meaning to her life by joining the Peace Corps. They sent her to Przeworsk to set up a proper bookkeeping system for the town council and the railway repair works. She was curious about my interest in Poland: it seemed a poor, sad country. How did she possibly spend her free time, even though the Beskids, a low but pretty range of the Tatry, lay to the south along the Slovak border. A heroine of progressive democracy and responsible capitalism.

What might be by now the meaning of those two terms was the reason that brought me again to Poland and to what was left of Czechoslovakia. I had friends to see, I enjoyed the puzzles of working with those two languages and the pleasures of walking through Kraków and Prague, but what was happening to their world? 1991's visit had left me disheartened by the cynicism, discouragement, confusion apparent everywhere.

I had read an article in the London *Economist* praising the hard-boiled effectiveness of the Balcerowicz economic policy: shifting industrial concentration from coal, steel and armaments to decentralized factories in furniture, construction, food processing, and services like auto repair and restaurants, abolishing subsidies and price controls, holding firm against tempting welfare programs that would have broken all restraints against inflation. The *Warsaw Voice* wrote about a new shirt factory in Łódź that is exporting a steadily increasing production to high cost countries like Germany, Holland and Norway. The bloom of that rose fades as Western nations raise protective tariffs against those Mexican-wage-level imports. Since unemployed textile workers are predominately female, Łódź becomes known for its prostitutes. The new dynamism, however, turns again to the Ukraine—Poland's Poland—where the Poles send not cavalry but capitalists to set up textile factories with even lower wages. Procter and Gamble is opening a large Pampers factory, the supreme luxury for every Polish mother I knew. I am paying an excessive price to stay at the *Bristol*, newly remodeled by a British hotel chain, just to see what the new Poland is like. How do these macro-facts work out in micro-reality?

The day budgeted for Warsaw is spent with Anna Grocholska, Jacek Woźniakowski's younger daughter, married to Colonel Grocholski's youngest son. Her two generalizations are the fast rise in prices matched by the slow rise in wages and the fact that now the stores are filled with everything, there is no more need to send food parcels. All that is lacking is money.

Anna takes me to the Russian flea market where merchants from the former Soviet republics (many Asiatic faces) sell the sort of junk—shoddy clothing, cheap cosmetics and appliances, matryosha dolls and officers' caps—that Poles used to sell across the Odra to East Germany. These shabby peddlers are the Turk and Tatar invaders whom Sienkiewicz's heroes fought against, and bring with them reminders of Chernobyl and Siberia and prisons in just about every Russian city, and the warnings of an uncontrollable amount of refuse if that world falls apart. Since the Germans have sworn to expel any illegal alien back across the border, Poland, as usual, faces invaders from both East and West.

The newest fantasy structure comes from Russian patriots nostalgic for Tsarist days: We'll get back Finland, Alaska, perhaps, even, and Cossacks will trot once again down the Krakówski Przedmiescie in front of the *Bristol*.

Anna and I visit the new monument, forbidden by the Communists, to the heroes of the Powstanie: a mother and her baby climbing out of a sewer (the last communications link), with a priest and a boy soldier with machine gun and German helmet. We call upon her sons' public school, which she respects. For an American it is strange to meet the nun, a friend of Anna's, who teaches the boys religion, even stranger for me since the young woman has the face and demeanor of one of Commonwealth's staff who taught in Nicaragua for a year, in the dangerous highlands around Estelí and on the black, Creole-speaking Mosquito coast, in the same Christian calling, though she wouldn't have used that term.

In Warsaw, in any Polish city, there is never any hiding place from the war. That wall of polished marble in Washington with its 58,000 names is America's monument to the dead, the nearest we have to a pilgrimage shrine. Poland's number is about six million, half Jewish and half Gentile. On our walk through the Old Town, Anna takes me to half-a-dozen churches, at each she kneels and prays. One has a ceiling painted by her sister-in-law, Anna Sr., the 11-year-old messenger during the Powstanie. Another had been promised as a sanctuary for women and children, then blown up with every person killed. Warsaw is still a city of the dead.

I go with Anna to fetch her boys from choir practice at their parish church. Henryk is fascinated by history, Stefan by sports; he will become a wealthy athlete able to support his aged parents. They have lived all their lives in that one apartment which belonged to their grandparents, and which seems to be a place of order, with laughter as well as seriousness, without, so far as I ever saw, tension beyond the question of how do we pay the month's bills. There have been 45 years without a war. No one was ever arrested. Piotr's first wife died in childbirth. His daughter by her was almost killed in a car crash. That is life, but the boys have been reasonably protected from History.

What are changes? Western tourists used to come back from safari in Warsaw with imagery of Communist oppression and brave, clever resistance. Now it is examples of Americanization: a monumental red and white can of Campbell's zupa condensowana at the bus stop. Your first McDonald's. The exciting gourmet restaurants that other people find while I am eating toasted cheese sandwiches in Anna's kitchen. Besides the traditional drunks, there are now narkomany, gaunt, vague, whining, drifting along the Krakowskie Przedmiescie. How do the old stereotypes about the protection of integrity through faith fit in with the new Christian National party whose interpretation of Catholic belief is to pass the strictest possible anti-abortion law, leaving the greedy and the cruel alone, while they concentrate on the pregnant woman? Another new law requires the media to adhere to 'the Christian system of values.' 'Real' American Christianity, not the attenuated faith of liberals, leading its own holy wars sustained by a Slovak/Croat patriotism, would feel at home.

The female prime minister, Poland's first, Hanna Suchocka (the fifth prime minister since 1989), is admired as honest and capable, but with twenty-nine parties represented in the Sejm it is hard to get anything accomplished. This is a Polish custom: in the 1920s over ninety political parties were registered. Unemployment for the unlucky, motionless wages and rising prices for the fortunate mean a short fuse before a popular explosion, but the amateur deputies identify democratic politics as the freedom to speak and speak whether anything they say is useful or relevant.

In the fall the new elections will be won by neo-Communists, replacing Pani Suchocka with an aggressive young ex-apparatchik. If you knew the faces and stories of those who lost and those who won seats in the Sejm, this election could be an ugly sign of turning the clock back. But perhaps a hardcore optimist could see it as a human sort of protest against that return of authoritarian Catholicism A human reaction to the victories of Milton Friedman monetarism at the expense of one's job and one's children's school. To too much Americanization too fast. Underemployed American political scientists travel here to give helpful seminars on democracy. Maybe they should stay home. Besides the skills of raising vast sums of money to pay for television commercials that substitute image for reality, what do American politics stand for?

Poles and Czechs and those others should learn English and the skills for handling computers and word processors. Very nice. In order to do what? That will be revealed later.

A certain black comedy plays out in the efforts of the Sapieha, Wisnowiecki, Radziwill, Czartoryski, Zamoyski families (beautiful names!) to recover their vast properties which they will turn into resort hotels or condominiums for wealthy Germans. Put that to one side, but the self-assured Western missionaries prefer to overlook the shark-and-seagull quality of Eastern European capitalism, without safety nets, without ideals of tolerance and civility that the more established democracies used to possess. "We fought for socialism with a human face,"—the hope in 1968. And capitalism?

In contrast with the rapid rise in the Polish birthrate in the 1980s as a retreat within the family against the misery of martial law, there comes in the 1990s a disastrous fall, down by almost 30% in the last decade, the lowest since the war, and with the death rate at its highest since 1945, signs of an unhealthy and fearful society.

. . . .

He would like to remain faithful
to uncertain clarity.
    Zbigniew Herbert *Mr. Cogito and the Imagination*

It must be borne in mind that the tragedy of life doesn't lie in not
reaching your goal. The tragedy lies in having no goal to reach.
    Benjamin Mays, President of Morehouse College, Atlanta

In Kraków again, leaving the train from Przemysl for the *Pod Różą*, where from my bedroom I can see the towers of the Mariacki and faintly hear the trumpet call cut short by that Tatar arrow. No one is yet aware that I have arrived and I am free to circle the great rynek, to enjoy that dignified beauty, noticing new painting, new stores, yes, sex shops and peep shows. Down the central aisle of the ancient cloth hall past the little stalls of painted eggs, mountaineer axes, chess sets, linen table cloths, felt slippers. The lady did not have my size and introduced me to a competitor who did. There is a natural courtesy one can encounter in this land. In the 1970s came an interesting pattern for a while of retired Americans settling around Gdańsk, not simply those from Polish parentage or because a Social Security check in five-dollar bills went farther than in New Jersey, but because the senior citizens found there a respect toward the old lacking at home.

I shelter myself from large questions by small usefulnesses. Grazyna Kaminska had raised private money for a new electric stove at her school in the impoverished suburb of Podgorze: children should get at least one decent hot meal a day. Now she has taken on a tougher job: looking for $25,000 with which to construct a gym. Poor food and hygiene, the efforts of cumulative pollution including an increasing number of birth defects, too much television, the motionlessness that unhappy families sink into produce children coming to school almost misshapen. The weather is too harsh, the ground muddy or frozen—they don't have good shoes—for playing outside during the long winters. Formal, guided exercise is much more important than one would ever imagine. Under Communism there were state-funded activities in after school hours for children of poor communities. These are ended. In the post-war years a heavy-handed form of affirmative action tried to ensure that proletarian students, children of workers, peasants, miners, obtained entrance to the university, no matter whether a Woźniakowski or Grocholski had far better grades. Good or bad, any efforts to counterbalance the inequalities of society are ended.

A colleague of Pani Kaminska's is a good interpreter, and I am impressed by how readily we are able to share information and conclusions at our breakfast meeting at the hotel. The chaos of post-Communist times has badly hurt her fragile community, and in this new world of Social Darwinism Podgorze is not high in the survival-of-the-fittest sweepstakes. On the other hand, under Stalinism Grazyna's personal status would have been precarious. Put to one side that she is asking help from foreigners—I am already making a list of generous relatives, Poles, loyal ex-students, people I have helped, from whom a small check would show gratitude—Pan Merrill dangerous because he knows more than he should. For her efforts to improve her school she would receive a medal.

Nevertheless, her fierce determination and self-reliance (she has organized volunteer parent committees, not a Polish custom, to repaint the classrooms) reveal an alarming individualism, following her own analyses of social reality rather than seeking to interpret the judgments of Party leadership. That electric stove project, whether or not Pani Kaminska consciously meant to, encourages reactionaries to discuss malnutrition in socialist Poland—*which does not exist!* Subjectively she is socialist, objectively she is counter revolutionary. Her very sincerity and effectiveness make her a dangerous role model—and she must be stopped!

It would not be hard to find officials within American school systems equally threatened by Grazyna's independence.

Then to Dr. Fialkowska's private school and a discussion of the problems of the whole confederation of little schools that she represents. The first need is money for salaries. A teacher is paid $250 a month and prices never stop increasing. Who can ask *anyone*, unless she possesses a well-paid husband, to enter the profession? Communism is done with, but the same teachers sit behind the same desks, using new words to enforce old attitudes. A need back in 1989 for starting these schools was to insist on the right to teach religion. Now religion is official and, with certain modifications according to the principal, becoming compulsory, taught often enough in the authoritarian style used for Marxism. Will schools like these insist on the freedom to *not* teach religion?

A call on Krzysztof Skórczewski, probably the most technically brilliant and imaginative copperplate graphic artist I know. No Pole can afford now to buy any form of art. Spare change goes for a VCR, computer, word processor, auto. Skórczewski's subjects are apt to be menacing biblical themes—the ark, the tower of Babel, the deluge—where the monstrous focal object is surrounded by clutter and wreckage, what accompanied every great grim project that its masters foisted off on this unhappy country. My errand today is to pick up an etching by him for Dr. Jařab, the rector of Palacky University in Olomouc, my tiny blow against American hegemony.

Supper with Jacek and Maja. Yes, we are free, which depends now upon constant fund raising. Dr. Woźniakowski is most valuable to the new Poland by making use of his many, many contacts to raise money for this museum and that conference, and he is wearily packing for a lecture tour through a dozen American university towns.

At Henryk and Barbara's apartment both Urszulka and asparagus-tall Justyna are ill again with chest trouble. He appears tired and disheartened. The defense of integrity, the central core of my reflections, which to him often seem naive, was easier a few years ago, when there was only one enemy. Can *Znak*, his monthly, be kept alive not against censorship, but against mass-circulation journalism, the need for new equipment, rising paper costs? Will the partnership with a French publisher bring in extra working capital while still allowing independence? What are the priorities of a liberal journal when the most dangerous enemies are now the Catholic fundamentalists, angered by those intellectuals' lack of simple loyalties? In Stalinist times the oldest friendship might become a luxury if the other were suspected by the police, in capitalist times if the other's salary doesn't fit the budget. And, of course, the new ruling class, polite and callous, whose command post is the cocktail lounge of the *Hotel Bristol*, has no interest in such matters.

Arise, ye prisoners of starvation,
Arise, ye wretched of the earth,
For Justice thunders condemnation,
A grand new world's in birth!
　　The International

It's a good song, worth singing now when Justice has become a forbidden word and when more people than ever before are wretched and starving.

Is Poland to be saved by small actions done well: the cleaning woman returning from a month in Boston with $1500 in ten-dollar bills, Grazyna Kaminska building a gym for the school in Podgorze, Henryk Woźniakowski's efforts to keep his honest, thoughtful monthly alive? Given the magnitude of the problems, do these miniature accomplishments offer hope or simply self-delusion? What mix of the tragic and the ridiculous lies ahead?

Someone, broom in hand,
still remembers how it was.
Someone else listens, nodding
his unshattered head.
But others are bound to be bustling nearby
who'll find all that
a little boring.

From time to time someone still must
dig up a rusted argument
from underneath a bush
and haul it off to the dump.
Those who knew
what this was all about
must make way for those
who know little.
And less than that.
And at last nothing less
than nothing.
　　Wisława Szymborska *The End and the Beginning*

At this point I am not sure whether I care to return. A sense of sadness stays with me as I head home. I'll raise as much money as I can for that gymnasium—I read somewhere that Podgorze was the site of a ghetto transit camp under the occupation. But what are the odds? No one has been firm enough yet to shut down Nova Huta and tell its 30,000 employees to go and solve their own problems, like the employees of General Motors and Eastern Airlines. The world is no longer run by the commissars of the Communist Party or the generals of the U.S. Strategic Air Command, but by the bankers of the International Monetary Fund. Their vision of civilization is the solvency of the central banks in New York, London, Zurich. Poland, Brazil, Nigeria, Philippines wasted most of the money lent to them—saloon-keepers selling drinks on credit to alcoholics. Now these profligates must lead sober lives and stop the printing presses from churning out 100,000,000 dinar and cruzeiro notes.

Money should be spent only to encourage economic development: helping the rich become richer. Imports must be cut, exports—mahogany forests, tiger skins, adolescent girls—pushed at any price. "Austerity," "rejection of demagogic populism" are words for slashing health, education and environmental budgets even if the improved balance of payments will be paid for with higher rates of malnutrition, illiteracy, prostitution, drug use, and violence. The police budget, of course, is increased. *Demodernization* is an interesting term used for Nigeria and Nicaragua and—yes and no—for Poland as well as the inner cities of United States and Britain.

If the dream of most Poles is to have their country be like the United States, then what, beyond the great liberating slogan—Get Rich!—of the 1980s, is the United States?

Each week over the last few years I receive about twenty letters, mainly from black single mothers, originally living in communities of inner-city Boston—Roxbury, Dorchester, Mattapan—a widening out area, as a woman tells her cousin, a sister-in-law, a friend, to Brockton and New Bedford, Savannah, even Middletown, a rustbelt Ohio city I have never been to, where in a couple of end-of-the-road shelters my address is passed around as currency. I send along a check, a few words of sympathy and apology. This level of arbitrary charity is meaningless, as any sociologist will remind you, but in a country as callous as ours where are the alternatives?

Hi My name is Kenza Jones and I am living in a shelter, and I am having a hard time with feeding me and my kids and our time is almost up at the shelter and I do not know what to do could you help me out I would hate for me and my kids be homeless.

The childrens' father kicked his way into the apartment. He was drunk and I gave him $5 hoping he'd go away but he hit me in the face and cracked my jaw then he knocked me down and kicked me *and took the rest of the money and he even took all the children's clothes I suppose to sell them and buy more booze. I don't know what to do.*

They cut off my gas and electricity and last week they cut off my water. I go around to the neighbor lady with a bucket once a day for me and the three kids but I'm afraid if I ask for more she'll get cross at me. One bucket of water for three little children for a whole day that's rough.

Me and my sister go down at night to climb around the dumpsters outside the restaurants to look for a piece of food or clothing to take home to the kids. Sometimes I go out and collect cans to sell, but I feel confused and very sad.

I am sorry I have to ask you again for help. But I need help so bad My childrens need things and food I cant help them or me I am sick My bills so high I cant even give them the food they need or clothes its so cold at night We all bundle up together to stay warm. Sometimes I wish I was dead but that would only solve my problems and cause a bigger one for my children

I don't have any money and I am very poor.

I'm a single parent with 4 kids at the age of 24 despert need. I am wrighting you because my husband has been in prison since May and he left me with 4 children to take care of alone. It is been impossible to make ends meet. My children are everything in this world to me.

I have 5 children from ages 5-12. I am 2 months behind on rent. My lights are about to get cut off again and I have not been able to buy a single gift for my children for Christmas. My children are in desparate need of shoes and boots.

My son James was killed last year over a pair of sunglasses.

Poverty is worse, of course, in Calcutta, more dangerous in Soweto; and in Rio and São Paulo the police handle the problem of lawless street boys by shooting them. I know that.

Most of us who grew up together
are dead, pulling hard time, crazy
or strung out. i who have survived
the soft holocaust of the fifties
and sixties long ago learned that
words do kill whether spoken
or unspoken, printed or censored.
  Gary Hicks *Crates Boston 1993*

25

Auschwitz

Hopes faiths philosophies
tossed on the trash heap doused
with gas for the holocaust
Hopes faiths philosophies
sprinkled with quicklime to prevent
spreading of pestilence and plague.
. . . .
    Tadeusz Nowak *Psalm on a Dumpheap*

How many gold teeth from the mouths of Turkish Gastarbeiter
    are needed to buy enough gas to terminate x Gypsies?
    German board game, 1992.

Our heads are shaved, our fists hard as steel
Our hearts beat true for the Fatherland
We are the force, the force to clean up Germany
—Germany awake!
    Stoerkraft*

HENRYK OFFERED TO BE MY DRIVER, and we headed southwest over snow-slick roads through a drab landscape neither city nor country. The way to Oswiecim, its Polish name, is clearly marked, as if it were Montclair. In actuality it was two camps: Auschwitz, where the prisoners lived in brick barracks, hemmed around by electrified barbed wire—lebensgefahrlich—as I had seen at Mauthausen and Majdanek, and a few hundred meters away the gas chambers and crematoria with their giant chimney, of Birkenau.

For my entire adult life the death camps, of which Auschwitz was the worst, have been a part of my thinking: who existed inside them and how, who helped create them, how would I have acted? And when a 'revisionist' says these camps never existed, I can call him a liar.

* Disruptive Force, a skinhead rock group

Yes, over the main gate is "Arbeit macht Frei." "Through Flames to Truth" was, I think, Dachau's motto. The camp has been redesigned as a total learning experience, with endless variations of the photograph, a frightened child holding on to its mother's hand, and in each barracks a pile of artifacts behind glass walls: shoes, suitcases, eyeglasses, empty canisters for Zyklon B, women's hair, including a coat cleverly woven of such hair, used to make socks for submarine crews and felt insulators for the boots of railway workers. The gold teeth have been recycled, but what struck me was a little hill of shaving brushes. The prisoners wanted to look neat.

What did the British and Americans know? I heard the story of a high officer in the Home Army, Jan Karski, who, at great danger and expense (the Germans responded to *large* bribes), was smuggled into the Warsaw ghetto and then into the camp at Belzec, near Lwów, smuggled out again, and then smuggled to London to tell the truth to Churchill, who was busy and shared no doubt, like Roosevelt, Sunday-dinner-at-Southampton attitudes about Jews, and for whom Poles were, let's face it, a damn nuisance.

What could have been done? Small bombs dropped at low level would have smashed the railroad yards, the gates, the power station, and the Birkenau death complex. Parachute scatter drops of thousands of little Sten guns (very cheap) would have caused a lot of trouble. There weren't even warnings that those who drew up the plans and gave the orders and those who enforced them would be tracked down and personally punished.

Pope Pius XII, who played a sleazy role during the war, showed no concern, of course, for the Jews murdered, but also did nothing angry or specific about the Poles, including their 4000 or so murdered priests, and had his spokesmen explain that protests with any bite would have provoked expensive retaliation against church property.

We are back to Miłosz's description of the Warsaw citizens watching from their rooftops as dive bombers swooped over the burning ghetto: "You've got to hand it to the Germans—they're cleaning up Poland!" The spirit lives on among whites reading about young blacks killing young blacks. "You can't blame us."

Auschwitz's messages keep changing. A certain type of American male may well envy the SS officer who picked out a pretty Jewish girl, fucked her all night, and shot her the next morning. Maybe it serves as an antidote to the belief in Progress.

A relevant observation came from the German-American psychiatrist Bruno Bettelheim out of his own years in Dachau and Buchenwald,* facing the question of who survived and how. The most obvious survivors were Communists and Seventh Day Adventists who possessed a rigid internal structure of discipline and identity. The most quickly doomed allowed their environment total control, retreated into a childlike dependence on their guards, exercising neither feeling nor comprehension. In effect they had become walking corpses and for this lethal passivity were nicknamed Mohammedans. On the other hand, because the SS recognized active awareness as a form of resistance, any remark or even expression of the eyes which betrayed that could have a prisoner shot. Ditto for a black male in ghetto Boston. Back to old-time Mississippi where Negro boys were carefully schooled to be stupid. Or to the collapse of the Paris Commune in 1871, where the Versailles forces who could not execute every one of their thousands of prisoners limited themselves to those who seemed intelligent or carried some sign of distinction like a wristwatch. In Cambodia during the 1970s when the Khmer Rouge were enforcing a national socialist democracy, a fountain pen revealed foreign contamination and marked its wearer for death.

The erection of a Carmelite convent within the walls a few years ago provoked an ugly 'we suffered worse than you did' confrontation between Jews and Poles. Now a compromise convent outside the wall has been built, new plaques affixed stating that 90% of the 1.5 million dead were Jews, taboo to mention in Communist days. The Jewish Historical Institute in Warsaw was recently asked by a bishops' conference to run classes for religious-instruction teachers: "No, dear, Jews did not use blood from Christian children to make their matzohs." There is even a Hollywood millionaire making a film about a heroic German industrialist who saved hundreds of Jews. 1500 extras are hired, and the Americans at the *Forum Hotel* pour cash into the Kraków economy.

Bosnia offers the closest comparison. There is the same frightened child. The same officers who measure themselves by the misery they can cause others. 'Ethnic cleansing' is as good as 'final solution.' The outside world is less ignorant but just as ineffectual. The Serbs, too, use History as a faithful employee. "You should have seen what the Croats did to *us* fifty years ago. The Germans raised an SS division out of Bosnian Moslems [Yes, they did.] and let me tell you

---

* *The Informed Heart* (1960), quoted in Stanley Benn, *A Theory of Freedom*, Cambridge University Press, N.Y., 1988, pp. 192–196

how *they* acted. The Turks massacred *us* at Kosovo in 1389." Rape was common enough within the Wehrmacht and Red Army, but spontaneous. Official use of rape as a way to build fighting spirit is an innovation.*

> *Hatred—One religion or another—*
> *whatever gets it ready, in position.*
> *One fatherland or another—*
> *whatsoever helps it get a running start.*
> *Justice also works well at the outset*
> *until hate gets its own momentum going.*
> *Hatred. Hatred.*
> *Its face twisted in a grimace*
> *of erotic ecstasy.*
>   Wisława Szymborska, *Hatred*

Almost every city I have visited was in Auschwitz's catchment area. The Teich family in their empty Berlin apartment back in 1939, and the four people seated on the yellow bench in Vienna's Stadtpark. There was a crazy Italian in Budapest pretending to be the Spanish consul who insisted that Sephardic Jews were descendants of those expelled from Granada in 1492 and could rightfully claim Spanish citizenship and passports, and thereby cheated the Nazis of some hundreds.† In Modena I saw the brittle survivors with numbers tattooed on their arms. Our interrogation team was quartered in the Palazzo Ducale on a Sabbath eve, and soldiers of the 8th Army's Jewish Brigade who had trucked these men, boys and a few females down from Austria led one hora after another in the courtyard. The ex-prisoners threw themselves at those Sabras in their heavy boots, seizing their arms to share their strength.

My family and I lived for two years in Paris, which was quite accommodating to German demands, supplying more bodies than were asked for. Amsterdam was the home of Anne Frank, whose story was acted out in my school's gym. Many of our Jewish parents had been exactly her age then, I taught many girls like Anne.

---

* "A soldier who won't fuck won't fight"—General George Patton, 1943.

† In Kaunas, 1940, an even odder consul, who was Japanese, gave out hundreds of transit visas to Lithuanian and Polish Jews, who then could reach safety by way of the Trans-Siberian railroad. On the other side, in northeastern Italy after war's end, was a British major in charge of a camp of ex-Red Army prisoners in Wehrmacht uniforms due for repatriation to Odessa and almost immediate execution who forgot to lock the gates of his camp at night until most of the men vanished. (Norman Davies, *The New York Review of Books*, May 25, 1995, p. 11)

The claustrophobic confinement of that apartment accumulated its own silence around us until the final pounding upon the door by the Germans. My liberal school has a strongly Jewish flavor, and I asked myself over and over, suppose we had been in Paris or Amsterdam.*

"How many Jewish kids you got?"

"I don't know. I don't take a census."

"Don't fool around, mister. Show me your name list. Apfelbaum. Goldberg. Hirschfeld. Kaplan. Look at those! What sort of place you run? You got a grandmother hidden someplace yourself, Mr. Merrill?"

What sort of German would have showed up? A thug? An officer like the man who came to the children's home in Warsaw? The beautiful Viennese at Verona? What could I do? Whom could I protect? My secretary has blond hair and a non-Jewish name. How firm was the loyalty of our gentiles— would they finger the classmates who had been overlooked?

A week later, close to midnight, our apartment bell rings. Sharon.

"They came for my parents but I hid in the laundry. I don't have any money. I haven't had a bite in two days. What'll I do? Help me!"

"Stay with us."

Can I say that? The apartment building is porous. The cleaning lady comes tomorrow. Will our twelve-year-old tell her best friend? Sweet-natured, hard-working, anxious Sharon Haas is the Angel of Death.

⟐

What was God doing? If Abraham accepts Yahweh as his lord and master and swears allegiance to Him alone, the Lord will protect and cherish him, and his descendants will be as the sands of the sea. All right, the Jews of Paris and Amsterdam had other things on their minds. But the Jews of Kasrilewke and Tyszowce? They had nothing else, only the conviction that as He had led His people out of bondage in Egypt and across the Red Sea, once again, when He was needed, He would lead the faithful to safety.

He didn't.

Why?

---

* I found a recent article in a Jewish magazine of a Belsen survivor who had seen Anne's naked body on the ground outside her barracks, dead of starvation and disease, and felt it terribly important that people be aware of this actual female Jewish corpse, not of the beloved abstraction we have made of Anne. And in California the religious Right has placed the Diary on its taboo list: Anne's belief that one can find God through every religion might disturb a Christian child.

The story is a simple one, the argument obvious, and whatever conclusion you accept—there are many—devastating.

A friend of mine, a former rabbi, had worked out a totally logical line of reasoning that the historical God of Abraham was dead, and that any theology worthy of respect had to start from that conclusion. We wander upon a dark plain without guideposts, and we maintain our courage by holding each other's hands and following the symbols and ceremonies that remind us who we are and where we come from, and that is the most we can expect.

Dr. R. delivered such a lecture in Commonwealth's library one year, and even those youngsters who boasted that they didn't care listened in a frozen silence. One little creature suggested, as he had been taught, that at least the Holocaust had led the Jews to possession of their own state. The lecture ended and the silent boys and girls filed off to class. I taught a tenth grade Bible course then but thought it better to keep my mouth shut.

"Michael," one of the students asked, one might almost use *implored*.

Michael was a serious boy, at 15 holding a position of moral respect among his schoolmates and not just among Jews.

"No. I won't buy that. We Jews have been through rough times. God hasn't quit on us, we don't quit on Him."

Every face brightened. Michael's logic could not compete with Dr. R's, but it made no difference.

God, of course, is always silent, though some people claim that they hear His voice. As a teacher, what should I say? Somehow His authority is higher than Lenin's, a new Mercedes, the force of AIDS, the death of your child? The beauty of every living thing reflects His creation—a deer running, a flight of parrots over a rain-forest clearing as once I saw in Guyana on my way home at war's end. So what happens when deer and bright-colored parrots are replaced by rats and cockroaches? Justice—the powerful are brought low, the evil punished. Not exactly. I cry unto Thee and Thou dost not hear me, a modern reflection by Job. In Mr. Spielberg's movie about Auschwitz, how seriously will he discuss this problem?

⁘

In the Soviet bloc societies, the line of conflict ran through each person, for everyone in his or her own way was both a victim and a supporter of the system.
   Vaclav Havel *The Power of the Powerless*

At the Cieszyn border post, Henryk simply hands my bags over the railing to the Czech side where Jiři is waiting. Gone are all the interesting searches and questions, and this, of course, makes the traffic in drugs, explosives, weapons, stolen icons, even black market eggs tediously easy. Jiři drives me across the Hana plain with its cloud castles and shifting light to a village outside Přerov where live Jitka Zehnalova (my translator for the Czech version of *Emily's Year*), her husband Otto, and two-week-old Natalie. Jitka I had met as a serious, reserved student at St. Andrew's Presbyterian in southeastern North Carolina, chosen because it was the only college any place where every single room was wheelchair accessible. We sit together watching Natalie sleep, her bud-like mouth half open. "She's a little angel!" Mom points out her perfect little ear, her little hand. To sit silently beside the new mother, overflowing with love and awe before her baby, is some balance to Auschwitz.

At Žilinska 11 the excitement is about Jana's wedding in August. Tom (Vlach) is worthy of their darling, their sunshine. The house is filled with smiles. His father, unlike an earlier boyfriend's, was never a Communist—no Montagues and Capulets. Jiři has always felt strongly about the evil of young people who cannot afford a home of their own and have to live with their parents, a major cause of divorce. Any male who can handle a hammer and a saw has been conscripted to rebuild the attic into a spacious private apartment. Tom and Jana will go to Frankfort or Stuttgart and get jobs at McDonald's to earn enough money to buy a stove and a refrigerator. Her ambition is to run a nursery school where children will learn English from the earliest years, and say, I tease her, 'dese tinks,' like their teacher. She helps me practice the Czech introduction to Wednesday's lecture, but I am too old now to pronounce 'čtvrt' (fourth).

The shadow behind all this, nevertheless, is the breakup of their country. For years Jiři has been angry at what he considered blackmail by the Slovaks, who won't work properly and then blame everyone else for the results. (Like most Bostonians, I've always thought of Arkansas as a typical Slovak province and Clinton has many of the traits of a Slovak politician.) As their whining about Czech dominance acquired a sharper edge, Jiři's own responses hardened: "Let them go out on their own and see how the world treats them."

The arguments, on both sides, were not totally honest. Mečiar attacked the hard-line free market doctrines of Havel's Minister of Finance, now Prime Minister, Vaclav Klaus, for the unemployment these were causing in Slovakia, but he was clearly enjoying his coming role as Boss, promising vengeance on those who criticized him irresponsibly. Already in January the first refugee intellectuals were arriving from Bratislava, and the clever had transferred their Slovak korun into Czech banks. It is intriguing to watch the creation of a new state. One of the first events was the visit of a group of Hong Kong businessmen: in exchange for sizable investment now, might they receive some fall-back assurance of Slovak citizenship after the Communists take over in 1997? Shades of 1939. (You can buy Peruvian citizenship for $25,000.) Independence hasn't halted the rise in unemployment. By summer the figure for health care will be cut in half, and the reserves set aside for teachers' salaries will not last beyond November. No one had really figured out the details of how to divide up railway, banking, pension, electricity systems in what was a very centralized Czechoslovak state. Prague possesses the atmosphere as well as the mechanics of a European capital. Bratislava is a provincial town. As a popular little insult, a Czech entrepreneur is marketing a new brand of chewing gum with the design of a miniature Slovak 100 korun note.

A friend sends me the first Slovak stamp: the outline of three hills in dark blue, a gold double cross against a red background. What a high price has been paid, will be paid, to print that pretty stamp. Can the old nation be glued back together? Probably not. With each passing month it will be harder, unless Slovakia blows apart, as the new ruling class digs its way ever more firmly into office and the two state structures harden.

Klaus has his own agenda. If his deflationary policies attract foreign investment without too much disorder (the ghost of Pinochet again), he may replace Havel as the next president. And if, instead of building a cooperative entity with Poland, Hungary and Slovakia, he insists on the Czech Republic's standing totally on its own, a grade B Austria, he may bring it into the European Economic Community and, as the first leader of an ex-Communist country to do so, win all sorts of prestige.

The sad part of this soap opera is that the divorce, until the end, was never inevitable. Both sides wanted adjustments and compromises, and the Slovaks, in worse shape, wanted concessions that would require some skillful negotiation; but in poll after poll neither half of the country wanted separation. Here I blame Vaclav Havel. He is an articulate, decent, intelligent man, but he is lazy. Nor did he listen to Machiavelli and reward his friends and punish his enemies.

Likewise, Havel might have done more than he ever attempted to try and enforce civilized rules of behavior upon a disintegrating Yugoslavia. No leader in Central Europe held a higher moral stature. He was the heir to Tomaš Masaryk, who had built a name for himself in the Habsburg parliament as an impassioned defender of Serb and Croat rights. Everyone blames everyone else for the Bosnian horror, but Havel was closer to the scene than any leader in Bonn, London, Washington, and he might have insisted that Europe could not tolerate again the sort of savagery it experienced with Hitler and Stalin. Nor the new brutalities against Gypsies, Turks and all the other outsiders. He was the only man in Central Europe who might have acted effectively, and he didn't.

> *That night,*
> *when the seven of them*
> *raped me at the camp,*
> *I prayed for You to spit*
> *from my womb the seed of that dog's sort,*
> *why did you not heed my prayers, oh Lord,*
> *when I have done You no wrong?*
> *I prayed to You*
> *to free me, if but an instant,*
> *from the vigil of my captors,*
> *so that with my fingernails*
> *I could scrape out my womb.*
>   Enes Kisevic *Hava's Plea, Bosnia*
>   (translated from the Croat by Ellen Elias-Bursać)

The stay in Olomouc was laden with obligations. My first stop was at a school for deaf children at Kopeček in a convent-owned building (the nuns want it back) on a hilltop outside town. Jiři, who had run across the institution in his new job as school inspector and admired its director, had discussed with me the possibility of sending one of its staff for advanced training at the Clarke School in Northampton, Massachusetts, our country's leader in the field. The price would come to more than $20,000, and though I had set up interviews with two possible candidates and considered names of possible contacts who might share that sum, it did not meet any cost-benefit analysis. Two hours at Kopeček, moreover, looking at the advanced technology, the small classes, the careful, patient, cheerful teaching which turned little animals who grunted and gurgled into humans able to carry on practical conversations and support themselves in mainstream society made me change my mind. A tenth of that figure would pay for extra services and equipment, a broader range of teacher training. That would be sufficient. It was a good school.

The next day was spent at Palacky's rektorat dating from the graceful age of Maria Theresa, at one of the palaces of the archbishop, who wants it back. I met first with the two women who administer this scholarship program.

Thirteen students will be heading for America in September—how about exploiting Dr. Jařab's contacts with Carleton University in Ottawa? The Canadian variant would be stimulating. How might Palacky better integrate students from the other direction into Olomouc? Curtrice from Chicago and Spelman College, with a black father and a Czech mother, self-reliant, inquisitive, (light enough to escape one prejudice, dark enough to attract another, as a gypsy—Czech society has the homogeneity of Ivory Soap) was the first such adventurer last semester and was left pretty much on her own.

How to find more applicants with a science background, particularly in the field of pollution control? I know an inspired environmentalist in Ankara, a disaster area as awful as any place in Silesia. A Turk would have a lot to share with any serious student from Palacky, again the effort to build linkages that need not go through American channels. When the Russian garrison abandoned Olomouc, they left every square meter of their camp poisoned: waste metal and barbed wire, oil refuse and battery acids, combining genetic slovenliness and bloody-minded spite.

This whole belief in student exchange is quite old-fashioned. Can young people who live and work together for a year learn to trust each other, make what they have found a permanent part of their own lives, and stand against the trend worldwide of ever uglier confrontations between races, nations, and religions? When I was a boy I believed that when young people got rid of their parents' generation, the world would be run in 'progressive' ways. Not really. The young militant is proud of his hatreds. In contrast, Dr. Jařab's belief in reason comes out of the nineteenth century, similar to the steam locomotives that set the rhythms of Dvořak's chamber music.

The lecture hall has a good-sized audience for my evangelism: "In the years when this part of the world was under Communist control, we all dreamed of what it would be like to be free once more, free as individuals, free as a society. Instead we have found, everywhere, that freedom (svoboda) can be more troubling even than the old days . . . The purpose of these scholarships is not simply to learn English (Angličtina) and computer skills, but to see another society from the inside and from that experience to gain new experience of looking at your own culture and your own life—vaše vlastní kultura a život."

The night before, I had been troubled by Jana's protest that three out of her four courses had been with American teachers on the American legal and economic systems and culture when she knew zero about her own country—no one had wasted time on Communist history courses. So, in the English part of my lecture I tried to irritate the audience by stating that in the nineteenth century a good Czech had been a second-rate Austrian, that under Gottwald, Novotny, Husak and Co. he had been a second-rate Russian, and today are you satisfied . . . ? A sense of national identity does not have to be based on the vulgar resentments of a Mečiar.

The speaker plays for laughs: "America makes the finest toilet paper in the world, but is that enough . . . ? Hillary Clinton, like most women, is smarter than her husband."

Silence. No one in all Czech history has ever made such a statement.

At day's end Dr. Jařab walks me to Žilinska Ulica from Maria Theresa's palace, past the Habsburg façades of downtown Olmütz. We discuss the Czech edition of a book I wrote ten years ago about Commonwealth—*The Walled Garden*—that Palacky is sponsoring. Granted, nothing is less relevant to Czech needs today than the ordeals and little victories of some miniscule school in Boston, but just because everything in this country, including its educational system, is in such a state of confusion, perhaps even that. . . . I am not interested in discussions of ideology and curriculum, the preoccupations of every Minister of Education. Originally I had planned for Commonwealth to teach Russian as its primary foreign language so that our graduates could interrogate Soviet PWs and argue with passersby on Red Square. To my dismay, though, I kept hiring Latin teachers of better quality, and the students chose that obsolete language instead.

Who are these young people and teachers, and parents? What do they believe? How can they speak honestly to each other? When other objectives fade—mine had started out as training up an élite that would change the direction of American society—can they hold onto old Dr. Freud's ideal of love and work? How can adult authority free youngsters from the tyranny of their pals? How does the school referee the never-ending boxing match between justice and mercy? Between freedom and responsibility? Is salvation by grace or by works?

I had added on a conclusion to this edition, commenting on the book's message at this time of disillusionment and cynicism, worsened by the meretriciousness of American examples. Dr. Jařab urges me to write something else: it is too close to the Communist line. At this moment Czechs cannot enjoy the luxury of totally free criticism. People are so disheartened that they must be encouraged to recognize and then build upon their strengths. I see his point, though I am reminded that the Communists used the same message to justify their own 'temporary' rules of censorship.

President Havel announced that he would be the president for education, public health, and environment, and then slashed the budgets of all three ministries. Sounds familiar? Nevertheless, somehow Dr. Jařab finds money for one new idea after another: a course in Jewish studies, once taboo, language classes in Chinese and Japanese, an African American Institute, the critical new school of environmental studies.

These additions are useful ways of giving his community a sense of change and movement, but they aren't what is most needed. It isn't enough to dismantle the institutes of Marxism-Leninism and the centralized governance (Josef II again) of the education system. Communist indoctrination set not only the content, but even more important, the methods of learning and teaching. As important as spreading its dogmas of absolute truth was preventing the cultivation of critical thinking, keeping its students from even understanding what was meant by independent thought. If this amputated nation of Bohemia and Moravia is to acquire any self-confidence, then it has to build a sense of honor out of a respect for truth.

So here Josef Jařab and I are tramping across the February streets of Olomouc sharing the words of Vaclav Havel, even those of old Professor Masaryk, insisting that the new nation must be based upon a basic change in its people's moral values.

Jiři's embittered conclusion is that you cannot play fair and still hope to win. Perhaps that doesn't have to be true.

༺༻

I take the early train to Prague that I have ridden on a half-dozen times. Under fog and fresh snow the city looks as romantic as it does in the postcards. Last week, however, a thermal inversion carried enough sulfur dioxide from the northern mines for the city to be called a disaster area with schools closed and people warned, as in Ankara, to stop breathing. Nevertheless, I have two and a half days to myself—no one to see, no appointments.

"There are 50,000 Americans in Prague!"

That's three infantry divisions, all the schlurfy riffraff that littered up Paris and Amsterdam, here now where it's cheaper. Will they write novels about the adventure as their aunts and great-uncles did about Barcelona and Athens? Neither the experiences nor the novels of instant intimacy are worth much.

They are far from home. Nobody knows them. In September they'll be back in college or work in Dad's office if nothing better turns up. Miroslav has a cute smile. Irena has a neat figure. If you say "Pivo, prosim," the waiter brings another beer. You've made it into the middle of Czech life. Not like those dumb tourists who hang out on the Charles Bridge. Where is Indianapolis? Is it true what they say about Americans? What do you mean by 'what'? Family and History: Miroslav's uncle was arrested by the security police and had to work as a window washer; Brenda's uncle was wounded in Vietnam and after he came home just sat around and smoked pot. The first sincere glance into the other's eyes, the first real kiss, the first long night walk, the first bed. I can waitress at Miroslav's café overlooking the Vltava. (Tell me again how you pronounce it?) If she gets pregnant and we get married I'll get a green card and her father will get me a job. Brenda and Kevin, Miroslav and Irena open small accounts in their memory banks to deposit these anecdotes, but there's a quarrel about money, a silly wisecrack about Elvis Presley goes out of control, for a moment one woman or the other thinks she's pregnant, the men say it's not me. The visitors suddenly go home and sit themselves down in front of their computers.

The *Hotel Paríz* is under noisy repair, which lowers the cost of my over-priced room but dampens my hopes for silence and the means to think through my conclusions about this country and what I wish to say in this book. So, out into the streets to walk slowly around that most beautiful of all city squares. Across the bridge, up curving Nerudova Ulica to the Hradčany Castle and the Cathedral and the view over the still snow-covered roofs and the spires and domes. In the *Narodni Galerie* is the glorious wheatfield painted in Van Gogh's last frantic year at Arles, which I call upon on each visit, a universal, removed from any time or place.

That night I chance upon a ticket to Verdi's *Masked Ball*, an intense, gorgeous performance. More German and even English appear spoken than Czech: we foreigners keep musicians alive who otherwise become computer technicians. By Western measurement the prices are reasonable, but almost impossible, now that subsidies are removed, for natives.

One walks towards home from the State Opera down Vaclavske Namesti, past the *Europa's* smoky art nouveau café, the shabby four-star *Ambassador* for the nouveaux riches of the 1920s and important Soviet visitors. Next to it is a McDonald's that attracts a different clientele and along the wall a sequence of aging prostitutes. "Be careful, a great deal of street crime"— from the newly unemployed, the new get-rich-quick spirit for drugs and other luxuries, a new Russian mafia, an Italian mafia, the drop in both numbers and prestige of the police.

New poverty encourages crime, here and in Warsaw, but new prosperity may make crime worse from the envy and spite of those who know they will always be left behind. In his search for silver linings, Jacek Woźniakowski used to say that at least their police state slowed down the spread of drugs and Polish poverty limited the numbers of drunk drivers. Now these compensations are eroding.

In May Jiři would be sent to Amsterdam for a quick look at the Dutch primary-school system, which is very good. Amsterdam has always been a favorite city of mine: harmonious, elegant, with the discipline to withstand hard times and a tradition of tolerance and civic responsibility. Yet he was shocked by the trashy streets, the drug sickness, the blatant vitrineuses.* When you come out of the railroad station and look toward the royal palace, just to the right is the sign "Gay Escort Service." During the 1960s an older friend of his whose father was the colonel of a tank regiment was offered a trip to North Korea. The dehumanized, leaden conformity of Pyongyang appalled her: was this ant-heap Communism the future for her country? Will Prague turn into Amsterdam?

The very rapidity of the fall of Communism and the vanishing of its symbols (if not its supporters) lead to fear. Everywhere, once, not a single word of Lenin could be questioned, not a single boss who gave directives in his name could be called a fool or a brute, nor a word of doubt about the eternal comradeship with our elder brothers in Moscow—and suddenly all this ceases to exist. Is there anything that can be trusted?

In the postwar Italy I saw in 1945 the easiest change was for low-grade Fascists to turn themselves into Communists—gestures and costumes were different, personality much the same. In the 1990s, from France and Germany deep into Russia, the Communists turn into fascists (F not capitalized). No big deal. Hitler has won.

⁓∞⁓

The second night I take the gamble of attending *Kral Lear*. This permits a visit to the National Theatre—*Narodni Divadlo*—built in the 1870s as a thrust of patriotic pride: culture need not be German. Shakespeare was always popular in Prague. Just as it was completed in 1881 it burnt down, but in a surge of angry determination was rapidly rebuilt and became a picture gallery of Czech ideals of nature and womanhood. I have read, taught, seen *Lear* often enough to be challenged by how much comes across.

The costumes and sets are late Communist, fitting enough for all the apprehensive, self-absorbed old men in authority, shop-worn apparatchiks like Gloucester who perhaps had been truncheoned by Masaryk's police or imprisoned by the Nazis and had exploited those credentials for 40 years,

---

* Vitrine—shop window. In the widespread red-light district, the professionally clad prostitutes—many of them now Czechs and Poles—sit in their windows, smiling at possible customers, drawing the shades during business.

scheming careerists like Edmund and the two sisters, the king's knights in black leather jackets. Shakespeare is obsessed by the conflict between loyalty and betrayal, and there were Communists who, like Kent, believed in the honor of the system and the fealty they had sworn to their leaders, and who often paid for this with their lives. Any Lear in Prague will still recall old Dr. Husak, at one time a reasonably honest man, imprisoned in the 1950s, put in office in 1968 and kept there for 20 years by Brezhnev; two tired, ailing senior citizens trying just to get from morning to night. The arrival of Gorbachev and all his unnecessary novelties was very disturbing at the Hradčany.

In Shakespeare, tragedy ends with resolution. The evil meet their proper fate in Act V and, either humbly or defiantly, admit their guilt while dying. Order is restored. In Czechoslovakia after 1989 with its all-pervasive miasma of collaboration, nothing is firmly resolved, which fits Havel's theatre of the absurd but is not what the audience needs.

Many grandparents in the audience believe, as did the Communists, that a classic is a classic, of universal value like vitamins, and have brought along velvet-dressed little girls and mini-skirted adolescents, not really the audience Shakespeare had in mind when Cornwall and Regan pierce old Gloucester's eyes — "Out, vile jelly! Where is thy lustre now?" More shouting and rushing about take place than I can decipher, and at mid-break I admit defeat.

"Sex & drugs & rock 'n roll" are scrawled beside the street up to the Hradčany to show who has won. On a wall elsewhere, "Wir kommen wieder." Is that a friendly assurance that the visitors will return to buy more beer and souvenirs, or a reminder that under the Greater Rationality this dwarf nation is destined to be and ever remain German?

How well can a national economy be sustained by the sale of postcards and T-shirts, a puppet for my grandson and a pretty Slovak vase for my sister? Well, the bazaar is fueling thousands of jobs, paying taxes, strengthening an immature capitalism, bringing thousands of new visitors to this beautiful old city. What happens to a city's integrity when the competition for foreign currency reaches such a frantic level? Venice, Paris, Rome, for example, do achieve an equilibrium, and Prague is protected by its language and its mediocre restaurants.

Czechs turn into Mexicans. In a border town, as Jiři recounted, teachers and others of that social level would cross over to Germany or Austria on Saturdays to work as street cleaners. Or German-speaking tourists on their way to Karlsbad would, like Californians in Tijuana, make a sex-stop at the brothels of Cheb.

In the life of any institution, whether a nation or a small private school, the opening for serious thought is surprisingly narrow. When things are going well, anyone who questions the operating procedures is a gloom-and-doom troublemaker. When things are going badly, the problem of finding enough cash to pay the janitor on Thursday makes thought a luxury. Slovakia is almost there. Selling those T-shirts may give Vaclav Havel a bit more time if he moves expeditiously.

What to do? He and Vaclav Klaus are trying to involve citizens in the privatization and further capitalization of the dinosaur-style state enterprises. Each individual receives a certain number of mini-shares, foundation of an embryonic stock market where the investors are encouraged to watch the rise and fall of share prices and dream of how they will spend their $10 dividend. A semi-American go-getter with his Harvard Investment Company and exciting TV commercials has already built up a sizable mutual fund guaranteed to make its investors 'rich.' Interest the first year is 28%, paid for, I assume, as with American railways in the nineteenth century, by subsequent stock sales, which drive up the share price, and then just before everyone realizes that no business activity exists behind all this, the financier moves to Istanbul.

Even if there had been no workmen hammering away in the corridors of the *Paríz* and the hotel bar had been open for a small slivovitz when the eyes blurred, a proper conclusion to this journey would have been hard to work out. It is still only ten minutes from my room to the Charles Bridge and the view over the river up to the castle, but they have lost their magic, like the *Eroica*, like Christmas.

Nazism, which the trip to Auschwitz recalled, and Communism were supposed to last forever. Now both of them, more or less, are done with. Why isn't there a greater sense of joy in the conversations I have been sharing these past two weeks? Is the democratic alternative to police state totalitarianism simply not sharp enough? This gloomy reasoning somehow calls up the frustrations that nag me about Commonwealth and its black students. The school I started 35 years ago was never to be merely a demanding, bright, humane place but one that would supply honest leadership in reconciling our two races, bringing in not only the children of black doctors and teachers but of carpenters and janitors.

The passage of time did not make, as we'd hoped, this process any easier. Though a fair number of girls were pragmatic enough to enjoy what Commonwealth offered, it was always difficult to attract boys. The deterioration of Boston's inner city schools, the alienation not simply from white models of schooling but from the belief that any educational institution could offer *anything* that might make life tangibly better stopped almost any chance of interesting boys. And add Fear.

It has never been easy, in any culture, for young men from a lower social level—even Masaryk, I am sure—to take advantage of an invitation to compete for entrance into the upper class. "You think you're better than the rest of us!" Even the cheering pals and cousins secretly hope that the adventurer will fail. There was always a gauntlet of jeers and taunts to run. Nevertheless, in black American cities today where the only way for an ambitious boy to obtain money is through selling drugs or status through owning a gun, if someone his age shows by his dress, his walk, his eyes (back to Auschwitz) that he expects to succeed by a channel as contemptible as going to a white school, he is a traitor who deserves to be killed. And may be.

Marxism offered certain useful, forgotten disciplines, such as the habit of looking for basic economic causation. Those street-corner killers are not simply animals. They have been dumped into a dead end where the current level of capitalism offers few of the unskilled jobs which used to mean survival and a bit of self-respect. Marxism set up certain minimum standards—every Polish child should own a pair of shoes. Your own salvation was less important than that of your class. Your enemies were your economic oppressors, not your neighbors of a different race or nationality.

The lies, corruption, paralysis, the humiliation of having to praise leaders you despised, the ever-present fear of the police (though the obsessed historian forces himself to repeat that nothing those Czech and Polish Communists did was as cruel as the fire bombing of Vietnamese villages or as sadistic as the tortures employed by our Latin American clients), these, of course, show the realities of Communism's hijack of Socialism—which Marxism was unable to prevent.

What are alternatives? What are reasons for hope? I try to discipline my weakness for simple, sentimental examples as when I sat beside Jitka Zehnalova while we watched little Natalie sleeping. I talked and laughed with Jana Kořinkova, who is filled with the most old-fashioned joy, hope, apprehension, sureness about her marriage and the life she will share with Tom in the brand-new apartment her father has been building with its corner room for the two rational babies who will show up after a while. These are small, clean, good facts.

And one set of measurements can show that this Czech republic has been handling its affairs pretty well. It is the only country in Eastern Europe whose currency has not collapsed. It has a balanced budget. Its unemployment rate, 3.5%, is, after Luxembourg's, the lowest in Europe. This figure disturbs, even angers American economists, who see it as a sign of poor discipline, lacking the proper lean and mean ethic. (American economists are a luxury import?) Anyone who tries to write about this part of Europe develops a maddening habit of preaching in opposite directions at the same time. He warns against the old-fashioned Catholic authoritarianism of Poland's anti-abortion law and against the anything-goes ethic of Amsterdam and Los Angeles. Free the economy from crippling restraints but still retain awareness of the needs of a wholesome society, of mothers, children, violinists, foresters.

What does democracy stand for? What makes it worth respect? Does it have to be tied to an American-style, free-market capitalism, which eats its children as Stalinism did?

26

Envoy—Spring 1995

The main task in the coming era is a radical renewal of our sense of responsibility. Our conscience must catch up to our reason, otherwise we are lost.
  Vaclav Havel*

If you so smart, boy, why ain't you rich?
  Texan proverb

IT WAS WORTH WHILE to use this concluding chapter as an excuse to go to Prague and to walk again across the Charles Bridge. The Hradćany, of course, stands for supreme state authority—Staatsmacht—while the more or less new *Intercontinental Hotel* facing it stands for the authority of My Right to get as rich as I can and buy whatever I want.

The trip was planned for November, the honest month to arrive in Warsaw, when the days are cold dark damp and laden with sulfur dioxide. At summer's end it had to be postponed after a B– heart attack treated by the costly gimmickry and saturation medication that Americans enjoy. A warning by Nature? By God? The interpretation is ambiguous. Do you lower your assumptions in a modest realism? "Unto thy hands I commend my spirit." In fact, if the budget of every Western nation is increasingly burdened by the demands of its old folk for pensions, medical care, housing, and amusement paid for by fewer resources available for their grandchildren, isn't it the duty of the aged Good Citizen to die? But when? How?

Or make the best of each remaining year, each week, evade the jaws of the medical industry, go to Warsaw!

The postponement allowed me to share the great liberal wipe-out of the 1994 elections. What went wrong? Does Our Side have nothing of value to offer any more? Does the liberal concept of a responsible society supported by fair taxes and reasonable regulations lead only to yet another version of the ideals of Emperor Josef II, who knew what his subjects needed whether they knew or not?

---

* At Harvard University commencement, June 8, 1995

Singing "Gimme that ole time religion!" as they marched to the polls, the voters demanded a return to familiar certainties and familiar enmities. More police on the streets, tougher laws and tougher judges to put the (darker-skinned) bad guys in more and more prisons even if that means less money for schools. Welfare mothers and their children will be disappeared—a transitive verb imported from Argentina and Chile. If worrying about destruction of the forests, fouling of the atmosphere is an obsession of liberals, get rid of the problem by getting rid of the liberals. Neat.

Warsaw

The tourist pamphlet on the KLM plane from Amsterdam advertises a new nightclub, *Arena*, where one can watch young ladies wrestle in mud or oil, or, if preferred, an artysta stryptizowich may be invited to take off her clothes beside one's table. "After an evening of relaxing entertainment, the guest will be discreetly escorted to a waiting taxi for return to his hotel." Or, with other tastes, one can visit the café of the *Bristol Hotel*, the most elegant spot in this Paris of the east, where the heavy fragrance of coffee and the spare-no-expense brass, marble, linen are enjoyable for a while, and the only Polish to be heard is muttered between a couple of the waitresses.

There is a reassuring new currency now, one new złoty (about forty-five cents) equal to 10,000 old, even metal coins that clink. New pizza parlors and Oriental restaurants, brighter clothes on the children, sex magazines. The taxi driver from the airport, however, complains that his father's pension covers only rent, his mother's only food. Everything else must be paid for by his sister and himself.

What is Poland? I feel obliged to pay a visit to the War Museum. The front yard is filled with aging artillery, tanks, fighter planes, the display cases with helmets, sabres, medals, horses and machine guns, paintings of our great adventures: rescuing Vienna from the Turks, scythe-armed peasants falling upon the Russians at Raclawice, a cavalry charge for Napoleon in Spain, Tobruk and Monte Cassino, the sewers of Warsaw. There are new displays about soldiers in Soviet prisons whose survivors I saw in Italy. Do boys still want to be cavalrymen when they grow up?

Despite the cardboard skyscrapers of the *Marriott Hotel* and its peers and the international brand-name stuff filling up the shop windows, there is still some sense of a Warsaw that I've been calling on for over fifty years, in the details of the building façades and the faces of the young women in their springtime dresses. I walk through the Stare Miasto, cheerfully crowded on a warm Saturday night, a part of town rebuilt out of the war's rubble with detail, color, workmanship of a human scale. Back at the *Europejski*, where I am staying, a wedding party led by two guitars and an accordion is dancing athletic waltzes, the middle-class love of a good time that always infuriated the Marxists.

Kraków

At a lunch with some Polish-Jewish acquaintances before I left Boston, I was warned to watch out for an ugly scrawl—Żydi do gazu*—on a wall beside the railroad tracks, and in Kraków graffiti of a star of David hanging from a gallows.

"The authorities should do something about that!"

"No, perhaps not. There aren't really many Jews still around to be offended," was a sober response, "and it's a useful reminder to Poles."

From my room I can see the tower of the Mariacki over the intervening rooftop and hear the same trumpet call each hour warning us against the Tatars of 1241. I hurry out to walk around this beloved square, but on the other side of the Sukiennice wade through a great basketball and sneaker festival put up by Adidas for teenagers, not art historians.

First stop will be with Henryk Woźniakowski at the *Znak* office. His spread of books on politics and economics, philosophy, theology is the most concrete proof of Poland's new freedom, even if a run may be 2000 copies instead of the 10,000 or 50,000 in the good old days when there wasn't much else to do besides read and the Communists subsidized book prices. Political jokes have died, Henryk complains (I'll hear the same in Olomouc), the oblique constructions about Russians and Communists that gave flavor to life. Who can make jokes about de-acceleration of mortgage rates?

At home Ursula is now the pianist, pounding out a sturdy Bach. Justyna is exhausted from overwork for university entrance examinations. Will she become an art historian like her grandfather or a sociologist?

As I walk about this city, small enough that most traffic is on foot, and revisit the churches I know, the courtyards, the patterns of roof angles, stone work, window design that appear at every street corner, I am reminded of Florence. There is the same architectural harmony, the same patina of learning and history, but never enough affluent art lovers, tourists, or maiden ladies from London and Boston to engage rooms with a view.

My major stop is at Szkola Podstawowa 116, across the Vistula in the discouraged suburb of Podgorze. I had been impressed at my first visit and by my long conversation with Grazyna Kaminska in 1993. If Poland is going to

* Jews to the gas chamber

find a sense of direction, then one might as well start with 116, and the money I've been able to raise has gone for repairs on the façade, a small gym for the littlest children, new plumbing. There are also two young friends from New Hampshire, Noah and Amy, who are teaching English and games because they made the mistake of asking me where could they find greater meaning for their lives.

In the new gym the kindly American painfully reads a little speech on the need to work hard, speak the truth, and build democracy by sharing decisions instead of merely obeying orders. Then everyone relaxes while the tiniest people, in Krakowiak costumes, sing and dance, and each class's representatives recite a poem and hand me a stuffed animal until the guest of honor staggers back to his hotel with an armload of teddy bears and dinosaurs.

Reality is more complicated than story books, and the past twelve months have been rougher than Noah and Amy ever imagined. Their own education had been in reasonable middle class schools—they never had to deal with either children or principals in inner-city Boston. A large number of the girls are won over by the Americans' good nature and obvious commitment to their job, but when both parents must work, or, worse, when father is newly unemployed and dulls or fuels his anger on vodka, and the after-school programs that the Communists used to run no longer exist, the kids are raised by the streets or by television (sound familiar?), and the result, particularly with boys, is apathy and chaos. This means throwing things, fighting in the hallways, calling your enemy a Jew, or answering questions with obscene words in the hope that teacher will copy them and make a fool of himself.

In every sense of the phrase, American and Polish teachers speak different languages. The visitors feel that their colleagues don't want to make any extra effort to enforce better discipline or work out imaginative projects to fill the terrible vacuum of the children's lives. The home team sees the Americans as ignorant trouble makers unfairly protected by their guest status. Noah has already quit and helps support the household by giving private lessons and teaching at a new private school with small classes of well-brought-up children. Amy stays at 116 out of loyalty to one class where teacher and pupils have learned to care for each other.

"What is post-Communist Poland?" I ask them, who by now know this country better than I.

"Well, if you're a member of the intelligentsia, you have your own passport."

In the old days you groveled at the Ministry of the Interior, the police, not at the Ministry of Foreign Affairs with its unreliable liberals, and when you

handed it back upon return that included a careful interview with one officer, in the presence of a second, who would ask why did your mouth twitch
when you answered that question.

"But if you're not a member of the intelligentsia? Losing your job? No
guarantee that your children will have shoes?"

"I don't know, fewer lies thrown at you?"

"Come off it, there aren't lies in Western countries?"

Then I am invited by Anna, an artist I have known for some years, to visit
the house that she and Marek have built in the outer suburbs. They have little money and, besides, good workmen are off earning good wages in Germany, so that most of the skilled work they must learn to do by themselves.
Anna, though, is fiercely proud of this well-built new home and of the
newly-planted tree in their yard. They have a friendly neighbor who owns a
cow.

They cannot obtain proper papers, however, so therefore the house does
not legally exist. Rich people solve their problems with bribes. Poor people
are not worth bothering about. In the new Poland, middle-class people are
convenient targets for every spiteful state employee.

"When the Russians used to run our lives, I used to believe that we Poles
were superior," I hear one day. "We worked harder, we were honest, we
cared for each other. Now I don't know."

History won't stand still. The book never ends. Fifty years ago the ruling
class of Poland represented by Colonel Grocholski was finished. Steel workers and coal miners (and their Communist guides) formed the new aristocracy. Now the honored workers use computers, and it is hard for the heroes
of coal and steel to realize that they have become almost welfare clients.
When American planes dumped jellied gasoline on Vietnamese villages, it
was incidental that children burned to death also. The Serbian snipers in the
suburbs of Sarajevo, however, deliberately targeted Moslem children as the
most effective way of arranging the future of Bosnia.

Olomouc

A smiling Jiři displays his brand new Škoda, which has an intensely Czech
history. Vera's grandfather had been a peasant in eastern Moravia. In 1948,
when ordered to join a collective farm he refused, and for that he was sent to
labor in the uranium mines along the Silesian border. After seven years he
died, more slowly than most prisoners. Under President Havel, who believes

in justice, a law has been passed paying the next of kin $110 for each month of such imprisonment, and Granny, 89, receives about $10,000. She, however, has put aside enough money for her funeral expenses and with her pension lives adequately in a little house off in a village. Nor does her daughter on the second floor of the Kořinek home need this windfall, so the money is passed down to Vera, the granddaughter, for the elegant new car.

This is my first visit to Olomouc in springtime, and every fruit tree in the Kořineks' hard-working garden is in blossom. The first disciplined lines of asparagus have appeared, a plot of adolescent lettuce, the tulip border. Jiři and Vera become nervous when they think of all the work there that they must get at immediately. I have supper with Jana and Tom in their almost-finished attic apartment. She is proud to be mistress of her own home. They have gone beyond working for McDonald's, and while she finishes her studies here, he will go to Leipzig as apprentice in a machine-tools factory. Her brother will prepare himself to become a business executive by serving as manager of his lacrosse team.

I pay a call on the school for deaf children on Kopeček's hill outside the city. The director is more subdued than I remember from my last visit, for the date is closer to the year 2000 when the nuns will reclaim their property, and Pan Langer is killing himself trying to raise money for a new building. To dismantle this school in order to make a home for thirty elderly women will be heartbreaking. Langer is struggling to hold on to the belief that things can be made better: he has located a Polish school he respects, and if some extra cash can be obtained he would like to start up a teacher exchange.

Jiři wants to show me the new Olomouc, bright with Neapolitan color: a pistachio bank, an orange hotel, a cerulean dress shop. Work crews are busily repairing the streets in preparation for Pope John Paul's visit—he'll be starting the sanctification of two new saints in three weeks. Then I must call on the Saturday market. It used to be the day when peasants brought in produce, meat, cheese, but now it belongs to Vietnamese, leftovers from the 'guest workers' imported in the early 1980s, who run their stands with Czech salesgirls. Though some cloth is Turkish and there are gadgets from Thailand, most of the stuff comes from China: flashlight batteries, underwear, plastic raincoats, sleazy T-shirts covered with American logos. Americans brood about Japanese aggression, but this market warns what the world will really be facing in 20 or 30 years.

At noon the Kořinek family and I are at Palacky University's 18th-century reception salon to share a luncheon for me and the past and future students to American colleges. A few I have met before, some I remember from letters. I have been impressed by their self-reliance, spirit of adventure, their appreciation of American freedom and friendliness, their good sense against accepting too much. David Skoupil, who attended Moravian College during the project's first year, is organizing a joint summer program with advanced computer students from two midwestern schools. He is proud that the Czechs and Americans will learn from each other: Americans will no longer be instructing grateful ex-Communists.

One of these Palacky students, Šarka Tulcova from Ostrava, a hopelessly polluted city on the Polish border, I had met while teaching at Spelman College this past February. She was our first genuine proletarian, her father an iron worker, her mother worked in a textile factory. Dad, however, had clashed with the Party boss at his plant, and accordingly his daughter would never have been allowed to enter Palacky had not Havel's revolution occurred just in time. Šarka is clearly very intelligent and speaks almost perfect English.

"But how did a worker's child become a member of the intelligentsia?" I ask in my kindly Boston manner.

Her answer was as Czech as the story of Jiři's new car. In third grade Šarka had a brilliant teacher of university quality, who had been ordered after a clash with *her* Party supervisor to teach in that wretched city of Ostrava. She fell in love with this eager, bright little girl with dark red hair, told her that she was brilliant, she was special. "So I became special." After 1989 the teacher was transferred to a university, where she belonged; but perhaps the Communists had not been completely wrong in forcing her to teach 8-year-olds in Ostrava. An American university would have forced her to publish papers on the feminist implications of post-modern deconstructionism.

And because Šarka's linguistic training had been so thorough, she was paid by Spelman to tutor her American classmates in English.

(For 1995–1996 Ivona Krejcova is studying Japanese at Earlham in Indiana. That was her major back in Olomouc, and she is pleased to find many Japanese students there with whom she can practice conversation—which would not have occurred under Communism. We have to keep reminding ourselves of such gains.)

After a lunch of salami and chocolate éclairs (what a culture for underemployed cardiologists!), I am asked to speak. Czechs must learn to rely upon and respect themselves, not swallow this American-German bath water and turn their country into a Mexico. They might even find it interesting to learn something about next-door Poland, how their neighbor's culture and economy resemble and are quite different from their own. Find their way to Zamość's gem-like rynek and the Baltic streets of Gdańsk. Make some Polish friends. (Zero response.) Instead of worrying only about their own destiny, how about, once this terrible war is over, setting themselves the task of helping to rebuild Bosnia. Learn Croat (Hrvatski) well, not difficult for a Czech. Learn the skills necessary to rebuild a school, a clinic, a home. Rebuild a child, as a Bosnian, as a Moslem if need be, not just as a miniature Czech, and help it learn how to love and trust and smile again. Caring for someone else will help anyone find a sense of identity. (Zero.) Nevertheless, it is rewarding to be with this group of bright, handsome young people.

A meeting of this dignity means gifts of picture books, not stuffed animals. In Warsaw I had received one by a painter of cavalry charges, in Olomouc a photo study of the Bata shoe works in the sister city of Zlin. Bata was not only the greatest shoe manufacturer in between-wars Europe, but also the most progressive example of totalitarian capitalism. Every worker's motion was planned as meticulously as on Henry Ford's assembly lines: "If you stuck a broom up my ass I could be sweeping the floor too." Bata's culture in Zlin, however, was more nearly total than Ford's in Detroit. A T-square architecture designed the identical apartment blocks where every family lived and every other building they might wander into: stores, schools, gym and swimming pool, two churches—Catholic and Protestant, theatre, social center. Without a hitch Zlin's citizens passed from nursery to pensioners' club to crematorium. The photos show no close-ups of individuals. Were their lives equally geometricalized? Sex at 10:30 Saturdays? Josef II would have been bored by Zlin's architecture, but he must have envied Bata's authoritarian rationality.

Except for a bombing raid by Allied planes in August of 1944, support perhaps for the Slovak uprising—the eye welcomes the anarchic clouds of black smoke in the photo—history does not intrude. There seems no acknowledgment of conflict with the Germans after 1939—the machines simply convert themselves into turning out boots for the Wehrmacht—nor of disharmony when the Communists take control in 1948.

This is a digression, but I am fascinated by how easy it is for most people, in Zlin or anywhere else, to slip from one system to another. At what points do they feel inconvenienced? When do they start causing trouble?

Jiři is still unimpressed by Progress. In Freedom now the only way you measure a neighbor is by the car he drives: Mercedes or BMW, no longer Honda or Saab. Under the Communists Czechs were almost as slovenly as Russians; now you'll find ones who work 16, 18 hours a day until their wives slam the door—"I want a Life!"—and go off with another man. He complains about a new custom, contract murder: your wife for 50,000 korun ($2000—cheap), your business partner for 150,000 to 200,000. I tell him not to be judgmental. Few banks offer low-interest commercial loans, and it is only natural for an ambitious businessman to try any means he can to raise start-up capital.

Brno

In Habsburg days the Viennese resented the artistic and political pushiness of Prague. Brünn was a proper provincial city. Like Manchester it supplied the industrial motor of the empire with textile and machine factories, breweries, sugar beet refineries, everything prosaic and useful. I first ran across the city's authority on Thursday evening in Sarajevo, back when my wife and I lived in Graz. Bosnian Moslems who wanted to look neat at Friday mosque patronized an antique contrivance labeled *Brünn 1913* near our hotel, where their fezzes would be placed within a pair of cylinders and a burst of steam had them emerge gleaming new. The empire served all its people.

Even in Olomouc folks yawn when you mention Brno, but the sausage of my days has been so finely sliced there and in Kraków, that I am glad to have a silent room across from the railroad station. True, the streets are undramatic, but one can be grateful for the façade of a church from Maria Theresa's time and tolerant of the monuments to order and hierarchy and the innocent, Chicago-style arrogance of 1890s' prosperity: gables, balconies and towers, Oriental rugs, cigars, landscapes with cows. It was a city whose concept of progress—extension of suffrage and railroad mileage, literacy, use of soap—was expressed in simple Manchester-Chicago terms. Plus teaching the Moravian underclass to obey orders in German. This century's alternatives—Zlin's dehumanization, Dresden and Warsaw's rubble, Sarajevo's unending torture—make one less critical of a city run by and for old-fashioned bureaucrats and businessmen. Overlooking that bourgeois center, however, were the Austrian fortress-prison of Spielberg recycled later by the Nazis, and mile after mile of post-war concrete-slab apartment houses.

Prague

Highways all too readily acquire an American flavor, but railroads remain European, and we roll past pine woods, bare fields starting to green, flowering orchards, villages of red-tiled roofs clustered around a church with its onion-topped tower not all that different from when Dvořak was taking this same train.

At Prague my first chore is to call on a forthcoming school for teachers of religion in a tiny village about fifteen kilometers southwest. Shortly after the Communists had been driven from power, Professor Jana Fellnerova had appeared on television to ask if any parents who might be interested in some form of religious education for their children would write to her and had received twenty five kilos of affirmative answers. With the Ministry of Education's approval, Pani Fellnerova and her husband, a professor of mycology, set about planning a college for teachers of religion at church-related schools, making use of the shell of a Benedictine monastery, shut down of course by Josef II, then employed during the Communist period first as a prison for former landowners, later as a police school.

Now, if the Fellners can take care of plumbing, electricity, heat, beds, classroom furniture, books, they will open St. John under the Rock—*Svaty Jan pod Skalou*—(a tremendous cliff looms over them) in September for about fifty men and women of any religious background, who will be taught music, ecology, pedagogy, Old and New Testaments. The students, eventually to reach 130, will come straight from gymnasium, and though I have doubts about folks that young, with so little experience of history and suffering, serving as teachers of religion, they will deal with kids who know zero. Here is an example of the path I've been looking for, youngsters who aren't pledging allegiance simply to computers and English. Can I find out enough to start looking for support at Harvard and elsewhere?

At the simplest level, turning this vast dusty barracks into a school, warmed by a new furnace and a lot of noisy young people will mean useful jobs. That's an honest objective. A Czech school of religion can operate in a climate of tolerance without facing the demand, as in Poland, that every expression be confined within the strictures of Roman Catholicism. Because the old-fashioned Stalinists who ran the country despised Protestant and Catholic equally, the old-fashioned barriers between the two became less important. It became easier to insist, as Pani Fellnerova explained, that the only term of value was *Christian*.

The nice young teachers who'll come out of Svaty Jan will run enjoyable classes, a leaven to standard Czech authoritarianism. How will they deal with troublemakers? "Why were the Communists bad? If they were so bad, why did everyone (Mom and Dad too) go along with them? You say God is good and all powerful, why didn't he do something?" The teacher talks about the need to be kind to small animals. In America, every children's picture includes smiling white and smiling black face, but no one can talk about rich and poor. At least the students will see in Jana Fellnerova a woman who *will* do something.

In the *Guardian* of London (November 4, 1994) I had been warned of new changes in Czech fashions: heroism, idealism, nuclear power, poetry readings, crosses in classrooms, popularity of Americans, glamour were *out*. Nostalgia, cynicism, nuclear smuggling, buying Polish, grunge, condoms in classrooms, crime, home-made garden gnomes were *in*. Vaclav Klaus, hard working and clever, who wants to establish the economy on a monetary basis and concrete power in the hands of himself and his supporters, is in. The intellectuals and their president, who lacked a disciplined hunger for power, a unifying ideology, and, like the Russian intelligentsia of 1917, any experience in administration, are out.

The Fellners drive me to my hotel at the base of the Charles Bridge, *At the Three Ostriches* (U Tri Pstrošu), an elegant little place named for an eighteenth-century merchant of ostrich feathers. From my window a thin slice of the distant river is visible, but mainly the noisy crowd, as at a Red Sox game in Boston, to and from the bridge. Nevertheless, once I am outside on *my* bridge above the Vltava with the explosion of towers, spires, domes on both sides, the castle above, then I am again in the most beautiful city of the world.

The pilgrim walks past the street musicians and postcard sellers to the Old Town Square to gaze once more at the arcaded houses and the spired towers of the Tyn church behind them. He pays respect to the statue of Jan Hus, who was burnt to death because he preached a reasonable, democratic, honest Christianity.

On Wenceslas Square/*Vaclavske Namesti*, the twentieth century begins in the Art Nouveau café of the *Hotel Europa*. I should have come in 1927. That was Prague's peak year. French banks, disenchanted with the financial prospects of the new republic, were beginning to withdraw their deposits, but the Czech, German, Jewish intellectuals arguing through the clouds of cigarette smoke and the fragrance of sweet black coffee were unaware of the fact. Would Leos Janaček's *Jenufa* free us from the pastels of Smetana and Dvořák? What did your wife think of that New Orleans combo at the *Alcron*? Does the Socialists' health insurance stand a chance? What'll be the effect on *us* of rapprochement between the French and Germans?

During the 1930s a tangible sign of the narrowing of Prague's spirit appeared when each of those three groups retreated to its own cafés. You didn't care to, you weren't encouraged to cross over. With the number of unemployed larger each month, the echoes of German brutality louder, old professor Masaryk's government less effectual, talk itself had less to offer. After the Nazis took over Prague in March of 1939, the *Europa's* clientele was among the first to be sent off to Dachau.

At war's end the Jews had disappeared, the Germans were soon to be expelled by President Beneš, and Gottwald's Communists rapidly cleaned up the Czech intellectuals who remained. Coffee was expensive; the papers weren't worth reading.

I have less than 24 hours budgeted for Prague, and these hours in this city are to supply, more or less, the conclusion for this book, which might as well be thought out in the café of the *Hotel Europa*. What are the relations between the individual and history, as they work themselves out in the 1994 United States elections, in the flounderings of Czech and Polish politicians seeking to control their new economic systems, in the ethnic savageries that have broken out almost everywhere? Do you go back as far as Habsburg times? For my entire life, since senior-year history at Deerfield Academy, Habsburg Europe has supplied one framework to my understanding of history. From Vienna and Graz to Kraków and Prague, Lemberg/Lvov, Budapest, Triest, unimaginative, middle-class Brno, the hotels, post offices, churches, railroad stations, bookstores, cafés, concert halls out of that world presented the background for what I saw and thought about.

The Habsburg system worked pretty well, and not simply because we may compare it with what has gone on, far, far worse, since then. Its railway schedules were about as efficient in 1895 as a century later. A letter arrived as promptly. Its education system, at least in the Austrian half, allowed a bright peasant boy like Masaryk to get to the very top. There were the beginnings of a social security system. Industrial goods and commercial services moved across Central Europe without duties or quotas. In almost every city there existed a richly cultured tradition.

Also—misery, prejudice, and the desire to escape military conscription impelled the millions who came to the New World through Ellis Island. A dusty, heavy-handed control system in Vienna could not deal with change and criticism. The aged emperor, icon of unity for all this conglomeration, was frozen in ceremony and tradition and his own character. The forces of nationalism that could paralyze the system in Prague and Budapest caused it to explode in Sarajevo. More important probably than any individual weakness was the loss of the empire's confidence in itself and its values, the loss of *Will*.

Masaryk tried to put together a nation based on identity, reason, democracy, and morality, but the nation's resources and his own were not strong enough to deal with the resentments of its component groups, the devastation of a world-wide depression, and the rise of a far more brutal nationalism than he had ever known.

A café is the place where you write to friends, and it was almost dark by the time I left the *Europa*. A few buildings down the street is McDonald's, whose sidewalk is the narrow turf for Prague's prostitutes. One isn't prepared for this, whether it is the properly dressed coffee drinker eyeing the elderly tourist or the frantic girl who asks me for a cigarette.

This very day fifty years ago the Russians had broken the last German resistance around Olomouc and were racing for Prague. On May 5, 1945, a spontaneous uprising had exploded against the Wehrmacht garrison, by then occupied mainly by Ukrainians, to seize the city before any mass destruction could be carried out, and to allow Czechs of Prague to insist that they had fought for their own liberation, like the citizens of Paris and the north Italian cities, after their years of humiliation—therapy.

The approaches to V-E day are being marked with emotional nostalgia in England, France, Russia, even Germany, but here not a whisper. From anyone I met in Olomouc, not a word. In Warsaw there had been genuine anger that the Poles, who had truly been Hitler's first victims, who had suffered the most, had not been considered important enough to join the celebration in Germany. They certainly wouldn't consider an invitation from the Russians. Their record, their memories, however, were clear.

Perhaps the war years were so filled with memories of betrayal that the Czechs had little to celebrate. In 1938 the French and English had refused to help defend the Sudeten borders, and Roosevelt wrote to President Beneš imploring him to come to some agreement with Hitler.* The following year not a soldier in Prague or Olomouc had fired a shot against the country's complete surrender. There had been, at heavy cost, acts of resistance and the murderous uprising in Slovakia, but total credit for any heroism was stolen by the Communists. The soldiers who had fought in France in 1940, again in 1944–1945, the pilots who fought in the RAF were treated as badly as any collaborator.

The Communists appropriated every item of national history. The vigor of Smetana's *Bartered Bride* expresses the spirit of the Czech peasant, but it was impossible to keep reminding oneself, and still keep sane, that a few decades later those colorful peasants would have had to join a collective farm or be sent like Vera's grandfather to work in the uranium mines till they died. It is simply common sense to forget history.

Before leaving for the airport I have a couple of hours next morning to walk up the Hradčany and look over the city. President Havel will be the

---

* Vaclav Havel at Harvard University commencement, June 8, 1995

main speaker at Harvard's commencement this June. He'll be putting out feelers for a position in the political science department—better job security? He'll hardly tolerate Cambridge's prejudices against smoking.

At the top of Nerudova Ulica is a naive scrawl, "I love all the pretty girls in the whole world," and next to this the American victory cry, "sex & drugs & rock 'n roll." Some lout passes me with "Kill Everybody" printed on his black T-shirt. Put him in prison. If he means what he says, it will save trouble to lock him up now. If he is just trying to shock his parents, this might be a useful lesson that words have their consequences. He could be sent to clean toilets in AIDS clinics—that would give him a more focused idea of what he hated.

Oxford

To arrive at my son David's home almost at V-E day gives a special tone to the brick row houses along Hill View Road, their tiny spring gardens, the prams outside the front door. In the wartime movies the soldiers came from these row houses, their sober decency was what we were fighting for.

Lottie's school (she is five and a half now) has rehearsed a special program of seven and eight year olds as working-class evacuees. A double column of them turn into a train: "Sheep and cows, sheep and cows, pigs-pigs, pigs-pigs" is the railroad rhythm as they head off to the country. A dignified servant leads them to Lady Nose-in-the-Air. "You may put your toothbrushes in the bathroom—'Ain't got none!'—and your clean clothes in the cupboard—'Ain't got none!'—and now we'll have a lovely country lunch of milk and fresh vegetables." "Fish'n chips, fish'n chips!" the ungrateful kids chant while everyone bursts into laughter. A tape playing wartime songs comes to "There'll always be an England, and England shall be free, if England . . ." I find myself sobbing.

Why? I'm not sure. 1940 was a simpler time. Everyone else had been beaten or was still safely on the sidelines. Their own army had been broken. Now they had only the RAF fighter command (weaker than most people knew, losing pilots and planes that were not being replaced), Royal Navy destroyers, and an implacable conviction that they would never surrender. Other people eventually came along, including the 141st Infantry Regiment in southern Italy. The simplicity of the story got tangled. The RAF that saved England became the RAF that massacred Dresden. The stubborn pride that refused to consider even the thought of surrender became the stubbornness that refused to join in building a united Europe.

The Americans and Russians then fought each other for freedom or socialism or something by scattering landmines across Nicaragua and Angola and Afghanistan to blow off the legs of half-a-million kids. The courage of 1940 was wasted.

"Alienation is the beginning of education," I used to tell my students. It is only by distancing yourself from what you used to take for granted, from the measurements and values of the world you grew up in, that you become free enough to learn anything of importance. Then, later on, you can try to rebuild the bridges that allow you to return.

As a poor athlete in a schoolboy culture where skill at sports was the basis of worth and self-worth, as a student at Harvard, as a private in the 141st Infantry, as 75, I have had a fair amount of experience with distance. These pilgrimages to 'my' Europe became different ways of looking at my own country as well as learning about what was happening in Warsaw and Olomouc. If Americans had the freedom to express themselves freely in politics and work, in education and religion, as Czechs and Poles did not, then what did they do with their freedom?

Well, 'freedom' has come. Our Side has 'won.' I wish I did not feel compelled to use quotation marks. The alienation of thinking Poles and Czechs from Communist control fostered a useful objectivity on what is meant by society, economy, intellect. What distance can they maintain now from Success? It is rewarding to have a nice job in the new office of a corporation headquartered in Frankfort or Chicago, but what allows any conviction that one is more than an obedient employee?

With the war between West and East more or less tabled, almost immediately the war between North and South takes center stage. The ruling powers of the industrial middle-class and democratic North see the South, as Lenin wrote in *Imperialism the Highest State of Capitalism*, first published in Zurich in 1916, as the source of new markets: Avon ladies go from door to door in the Amazonian villages of Brazil to sell the skin cream that keeps women young and desirable. Raw materials: oil, anywhere. Labor. Lenin concluded that profits from the protected market and cheap labor of its Indian empire provided the foundation of Britain's comfortable standard of living and its complacent proletariat. The United States' empire in turn is supported by the 56 cents-an-hour labor of young women at the clothing apparel branch factories in Guatemala, Honduras, El Salvador, and the Dominican Republic.

As the Messerschmidt corporation used Jewish boys at Auschwitz to sort out nuts and bolts from wrecked fighter planes into accurate recycling categories, the manufacturers of brightly-colored children's clothes and sports jackets (American readers know which brands I mean, but the comparison with Auschwitz makes me afraid of lawsuits if I put their names on paper) enjoy the returns from these new concentration camps. The fifteen to twenty-five year olds work ten-to-twelve hour days in locked and guarded buildings, with two toilet permission chits per day—Auschwitz did not have that rule. When their eyes, fingers, backs give out, the girls are thrown away. There is no need for gas chambers. If they don't like the job, they can always quit—they couldn't do that at Auschwitz!—and become prostitutes.

American executives do not ask questions—"We're not social workers!"—about the work conditions of their girls as Messerschmidt executives and the average German did not about their boys. And if some do-good Honduran politician forced up that wage to $.65, the bosses on Madison Avenue would shut down the plant within 48 hours to reopen it in the Philippines, China, in West Africa, maybe even land a minimum wage of $.53.

In the good old days the Communists, even university Marxists, used to clamor at scenarios like these, but those trouble-makers have died out. Control is enforced by the central banks in New York, Zurich, Tokyo, who wrap up their clients, the dictators and ruling elites, in an impenetrable flypaper of debt. And if the undisciplined Southerners protest too irresponsibly, the United States ultimately enforces law and order. Sometimes those at the bottom possess enough hatred and courage to win out—after all, the Algerians expelled the French, the Vietnamese, enduring twice the load of bombs as were dropped on Hitler's Germany, defeated the Americans—but the cost is high.

Are there any vestigial memories as Hitler's helots, as cabbage growers, toilet cleaners, and prostitutes, to give Poles and Czechs a bit of sympathy for those at the bottom? And though the Russians and their agents employed a different vocabulary, the humiliation 'Our Friends' enforced was pretty much the same.

The memories, whatever they might be, elicit little moral distance. The former losers want to join the winners. The prime minister in Prague, Vaclav Klaus, is such a cold-blooded, Margaret-Thatcher monetarist that, if details about citizenship can be worked out, he may make a suitable compromise choice as Republican candidate in '96. He is smarter than the competition and isn't hung up on abortion.

Central European and American politics operate at a dishearteningly trivial level, but if one makes the mistake of thinking about real issues the result is a paralyzing pessimism. The bestial cruelty of the Serbs against the Bosnians destroys any assumption that Europeans, at last, have learned to treat each other in a civilized way. Europe falls into Africa. All the international mechanisms of mediation that we pretend to rely on turn into paper tigers of talk and talk, with the conviction left behind that in any other crisis there will be the same hollowness and cowardice.

Americans, first in everything, believed that the uneducated, unemployed, unemployable young man in their inner cities, dulled or enflamed by drugs and rap music, sets the model for everywhere else. Hitler, of course, recruited his followers from much the same genus. Although as war veterans they were older they were no less scarred and angry. The street corner lout in South Central Los Angeles starts out as a mugger, goes on to become a gangster. He has nothing to lose. If anyone, no matter who, gets killed, that's their problem—he'll be killed soon enough himself. If he's white he can shave his head and become a storm trooper. There's nostalgia to that: the poor guy was born 60 years too late to enter that magic kingdom of marches, songs, salutes, the pound of boots on pavement, the privilege, the duty of humiliating and beating up inferior people. In Paris and in North London, though, and now in Prague, there are still dark-skinned intruders for the new storm troopers to attack. In America he can buy an assault rifle and lose himself into a fantasy of defending his ungrateful country against United Nations troops and the Clintons' police.

Today Germany belongs to us.
tomorrow the world!

Liberia, Sierra Leone, Somalia, Afghanistan, boys are turned into soldiers before they learn to read and write. All they know—all they will ever know?—is how to kill.

My brother had died in February, a slow wasting ended by a mercifully sharp heart attack. James was a professional, had written fourteen books of poetry and won just about every American literary prize. I used to tease him in September about waiting by the phone for the call from Stockholm, but there were too many Bulgarians and Jamaicans in the queue ahead of him. He wrote with a subtle, witty, allusive, precise style, not easy to grasp, and though one critic called him the Mozart of American poetry, my image was the slow movement of Schubert's *Trout* quintet, with the piano's sunlight sparkling off the fish's scales, and that iridescence was Jimmy's music.

I was asked to speak at a couple of memorials in New York and Boston. "We shall not hear his voice again." What is there further to say about the death of a poet? He was not a writer for all seasons. But if the Poles and Russians who sustained themselves in Siberian prisons by reciting hundreds of lines from Mickiewicz and Pushkin they had memorized in school, elitist liberals rotting a few years from now in the basement cells of the Republicans' dread Christian Goodness Patriots might try to recall James Merrill as well as Robert Frost.

Nevertheless, there is a verse that begins one of Pushkin's last poems:

I have raised a monument to myself
Untouched by human hands—

to honor his life's work that could have been, worded somewhat more elliptically, my brother's. He broke through the constraints of money, power, fashion, correctness that other writers might have employed as limits or excuses.

What does a poet have to offer? Forget about muggers and storm troopers—how about the competition from 30-second spot commercials in an election year?

Any politician who wants to compete for the Republican presidential nomination in 1996 must start, common wisdom states, with a war chest of $18,000,000. Think of all the gratitude that will be expected for that amount of money. And since a slogan of the new politics is to break the power of government, the authority which fills that vacuum will be that of the great corporations which with their billion-dollar mergers become, as Karl Marx warned us, ever fewer and larger.

Since Safeway Stores, which my father financed, helped terminalize the high-cost, wasteful corner grocery and family farm, and Merrill Lynch for a while was the largest investment firm in the world, James and I should have taken some family pride in the process.

I am not sure to what extent does traditional American liberalism have the financial, even intellectual and moral resources to reverse this process. The enemy is too powerful. The New Deal, the Great Society are dead. The Habsburgs' meticulous administration, Josef II's inspired visions are discredited. Nor do I think we can rely on the traditional hope for change led by a new generation of idealistic young people. Young people are frightened. Can they get and keep a job (the firm survives by firing 5000 employees, from janitors to vice presidents, and by moving the plant to Manila), pay for their student loans, their mortgages, and save money for their children's own higher education? Don't rock the boat. Become even more conservative, more racist than the guy above you.

Are there any forces alienated, articulate enough to challenge this power structure? Hardly the moribund labor unions. The old black radicalism lacks the discipline and leadership to cause useful trouble. Black crime, real or imagined, is a handy way for conservatives to keep the television-dulled lower classes obedient. Perhaps the women's movement, at home, world wide, offers hope. Perhaps a common cynicism towards masculine rhetoric, the beginnings of a common understanding of each other's needs and humiliations can overcome barriers of culture and class. Exposure to a totalitarian police state in Beijing was educational. Within the family, within the workshop as well as within the office and the legislature, will this struggle for respect and equality go beyond threatening men, forcing them into angry, ever hysterical resistance? That's a question. The responses, whether from Algeria or America, are not reassuring.

Just the same, intellectuals, whether elitist or vulgar, may have to try harder than they do in looking for allies and digging up examples of things that actually work, going beyond the rationalization of resentment as their primary duty. In wartime Britain, rationing was so fair and so effective that even during the months most threatened by German submarines, children from the poorest families received more oranges than in peacetime. I remember the remark from my visit in Warsaw in 1957: "You know what I think of the Communists, but when our class ran things before the war, the poorest village children couldn't go to school in winter because they didn't have shoes. Now every child in Poland owns a pair of shoes." It is not impossible to hold a government to minimum measurements like these. A well-run university like Palacky can become an example of rebuilding an independent intellectual institution of quality after the degradation of totalitarian control. Sarajevo can be an example of reconstruction as well as devastation. And South Central Los Angeles.

The major theme of this book has been to look at how the individual and his family and society can maintain their sense of identity and integrity under the feet of History, whether those feet belong to Habsburgs, Nazis, Communists, or the current crop of businessmen, journalists, computer experts, Mercedes salesmen, sex queens, and Mafia gangsters. At the memorials for my brother James, I find myself forced into the same obsessive questions as to how does something as fragile as writing a poem have the slightest significance in the shadow of these power games. A poet is a pretty zoo animal. Or he may open a few hidden doors.

"Poland is not yet lost while we still live" begins the anthem sung by the soldiers who fought for and were betrayed by Napoleon, a song out of defeat, sung by men and women who were defeated again and again but returned to fight once more. Despite its banality "There'll always be an England" shares a bit of that. Out of the universality of defeat, betrayal, loss, that song reaches beyond its language and geography. There is no reason to give up.

> *Actually I should do something, warn them*
> *somehow, race to their rescue waving my arms, shout*
> *stop, that's crazy, but when I see how*
> *under a row of bare acacias in a gray wintry park*
> *the boy walking in front of me, half*
> *my age and twice as real, puts*
> *a bashful daring hand on the girl's hip, as*
> *   though nothing*
> *would ever threaten them, as if they too weren't*
> *   coming closer*
> *this instant, even they, to . . .*
> *then it seems to me that perhaps there's still some*
> *hope*
>> Stanisław Barańczak *Perhaps*

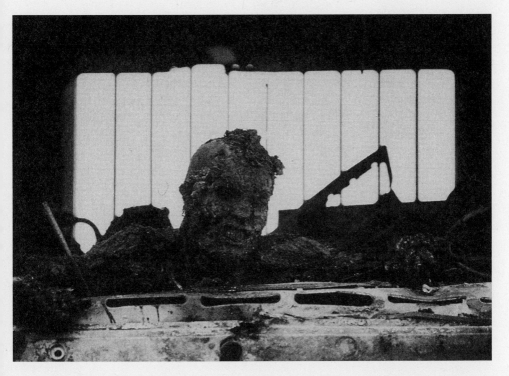

An Iraqi soldier who died trying to escape a burning truck, February 1991. Included instead of usual photos of dead Jews at Belsen or Auschwitz. This photo by Kenneth Jarecke, published July/August 1991 in American Photo *and reprinted courtesy Contact Press Images, New York City, never appeared in any American mainstream magazine. George Bush's censors were as careful as Hitler's to make sure that the home folks did not see the faces of the enemy dead.*

THE JOURNEY

Homage to James Merrill 1926–1995

THE CANADIAN ARMY back in 1942 was more old fashioned than the American and loved marching songs that made a fifteen mile slog more bearable. A favorite was *Colonel Bogey's March*, which middle-aged movie goers remember as the tune whistled by British prisoners in *Bridge on the River Kwai*. Spirited music, inadequate lyrics:

> *Bullshit*　　　*was all the band could play*
> *Bullshit*　　　*they played it every day*　　　*(ad infinitum)*

Fifty years later my brother, for whom Proust had been a lifelong mentor, offered better words:

> Swann's Way　*a book by Mar-cel Proust*
> *Tells how*　　*the hero took to roost*
> *Racy*
> *Odette de Crécy*
> *To whom his friends could not be in-*
> *Troduced*

—but by then too late to be picked up by the Canadian army.

Copyrights and Credits

Chapter 1: Excerpt from *Three Elegies*, by Bertolt Brecht, Routledge Publishers, New York. Excerpt from *Days of 1935*, by James Merrill, from *Braving the Elements*, Atheneum Publishers, New York, 1972. Excerpt from *Refugee Blues*, by W. H. Auden, Random House, New York.

Chapter 3: Excerpt from *September 1, 1939*, by W.H. Auden, Random House, New York.

Chapter 5: Excerpt from untitled poem by A. E. Housman, Alden Press, Oxford, 1936.

Chapter 6: Excerpt from *Lava*, by Adam Zagajewski, from *The Gothic Canvas*, Farrar, Straus, and Giroux, New York, 1991. Excerpt from *Report from the Besieged City*, by Zbigniew Herbert, from *Report from the Besieged City*, The Ecco Press, New York, 1985. Previously published by The New York Review of Books.

Chapter 7: Excerpt from *The Survivor*, by Tadeusz Różewicz, from *Holocaust Poetry*, St.Martin's Press, New York, 1995. Excerpt from *Bypassing Rue Descartes*, by Czesław Miłosz, translated by Renata Gorczynski and Robert Haas, from *The Collected Poems*, 1931–1987, The Ecco Press, New York, 1988. *But of Course*, by Julia Hartwig, from *Spoiling Cannibals' Fun, Polish Poetry of the Last Two Decades of Communist Rule*, edited and translated by Stanisław Barańczak & Clare Cavanaugh, © Northwestern University Press, Evanston, 1991. Previously published in *Tri-Quarterly*. Excerpt from *Dedication*, by Czesław Miłosz, from *Selected Poems*, The Ecco Press, New York, 1973. Excerpt from *Poème pour Adultes*, by Adam Ważyk, from *Anthologie de la Poesie Polonaise*, Editions du Seuil, Paris,1965. Excerpt from *The Power of Taste*, by Zbigniew Herbert, from *Report From the Besieged City*, The Ecco Press, New York, 1985.

Chapter 8: *Plans, Reports*, by Adam Zagajewski, from *Spoiling Cannibals' Fun*, Polish Poetry of the Last Two Decades of Communist Rule, edited and translated by Stanisław Barańczak & Clare Cavanaugh, © Northwestern University Press, Evanston, 1991. Excerpt from *A Little Song About the Censor*, by Adam Zagajewski, from *Humps & Wings: Polish Poetry Since 1968*, Red Hill Press. Excerpt from *Who Will Bear Witness to These Times?*, by Bronisław Maj, from *Spoiling Cannibals' Fun, Polish Poetry of the Last*

Tri-Quarterly. Excerpt from *The Gothic Canvas,* by Adam Zagajewski from *The Gothic Canvas,* Farrar, Straus and Giroux, New York, 1991. Excerpt from *The Weight of the Body,* by Stanisław Barańczak, from *The Weight of the Body,* Tri-Quarterly Books, Northwestern University Press, Evanston, 1989. Excerpt from *An Opinion on the Question of Pornography,* by Wisława Szymborska, from *Spoiling Cannibals' Fun, Polish Poetry of the Last Two Decades of Communist Rule,* edited and translated by Stanisław Barańczak & Clare Cavanaugh, Northwestern University Press, Evanston, 1991. Previously published in *Cross Currents: A Yearbook of Central European Culture.*

Chapter 13: *Someone Else,* by Artur Międzyrzecki from *Spoiling Cannibals' Fun, Polish Poetry of the Last Two Decades of Communist Rule,* edited and translated by Stanisław Barańczak & Clare Cavanaugh, © Northwestern University Press, Evanston, 1991.

Chapter 14: Excerpt from *Elegy X,* by Rainer Maria Rilke from *The Duino Elegies,* W.W. Norton, New York and London, 1939/1967.

Chapter 15: Excerpt from *Brief Reflections on Eyes,* by Miroslav Holub, from *Poems Before and After,* Bloodaxe Books, Newcastle-Upon-Tyne, 1991. Excerpt from *Evening Idyl with Protoplasm,* by Miroslav Holub, from *Poems Before and After,* Bloodaxe Books, Newcastle-Upon-Tyne, 1991.

Chapter 16: Excerpt from *By an Unknown Poet from Eastern Europe, 1995* by Gyorgy Petri, from *Child of Europe,* Penguin Books, London, New York, 1990.

Chapter 17: Excerpt from *United Flight 1011,* by Miroslav Holub, from *Poems Before and After,* Bloodaxe Books, Newcastle-Upon-Tyne, 1990.

Chapter 18: Excerpt from *Verses from an Old Tapestry,* by Jaroslav Seifert, from *Selected Poetry of Jaroslav Seifert,* MacMillan, New York, 1986.

Chapter 19: Excerpt from *To be a Poet,* by Jaroslav Seifert, from *Selected Poetry of Jaroslav Seifert,* MacMillan, New York, 1986. Excerpt from *To the Poet Franz Kafka,* by Lutz Rathenau, from *Child of Europe, A New Anthology of East European Poetry,* Penguin Books, London and New York, 1990. Excerpt from *A Song for the Feast of Purim, Terezin 1943* from *Music in Terezin,* Joza Karas, Editor, Beaufort Books, New York, 1985. Excerpt from *Lost Paradise,* by Jaroslav Seifert, from *Selected Poetry of Jaroslav Seifert,* MacMillan, New York, 1986. Excerpt from *After Auschwitz,* by Anne Sexton, from *Holocaust Poetry,* St. Martin's Press, New York, 1995. Excerpt from *Terezin 1944,* by Mif, from *Music in Terezin,* Joza Karas, Editor, Beaufort Books, New York, 1985.

Chapter 20: Excerpt from *An End to Idling,* by Peter Handke, from *Austrian Poetry Today,* Shocken, New York, 1985.

Chapter 22: From the *History of Journalism,* by Jerzy Ficowski, from *Spoiling Cannibals' Fun, Polish Poetry of the Last Two Decades of Communist Rule,* edited and translated by Stanisław Barańczak & Clare Cavanaugh, © Northwestern University Press, Evanston, 1991. Excerpt from *Hitler and the Generals,* by Michael Guttenbrunner, from *Austrian Poetry Today,* Schocken Books, New York, 1985.

Chapter 24: Excerpt from *To Go to Lvov,* by Adam Zagajewski, from *Spoiling Cannibals' Fun, Polish Poetry of the Last Two Decades of Communist Rule,* edited and translated by Stanisław Barańczak & Clare Cavanaugh, © Northwestern University Press, Evanston, 1991. Excerpt from *Mr. Cogito and the Imagination,* by Zbigniew Herbert from *Spoiling Cannibals' Fun, Polish Poetry of the Last Two Decades of Communist Rule,* edited and translated by Stanisław Barańczak & Clare Cavanaugh, © Northwestern University Press, Evanston, 1991. Excerpt from *The End and the Beginning,* in *View With a Grain of Sand: Selected Poems by Wisława Szymborska,* translated by Stanisław Barańczak and Clare Cavanagh. English translation © 1995 by Harcourt Brace & Company, reprinted by permission.

Chapter 25: Excerpt from *Psalm on a Dumpheap,* by Tadeusz Nowak, from *Spoiling Cannibals' Fun, Polish Poetry of the Last Two Decades of Communist Rule,* edited and translated by Stanisław Barańczak & Clare Cavanaugh, © Northwestern University Press, Evanston, 1991. Excerpt from *Hatred in View With a Grain of Sand: Selected Poems by Wisława Szymborska,* translated by Stanisław Barańczak and Clare Cavanagh. English translation © 1995 by Harcourt Brace & Company. reprinted by permission Excerpt from *Perhaps,* by Stanisław Barańczak, from *The Weight of the Body,* Tri-Quarterly Books, Northwestern University Press, Evanston, 1989.

Other books by Charles Merrill

The Great Ukrainian Partisan Movement and
   Other Tales of the Eisenhower Years

The Checkbook
   The Politics and Ethics of Foundation Philanthropy

The Walled Garden
   The Story of a School

Emily's Year
   A novel

Merrill's books have been published in German, Czech and Polish.

The Journey, as *Podróz,* is simultaneously being issued in Polish by ZNAK
Publishing Company of Kraków; Henryk Woźniakowski, CEO; Andrzej
Pawelec, translator.

Purchasing information for *The Journey* and *Podróz*:
Price for one copy $22 plus $4 for S & H (MA orders add $1.30)
Price for two copies $42 plus $4 for S & H (MA orders add $2.30)
Price for three copies $60 plus $4 for S & H (MA orders add $3.20)
Additional copies $18 each.

Make checks payable to and mail to:
BookCrafters
615 E Industrial Dr
Chelsea MI 48118

For further information call the Publisher at 212-727-7496.